Brain Mechanisms Underlying Speech and Language

Brain Mechanisms Underlying Speech and Language

Proceedings of a Conference held at
Princeton, New Jersey
November 9-12, 1965

Supported by a grant from the
NATIONAL INSTITUTE of NEUROLOGICAL
DISEASES and BLINDNESS

CLARK H. MILLIKAN, Chairman
FREDERIC L. DARLEY, Editor

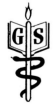

PUBLISHED BY
GRUNE AND STRATTON
NEW YORK and LONDON   1967

Library of Congress Catalog Card Number 67-13316

Printed in the U.S.A. (K-B)

Contents

Foreword

RECENT YEARS have seen impressive advances in our understanding of the nature of language and of the linguistic requirements for information processing, transfer, storage, and retrieval. There have been parallel, but, unfortunately, unrelated advances of our understanding of coding and decoding within the central nervous system, and of the neural mechanisms underlying sensation, movement, and even thought.

Probably because of the complexities of human communication, and especially of the underlying neurophysiological processes, there has been a tendency recently to overlook the interrelationship between the two. We have concentrated very heavily on the study of input and output, and have neglected the traditional effort to relate function to its underlying structure and neural mechanisms.

The purpose of this Conference has been to bring together those scientists who have been concerned with the language processes and those working with basic neurophysiological mechanisms in hopes that advances in these fields may permit us once again to attempt to develop a meaningful correlation. Certainly the ultimate understanding of the process of human communication will require a precise knowledge of the structures and mechanisms upon which this capability must be built.

RICHARD L. MASLAND, M.D.
Director, National Institute of
Neurological Diseases and Blindness
Bethesda, Maryland

Participants

BAIN, RICHARD C.: *Technical Specialist, American Council on Education, Washington, D. C.*

BENTON, ARTHUR L.: *Professor of Psychology and Neurology, University of Iowa, Iowa City, Iowa. (Neuropsychology)*

BOSMA, JAMES F.: *Oral and Pharyngeal Development Section, National Institute of Dental Research, National Institutes of Health, Bethesda, Maryland. (Pediatrics)*

BROSIN, HENRY W.: *Professor and Chairman, Department of Psychiatry, University of Pittsburgh School of Medicine; Director, Western Psychiatric Institute and Clinic, Pittsburgh, Pennsylvania. (Psychiatry)*

BROWN, JOE R.: *Consultant in Neurology, Mayo Clinic; Professor of Neurology, Mayo Graduate School of Medicine (University of Minnesota), Rochester, Minnesota. (Clinical Neurology)*

CARHART, RAYMOND: *Professor of Audiology, Auditory Research Laboratory, Northwestern University, Evanston, Illinois. (Audiology)*

CAVENESS, WILLIAM F.: *Associate Director for Collaborative and Field Research, National Institute of Neurological Diseases and Blindness, Bethesda, Maryland.*

CHASE, RICHARD ALLEN: *Assistant Professor, Psychiatry; Instructor, Otology and Laryngology, The Johns Hopkins University School of Medicine, Baltimore, Maryland. (Clinical Neurophysiology)*

CHOMSKY, NOAM: *Professor, Department of Modern Languages and Linguistics and Research Laboratory of Electronics, Massachusetts Institute of Technology, Cambridge, Massachusetts. (Linguistics)*

CURTIS, JAMES F.: *Head, Department of Speech Pathology and Audiology, University of Iowa, Iowa City, Iowa. (Speech and Voice Science)*

DARLEY, FREDERIC L.: *Consultant in Speech Pathology, Mayo Clinic; Associate Professor of Speech Pathology, Mayo Graduatae School of Medicine (University of Minnesota), Rochester, Minnesota. (Speech Pathology)*

EFRON, ROBERT: *Chief, Neurophysiology-Biophysics Research Unit, Veterans Administration Hospital, 150 South Huntington Avenue, Boston, Massachusetts. (Neurophysiology, Psychophysics)*

EISENSON, JON: *Professor, Speech Pathology and Audiology; Director Institute for Childhood Aphasia, School of Medicine, Stanford University, Palo Alto, California. (Speech Pathology)*

ETTLINGER, GEORGE: *Senior Lecturer, Department of Experimental Neurology, Institute of Psychiatry, London, England. (Neuropsychology)*

EVARTS, EDWARD V.: *Chief, Section on Physiology, Laboratory of Clinical Science, National Institute of Mental Health, Bethesda, Maryland. (Neurophysiology)*

FALCONER, MURRAY A.: *Director, Guy's Maudsley Neurological Unit, Maudsley Hospital, London, England. (Neurosurgery)*

GAZZANIGA, MICHAEL S.: *Research Fellow, Division of Biology, California Institute of Technology, Pasadena, California. (Psychobiology)*

GESCHWIND, NORMAN: *Chief, Neurology Service, Boston Veterans Administration Hospital; Associate Professor of Neurology, Boston University Medical School, Boston, Massachusetts. (Neurology)*

GOLDSTEIN, MURRAY: *Associate Director for Extramural Programs, National Institute of Neurological Diseases and Blindness, Bethesda, Maryland.*

GUTTER, FREDERICK J.: *Executive Secretary, Communicative Sciences Study Section, Division of Research Grants, National Institutes of Health, Bethesda, Maryland.*

HARDY, WILLIAM G.: *Director, Hearing and Speech Center; Associate Professor of Otolaryngology and Environmental Medicine, The Johns Hopkins Medical Institutions, Baltimore, Maryland. (Audiology, Speech Pathology)*

HARTMAN, ELIZABETH C.: *Chief, Training Grants and Awards Branch, Extramural Programs, National Institute of Neurological Diseases and Blindness, Bethesda, Maryland.*

HÉCAEN, HENRY: *Director, L'ecole Pratique des Hautes Etudes, Centre Neurochirurgical Ste Anne, Paris, France. (Neurology)*

HIRSH, IRA J.: *Director of Research, Central Institute for the Deaf, St. Louis, Missouri. (Psychoacoustics)*

KONIGSMARK, BRUCE W.: *Assistant Professor, Laryngology and Otology; Assistant Professor, Pathology, The Johns Hopkins School of Medicine, Baltimore, Maryland. (Neuropathology)*

LANSDELL, HERBERT C.: *Head, Section on Clinical Psychology, National Institute of Neurological Diseases and Blindness, Bethesda, Maryland. (Neuropsychology)*

LENNEBERG, ERIC H.: *Assistant Professor of Psychology, Harvard University and Children's Hospital Medical Center, Boston, Massachusetts. (Psychology)*

LILLY, JOHN C.: *Director, Communication Research Institute, Miami, Florida. (Psychoneurophysiology)*

MAGOUN, H. W.: *Dean, Graduate Division, University of California, Los Angeles, California. (Neurophysiology)*

MARUSZEWSKI, MARIUSZ: *Assistant Professor, Department of Psychology, University of Warsaw; Chief, Aphasia Unit, Centre of Neurological Rehabilitation, Konstancin near Warsaw, Poland.*

MASLAND, RICHARD L.: *Director, National Institute of Neurological Diseases and Blindness, National Institutes of Health, Bethesda, Maryland. (Neurology)*

MASLAND, MRS. MARY WOOTTON: *Lecturer, Johns Hopkins School of Hygiene and Public Health, Hearing and Speech Center, Johns Hopkins Hospital, Baltimore, Maryland. (Speech and Language Pathology)*

MASON, WILLIAM A.: *Head, Behavioral Sciences, Delta Regional Primate Research Center, Tulane University, Covington, Louisiana. (Psychology, Primatology)*

MILLIKAN, CLARK H.: *Consultant in Neurology, Mayo Clinic; Professor of Neurology, Mayo Graduate School of Medicine (University of Minnesota), Rochester, Minnesota. (Neurology)*

MILNER, BRENDA: *Associate Professor (Neuropsychiatry), Department of Neurology and Neurosurgery, McGill University; Canadian Medical Research Council Associate, Montreal Neurological Institute, Montreal, Quebec, Canada. (Neuropsychology)*

MOORE, G. PAUL: *Chairman, Department of Speech; Director, Communication Sciences Laboratory, University of Florida, Gainesville, Florida. (Speech Pathology)*

MORDELL, J. SOLON: *Executive Secretary, Communicative Disorder Research Training Committee, National Institute of Neurological Diseases and Blindness, National Institutes of Health, Bethesda, Maryland.*

MORRELL, FRANK: *Professor of Neurology, Stanford University School of Medicine, Palo Alto, California. (Neurology)*

MORRIS, WILLIAM E.: *Executive Secretary, Neurology "A" Study Section, Division of Research Grants, National Institutes of Health, Bethesda, Maryland.*

MYERS, RONALD E.: *Chief, Laboratory of Perinatal Physiology of the National Institute of Neurological Diseases and Blindness, San Juan, Puerto Rico. (Neurophysiology)*

O'BRIEN, THOMAS E.: *Executive Secretary, Neurology "B" Study Section, Division of Research Grants, National Institutes of Health, Bethesda, Maryland.*

POLLACK, IRWIN: *Research Psychologist, Mental Health Research Institute, Professor of Psychology, University of Michigan, Ann Arbor, Michigan. (Psychology)*

PURPURA, DOMINICK P.: *Associate Professor of Anatomy and Neurology, College of Physicians and Surgeons, Columbia University, New York, New York. (Neurophysiology)*

REED, L. DENO: *Consultant, Speech Pathology and Audiology, Vocational Rehabilitation Administration, Department of Health, Education and Welfare, Washington, D. C. (Speech Pathology)*

RICH, ROBERT P.: *Director of the Computing Center, The Johns Hopkins University, Baltimore, Maryland. (Mathematics)*

ROSADINI, GUIDO: *Chief Researcher, National Research Council; Neurosurgical Clinic, University of Genoa, Italy. (Neurophysiology)*

ROSENBLITH, WALTER A.: *Professor of Communications Biophysics, Department of Electrical Engineering and Center for Communication Sciences (Research Laboratory of Electronics), Massachusetts Institute of Technology, Cambridge, Massachusetts. (Biophysics)*

ROSSI, GIAN FRANCO: *Associate Professor, Neurosurgical Clinic, University of Genoa, Genoa, Italy. (Neurosurgery)*

SCHEVILL, WILLIAM E.: *Research Associate in Zoology, Harvard University; Associate in Oceanography, Woods Hole Oceanographic Institution, Woods Hole, Massachusetts. (Bioacoustics)*

SCHUELL, HILDRED M.: *Director, Aphasia Section, Division of Neurology, Minneapolis Veterans Administration Hospital; Professor, Neurology, University of Minnesota, Minneapolis, Minnesota. (Speech Pathology)*

SEBEOK, THOMAS A.: *Professor of Linguistics; Chairman, Research Center in Anthropology, Folklore, and Linguistics, Indiana University, Bloomington, Indiana. (Linguistics, Anthropology)*

SILVERMAN, S. RICHARD: *Director, Central Institute for the Deaf; Professor of Audiology Washington University, St. Louis, Missouri. (Audiology)*

SOLOWEY, MATHILDE: *Chief, Program-Project and Clinical Center Grants, Extramural Programs, National Institute of Neurological Diseases and Blindness, Bethesda, Maryland.*

SPERRY, R. W.: *Professor of Psychobiology, California Institute of Technology, Pasadena, California. (Psychobiology)*

TEUBER, HANS-LUKAS: *Professor and Chairman, Department of Psychology, Massachusetts Institute of Technology, Cambridge, Massachusetts. (Psychology)*

THORPE, WILLIAM H.: *Professor of Animal Ethology, Cambridge University, Cambridge, England. (Ethology)*

WALTER, W. GREY: *Head of the Physiological Department, Burden Neurological Institute, Bristol, England. (Neuropsychology)*

Introductory Remarks

CLARK H. MILLIKAN

Mayo Clinic
Rochester, Minnesota

WELCOME TO THIS PRINCETON CONFERENCE on *Brain Mechanisms Underlying Speech and Language.*

Since its inception the National Institute of Neurological Diseases and Blindness has addressed itself to an interest in, development of, and programming concerning a variety of aspects of speech and language. Dr. Richard Masland, the Director, has had great personal interest in these matters for two decades.

As the Council of the National Institute of Neurological Diseases and Blindness, in its advisory capacity to the permanent staff of the Institute and in its introspective functions as individuals, has looked at the subject of speech and language and at the extramural grants program of the Institute, it has noted that there is and has been relatively little crossover in the development of basic or clinical research concerning central mechanisms underlying normal or abnormal speech and language.

If one presumes that the substrate for speech and language is divided into three areas—input, output, and all of those central (brain) phenomena that have to do with reception, understanding, retention, integration, formulation, and expression—the neglected area has been the central one rather than input or output. Neurology, neurosurgery, neuropathology, neurophysiology, audiology, speech pathology, psychology, neurochemistry, the world of the computerist, the physicist—these things, these people, these disciplines have seldom been brought together in any effective attempt either to analyze or to do something about disorders of speech and language.

As the NINDB Council ruminated about this matter, it suggested that a conference—this Conference—attempt to bring together at one time representatives of a series of these disciplines to talk together about some of the problems; stimulate one another to some crossover of interest; produce a publication which, in its own right, might act as something of a stimulating mechanism nationally among the disciplines represented at this meeting; and update NINDB Council and staff personnel concerning activities about the basic brain mechanisms underlying speech and language.

It is with these purposes in mind that we have gathered. The rules for this Conference are simple. The presentations, as indicated in the individual letters to each of the essayists, will be limited in their duration, as will formal discussion, because some 55 per cent of the time theoretically available to us at this meeting has been allocated to open discussion. Perhaps the latter will produce some of the most stimulating phenomena or ideas to come out of this conference.

The first topic to open this Conference is "Animal Vocalization and Communication." Dr. Thorpe will begin the discussion of this subject.

1

Animal Vocalization and Communication

W. H. THORPE

University of Cambridge
Cambridge, England

I PROPOSE giving a general introduction to the subject of how animals communicate. In particular I want to discuss the subject with reference to birds, and I am going to include some quite recent work on birds which I think brings out some of the fundamental points, as I see them, concerning the communication systems of higher animals.

I begin by assuming that human language is primarily a series of actions performed with the intention of altering the behavior of another individual. Human language is thus a series of actions which are themselves symbolic, or, much more often, actions of the vocal cords and associated structures which result in symbolic sound signals used for the purpose of communication.

There have been, as you know, various classifications of the different types of linguistic expression. One of the simplest was that of Ogden and Richards.[300] These authors concluded that there are two forms of language: emotive and propositional.

Since then much more elaborate classifications of linguistic communication have been produced. I want to refer particularly to that of Morris,[289] and I would like here to acknowledge my indebtedness to Marler's[259] discussion of this subject, and in particular his 1961 paper.[260] Morris separates four different types of communication: (1) identifiors, (2) designators, (3) appraisors, and (4) prescriptors. Identifiors deal with location in space; designators give information about the characteristics of the environment; appraisors indicate preference; and prescriptors signify that specific responses are required. You will be able to tell me whether this is found to be a useful classification for human speech. Personally, I do not find it very helpful for analyzing animal communication. This is perhaps because the different categories seem to overlap so much that you can place almost any communicative act in two, or sometimes more, of them. So I find the older division, into emotive and propositional, a much more useful one.

I assume that the first function of language is to induce immediately a given behavior in the recipient or hearer, with or without a corresponding emotional state. The response can sometimes be so quick that it occurs before there has been time for an emotion to build up. But, secondly and more often, the effect of language is to induce an emotional readiness for behavior; and that is as true of animals as it is of men.

Then, of course, thirdly, language transmits information in the sense of being propositional; that is to say, it transmits definite numerical information about the environment or about a particular situation in the environment with which the organism is concerned.

In human language most communications are usually both propositional and emotive. In addition, they are purposive, in that there is nearly always in human speech a definite intention of getting something over to somebody else, altering his behavior, his thoughts, or his general attitude toward a situation. Finally, human language is very largely syntactic. So I propose to consider how far animal language fits in with this scheme.

I can deal with the question of purposiveness straightaway. Of course, with most examples of animal communication it is extremely difficult to know whether or not there is deliberate intent to communicate. But in the higher animals, whether in the wild (as in the chimpanzees) or with animals such as dogs and apes when kept as pets, it is quite certain that they have at times a deliberate intention to communicate. The evidence that under certain conditions the animals are trying to influence the behavior of their associates, is, I consider, beyond question, whether these associates are human, as in the case of a completely tamed animal, or whether they are other members of the species.

So I shall take it for granted that much animal communication can be purposive. It would, I believe, be rather sterile to discuss this in further detail.

When we study animal communication, we find that in the lower animals there is a good deal of what may be described as "all-or-none" signalling. Here we have discrete signals which change little if at all in form or intensity with the individual's changing emotional state. They are highly constant for the species, that is, very stereotyped. This is particularly true in certain groups of the lower animals, for example, the arthropods. Figure 1 shows three examples from the Arachnidae of the form of courtship, whereby the male spider ensures, before he comes too close to the female, that she is ready to respond in the right manner, that is, that she "recognizes" that this is a male of the species, not a fly or other appropriate food object. This is accomplished by a series of elaborate gestures. The male stands at a "safe" distance and goes through his motions with extreme precision, in each case the motion being characteristic of the species, so that there can be no mistake.

Figure 2 illustrates an even more remark-

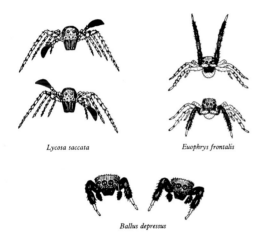

Lycosa saccata   *Euophrys frontalis*

Ballus depressus

Fig. 1. Gestures of male spiders of three different species. (From Bristowe.) Figs. 1, 2, 4-6 reprinted by permission of Cambridge University Press from *Darwin's Biological Work,* by P. R. Bell.

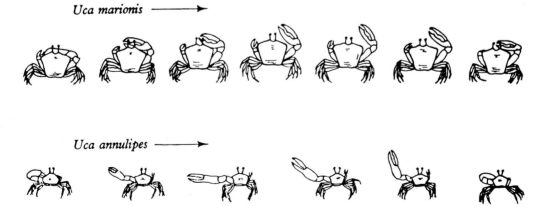

Fig. 2. Signalling gestures of two species of fiddler crabs (*Uca*). (From Crane.)

able case from the Crustacea. It shows the display of the males of two kinds of fiddler crabs (*Uca* species). There are about 40 species of this genus living on the tropical beaches of the oceans of the world. They have adopted a striking means of signalling to other members of the species by the use of a single large claw which has been specially developed in the course of evolution for sexual and agonistic displays. The claw is waved in a ritualistic way so as to provide a gesture absolutely characteristic of the species. The timing of the movement, the form of it, and the particular attitude which the claw takes in the course of this signalling are all so constant that by this alone an expert can distinguish the species of crab, whether it comes from the shores of Panama, Tahiti, or Bali. There must obviously be some very precise, presumably hormonal, mechanism which ensures that the individuals always do these gestures exactly at the right speed and amplitude and intensity; otherwise the whole system would break down.

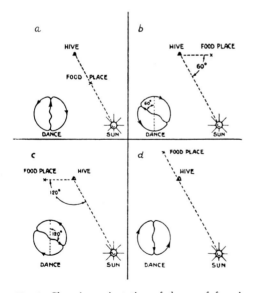

Fig. 3. Changing orientation of dance of foraging workers of the honey bee according to the direction of the food source in relation to the sun. (After von Frisch.) Reprinted by permission of *The Bulletin of Animal Behaviour.*

Figure 3 serves to recall a similar case in the honeybee where we have successful foragers giving a dance which provides indication to other members of the species where food has been found. Here again, there is practically no variation; the behavior is highly stereotyped. In this case, however, although the movements are characteristic of the species, details are variable according to the external situation, so that they transmit information about environmental circumstances according to a definite code. Thus the dance indicates that there is food in a given direction at a particular distance.

When, however, the dances of the honeybee are used for another kind of communication, we find that, besides by their orientation giving propositional information as to direction, the movements can be adjusted in both intensity and speed according to other types of information. Thus when scouts are out looking for a new hole for a swarm, those scout bees which have found a new home of very high quality dance with greater liveliness and vivacity, that is to say, at a higher overall speed and much more persistently, than those which have found a home of low quality[247] (pp. 39-54). In most cases the swarm will eventually, after inspection of the various sites by other scouts, choose to follow the most stimulating dancers—that is to say, the most vivacious and persistent ones—and this dance will direct them to the best place for the swarm to take shelter.

So here we have a graduation of signalling as a result of control of the intensity and duration of the movement. Perhaps the most remarkable thing about this very remarkable result is that in deciding the "quality" of a new site, the scout bees choose that site which is "the best" with respect to a number of different features. These include degree of shelter from the prevailing winds and rain, dryness, spaciousness (the new home must be large enough but not too large), and, finally, the distance from the temporary site of the newly emerged swarm.

It seems clear, then, that there must be

inherently coded in the bees' central nervous system some device which ensures that these various characteristics will be assessed and the results algebraically summed in such a manner that they can be adequately interpreted according to a specific scale of evaluation. Thus a new home in the alpha-plus class will be announced by dancing of the highest speed and persistence; another which is lacking in perhaps one or two respects will be placed lower down the scale, while at the bottom a home which is inferior in many respects will only be announced, if at all, by a sluggish and perfunctory performance. I know of no other case in the animal kingdom where fine gradations of perception are transmitted by a code to other members of the species—a code which is understood by all, which does not vary in scale from one population of the species to another (or only minimally), and, above all, which must be in the main standardized independently of individual experience. The recent discovery[403] of a sound component in the bees' communication system, not mentioned in my discussion above, does not affect this conclusion.

Figure 4 illustrates another feature of communication at a somewhat higher level. Very often movements are, in a sense, symbolic of the act concerning which communication is being made. Thus the attitudes are often appropriate to the beginning of an action. In this particular case, the female chaffinch (*Fringilla coelebs*) soliciting copulation, drops the wings and raises the tail. So effective is this posture that a male will copulate vigorously with a stuffed specimen provided

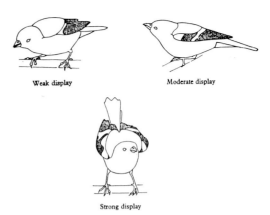

Weak display

Moderate display

Strong display

Fig. 5. Threatening postures of chaffinch. (From Marler.)

its attitude is correct. Figure 5 shows another chaffinch posture, this time threatening attack. The attitude is obviously appropriate for this purpose in that the head is down and directed forward. But note also that the intensity of the agonistic drive is expressed in the intensity of the postures threatening the intruder. These differences are certainly perceived by other birds and the appropriate response is given according to the intensity of the signals.

Figure 6 illustrates the principle of antithesis which was first described by Darwin. According to this principle the opposite of a given posture expresses the reverse of the drive in question. It is particularly evident in the blackheaded gull (*Larus ridibundus*), where the sight of the bird full-face shows aggression whereas, during the process of pair formation, the head is frequently turned away in a gesture of appeasement. This ap-

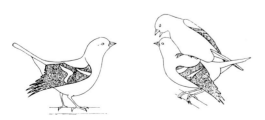

Fig. 4. Attitude of female chaffinch (*Fringilla coelebs*) inviting copulation. (From Marler.)

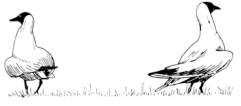

Fig. 6. Appeasement gesture of a pair of black headed gull (*Larus ridibundus*), displaying the white nape, which is reassuring, instead of the black face, which is threatening. (From Tinbergen.)

peasement gesture is enhanced by the fact that instead of the black face being presented, the white nape of the neck is shown; and the nape is the most vulnerable part of the bird. Presentation of the nape of the neck is very widespread in animals as an appeasement gesture. Similarly in the chaffinch, aggressive postures and submissive postures are, in detail, almost the exact opposite of each other.

When we come to a highly social animal like the wolf (*Canis lupus*), we find great flexibility of the communication system. Figures 7 and 8 show the various ways in which emotion can be expressed and the very fine gradations which can be indicated by the positions of the ears and the lips and by the different attitudes of the tail. It will be seen that there are 11 postures of the tail—each different and each with a definite meaning

to other members of the species. Here we have a complex and very subtle form of language, probably no detail of which escapes the attention of other members of the species.

Besides these gestures and postures there are, of course, many examples of chemical transmission of information, particularly in the insects and in animals such as the Ungulates, and the Urisidae and the Canidae. However, the chemical transmission of information is such a complex subject that I will not attempt to cover it today but will go straight to language of sounds because I think that is what most of us here are primarily interested in, and is a topic which has been greatly studied in recent years.

The great advantage of having a language of sounds is that sounds are very economical to produce. They are quick to decay, so that the field is clean for another communication almost immediately after the sound has been produced. Sound travels far and fast. It is independent of physical obstacles, it will "go round corners," and a great spectrum of fre-

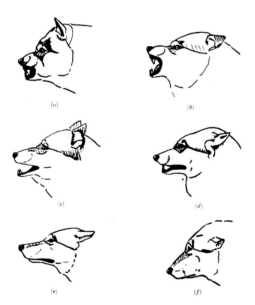

Fig. 7. Emotional expression in the wolf (*Canis lupus*). (*a*) Threat, high intensity, no uncertainty; (*b*) high intensity, slight uncertainty; (*c*) threat, low intensity with uncertainty; (*d*) weak threat with strong uncertainty; (*e*) anxiety; (*f*) uncertainty with suspicion in the face of an enemy. (After Schenkel, 1948.) Figs. 7 and 8 reprinted by permission of Methuen and Co. Ltd. from *Learning and Instinct in Animals*.

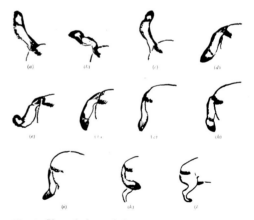

Fig. 8. Use of the tail for emotional expression in the wolf (*Canis lupus*). (*a*) Self-confidence in social group; (*b*) confident threat; (*c*) with wagging, imposing carriage; (*d*) normal carriage (in a situation without social tension); (*e*) somewhat uncertain threat; (*f*) similar to (*d*) but specially common in feeding and guarding; (*g*) depressed mood; (*h*) intermediate between threat and defense; (*i*) active submission (with wagging); (*k*) and (*l*) complete submission (After Schenkel, 1948.)

quency and intensity is available for use. For all these reasons, if you are going to have a really flexible and effective language, it is bound to be a language of sounds. There is no other way of reaching maximum efficiency and flexibility.

When we begin to study animal sounds, we find that they are very often highly complex. True, there are simple sounds with a single meaning just as there are simple gestures with a single meaning. But in the higher animals this is not the general rule. The question then arises: how much of this complexity is accidental and how much is meaningful?

As far as simple sounds go such as those which give warning of an attack or indication that there is food about, or that the group should keep together or scatter—it is a remarkable fact that the number of such "words" which are found in the language of widely different animals is usually about 20. Here are some examples: European wren (*Troglodytes troglodytes*)—20; chaffinch (*Fringilla coelebs*)—19; song sparrow (*Melospiza melodia*)—21; Lar gibbon (*Hylobates Lar.*)—12; rhesus monkey (*Macaca mulatta*) —between 20 and 30. With the higher animals the estimate arrived at may depend very largely on how precise one is about the distinction of the sounds. The person who has a very well attuned ear can, rightly or wrongly, argue that there are many more fine gradations and that the number should be higher. And it is certainly likely that a great many mammals and birds can learn to perceive fine gradations in tonal structure and quality and can learn to associate these with particular situations. But what does seem clear is that in mammals as a whole, and strikingly so in the primates, there is a remarkable absence of any ability to learn sounds by imitation.

When we come to a bird song, as distinct from the call notes which are the simple communication sounds discussed above, we find that the system is very complex indeed. We often have long sequences of notes, very

rapidly produced and, obviously, with great potentialities as carriers of information. The question is: how much is actually perceived and how far is it acted upon?

Recently two French workers, Busnel and Bremond[51,52,58] have been studying the effectiveness of the song of the European robin (*Erithacus rubecula*) as a signal for possession of a territory. The full song of birds, at any rate in the temperate regions of the world, seems usually to be a proclamation that the male bird is in charge of a territory and is prepared to defend it, and that he is prepared to receive a female and set up house in this territory. Now the song of the robin is quite complicated but Busnel and Bremond found that most of this complication has no effect whatever in the territorial situation. All that the rival bird pays attention to is the alternation between the high-pitched notes and low-pitched ones. It makes no difference whether the high ones come first and the others last, or vice versa; it is apparently the number of changes from low to high pitch in a given song which determines the intensity of the response.

I do not doubt that the work is correct, in the case of the robin and in this particular context of defending territory; but I suspect that it is not of general application to other species. When we come to study other birds in other situations, we find that there is a great deal more detail being attended to, and apparently affecting the behavior, than just the simple change from high frequencies to low and *vice versa*.[386,387] Now I think the important point here, the point that I am stressing particularly this evening, is the imitative ability that so many birds have. I believe it true to say that almost all the songbirds can at least copy the sounds of other members of their species to some extent.

In the chaffinch the song is characteristic of the species. The overall pattern is such that a field ornithologist, or another chaffinch, can recognize this signal at once as being that of a chaffinch. But there is sufficient complexity in the song for it to be varied greatly by the individual and yet be kept within the overall chaffinch pattern. So you can have variations which will specify particular individuals; and these variations can be learned, and are learned, while the birds are still in their first year, and in this way local dialects can be passed on from one generation to another. Thus, the ability to imitate the fine details of song is important in that it enables the song to be not merely a specific signature tune but an individual signature tune as well.

These birds, then, are imitating other members of their species. Of course, as you know, there are other species which are extremely good at imitating many sounds besides those of their own species. I am not tonight going to talk particularly about what are generally known as the talking birds—birds that can imitate human speech with astonishing exactness—though they are very remarkable indeed. Everyone knows that parrots can imitate. A parrot can learn to imitate exactly a hundred or more words, and some of the smaller parrot species, for example, the budgerigar (*Melopsittacus undulatus*) can do better than that. The Indian hill mynah (*Gracula religiosa*) can imitate a very large number of sounds with much greater exactitude and precision than the parrot. This does constitute a major problem! How and why is it that these birds can imitate so well when mammals are so incapable in this respect? From the point of view of this conference, it seems to me that the most significant point which I want to emphasize here is that one cannot imagine a true vocal language, flexible and adaptable as is even the simplest of human languages, having been evolved without a very high ability for vocal imitation. Imitation is, it seems to me, absolutely fundamental in the evolution, and in the learning, of language; and, apart from man, birds are incomparably better imitators than any other living beings.

Recently Konorski[207] has published a paper in which he discusses audioverbal aphasia in man resulting from certain types of brain damage. He says that lesions which have this effect are shown to have damaged either the posterosuperior part of the temporal lobe or to have severed the "arcuate bundle" which originates in this area and runs to the lateral frontal region. He points out (and no doubt you will have some comments to make on this) that there is nothing exactly comparable to this structure in nonhuman mammals. He regards the inability of nonhuman mammals to imitate as, in the main, the result of the absence of this structure and hence he concludes that this is the reason why mammals other than man are incapable of speech, since imitative powers are a *sine qua non* for the acquisition of a true language.

Now with birds we have only very meager neurological facts to go upon. The only bird species the brain of which has yet been studied sufficiently thoroughly is one of the doves (*Streptopelia risoria*). However, we have shown[211] that doves of this genus are unable to modify their vocalization by imitation. Consequently nothing can yet be said about any brain structures in birds which may be specifically concerned with powers of vocal mimicry.

I would like to discuss briefly some studies of my own, still in progress, which I think throw some light on the possible reasons for the development of these imitative powers in a number of the higher birds.[388,389] In the temperate zones most bird songs seem primarily to be a form of territorial proclamation. In the tropics, on the contrary, one finds a great deal of song which does not seem to fit that description. In a densely forested country like parts of East and Central Africa, you find that a great deal of song is of a very different kind.

In East Africa there are at least four unrelated groups of birds which go in for singing elaborate and very precisely organized duets in which one bird follows another with extraordinary precision. I call this antiphonal singing. In what follows I am going to discuss one of these species only—the tropical boubou shrike (*Laniarius aethiopicus*) which is found in Tanzania, Uganda, Kenya, and various other territories further south. The first point of importance about this antiphonal singing, or duetting, is that it seems a very good form of display for a species living in dense vegetation where the two members of a pair cannot keep one another in sight for long. So instead of being in visual communication, they maintain vocal communication by means of these precisely timed duets.

The duet seems to be worked out between the male and the female during a long practice period. The duet patterns themselves are composed of notes the quality of which is no doubt determined by hereditary constitution, but the pitch, timing and phrasing of which can be varied very exactly by the singers as a result of prolonged practice. For nearly every species we have studied so far, it seems that either sex can start and the other finish; or either sex can sing the whole tune, if the partner is absent; and when the partner returns, they can either duplicate in perfect time or, more usually, sing antiphonally again. As you will hear, some of these pairs work out quite precise little tunes. Each knows the other's contribution, which he or she does not normally sing unless the other is absent. When the mate returns, the first bird may relinquish the second half of the tune to the returning mate. So here you have rather elaborate patterns which have been worked out by practice, and each bird can take any part or the whole of the duet as required. Some of these patterns are quite widespread within the populations but, as they work them out by practices of the pair, the chances are that in any one area some of the duet patterns will be characteristic of that pair or, at any rate, the pattern of one pair will not coincide in every detail with that of another pair.

Figures 9 and 10, taken from a recent paper by Thorpe and North,[388] show a number of examples of these duet patterns which were recorded on tape and subsequently an-

alyzed by sound spectrograph. It so happens, however, that the notes of these birds are of such a pure flute-like quality that they can be represented quite accurately on a musical stave; and this is what I have done with these illustrations. The illustrations with their legends will, I think, be self-explanatory. But you will note that the last two illustrate not a duet but a trio! Thus in the last picture

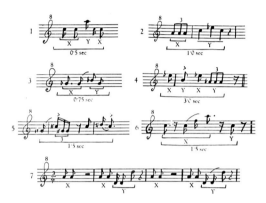

Fig. 9. Seven examples of antiphonal song of the tropical boubou shrike (*Laniarius aethiopicus*). Letters 'X' and 'Y' indicate the contribution of two different birds. (Reproduced by courtesy of the Editor of "Nature." From Thorpe and North.[388]) (1) *L. aethiopicus sublacteus.* Vipingo, Kilifi, Kenya, December 1954. *N.B.* All the illustrations are given at approximately scientific pitch (middle 'C' = 256 c/s). Unless otherwise stated, as here, all figures refer to race *major.* (2) *L. aethiopicus.* Dundori, Nakuru, Kenya, March 17, 1964. (3) *L. aethiopicus.* Kabale, Uganda, February 15, 1962. (4) *L. aethiopicus.* Meadow Point, Lake Nakuru, Kenya, March 17, 1964. (5) *L. aethiopicus.* Hippo Pool, Lake Nakuru, Kenya, March 17, 1964. Note that this is a rather more elaborate duet than the previous ones. The contribution of the two birds is not indicated in this case since it seemed to vary a good deal. (6) *L. aethiopicus mossambicus.* San Martino, Mozambique Coast (C. Haagner). The timing in this example is very precise, but the bar length might vary between 0.7 and 1.5 sec. (7) *L. aethiopicus mossambicus.* San Martino, Mozambique Coast (C. Haagner). This is a duet with a more complex time pattern. Bar length 1.5 sec.

(Fig. 10) you see that bird "X" sings a D-sharp, then bird "Z" sings three G-sharps, then "Y" sings a D-sharp, then "Z" sings three A's, and so on with perfect precision, the three birds together keeping perfect time. All I can say at present is that this phenomenon of trio singing is a challenge to future investigation!

But to return to the duets: it is clear that here we have elaborate mutual patterns worked out by practice. We also have some evidence that these duets are means of recognition and coordination of behavior between two members of a pair. They presumably enable the birds to keep in touch and recognize one another under conditions of life in dense vegetation.

I think observations such as these throw some light on the function of this imitative ability in birds in general. In 1903 two separate observations were published,[162,396] one from Germany and one from Australia, of

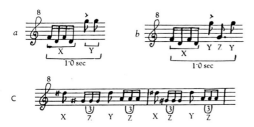

Fig. 10. Three further examples of antiphonal song in *Laniarius aethiopicus*. (Reproduced by courtesy of the Editor of "Nature." From Thorpe and North.[388]) (*a*) and (*b*) *L. aethiopicus*. Lake Bunyoni, Kabale, Uganda, February 14, 1962. (*a*) represents a duet pattern heard as a very long, precisely timed series. During one considerable stretch of this series a third bird 'Z' joined in. It was far away from the others, but nevertheless inserted its single note remarkably accurately (*b*). It tended to intervene in every second duet of 'X' and 'Y.' (*c*) *L. aethiopicus*. Dundori, Nakuru, Kenya, April 3, 1964. A remarkable trio. All 3 birds were in the same tree. Note that bird 'X' gave a *D* sharp every 2 seconds and bird 'Y' a *D* sharp every other 2 seconds, while bird 'Z' gave a *G* sharp and an *A* natural every other 2 seconds in alternation.

birds kept in captivity (in one case an Australian magpie (*Gymnorhina tibican*) and in the other case the European bullfinch (*Pyrrhula pyrrhula*) which had learned to sing antiphonally a melody taught them by human beings. They divided the theme between them, each normally restricting himself to his own contribution, but then when one of the birds was removed, the remaining bird would sing the whole pattern.

It has recently been found by Gwinner and Kneutgen,[146] using the Indian shama (*Copsychus malabaricus*) in captivity, that here again you have notes which are normally restricted to the male and others to the female.

If one of the birds goes away, the remaining bird sings the whole pattern (that is, the contribution of both sexes) until the mate comes back. In fact, it seems to be a way of calling the mate back! For, as Gwinner and Kneutgen suggest, if you go away and hear your own contribution being produced in your own territory, it must be a very strong incentive to return to see what is happening. My suggestion, then, is that this may be one of the mechanisms, perhaps quite widespread, which could be the basis on which this high learning ability has been evolved.

Finally, we come back to a very knotty problem: how is it that man achieved this extraordinarily perfect imitative ability, the ability immediately to imitate the sound which he hears? As far as we know, no other animal, apart from the birds, can do this. It looks, indeed, as if the birds are the group which ought to have been able to evolve language in the true sense, and not the mammals. What happened, then, to enable the ancestors of man suddenly to acquire the imitative ability without which they could not possibly have developed language as we know it?

CHAIRMAN MILLIKAN: Thank you, Dr. Thorpe. Dr. Schevill, will you open the discussion, please?

DR. WILLIAM E. SCHEVILL: I have the disadvantage of having arrived late, after Dr. Thorpe started speaking. I was impressed by a particular point in Dr. Thorpe's remarks, this allusion to a structure in the brain which, if I understood correctly, was reported only in *Homo* and not in other mammals. Is this correct, sir? I caught only something about the temporal lobe.

DR. THORPE: Yes! The "arcuate bundle," as such, is found only in man, and nothing quite comparable to it has been observed in the brain of the chimpanzee or of other primates that have been studied. I very much want to get the opinion of the conference about this. Konorski[207] argues that when, in human beings, you have this connection broken by lesion then, although speech can still be understood and the person can still speak, he cannot immediately reproduce sounds he hears. He displays audioverbal aphasia. For instance, he cannot possibly, as I understand it, repeat nonsense syllables. Konorski suggests that it is this mechanism which man alone possesses which enables him to imitate sound in such a way as to make true language possible.

DR. SCHEVILL: Yet the other mammals and other animals do pick up their ancestral tongue. In other words, I do not know how, for example, a dog learns to bark or how some of the whales and porpoises learn the particular notes which are characteristic of their species, but this is not what is ordinarily meant by mimicry; I gather it is learning by imitation. This arcuate bundle in the temporal lobe has nothing to do with that.

DR. THORPE: I do not think this is learning; I think this is instinctive ability. It is also true of the call notes of the birds in contrast to the song; these call notes do not have to be learned.

DR. SCHEVILL: I believe Dr. George Kelemen[195] felt the inability of the nonhuman primates to imitate human speech was as much as anything due to—he likes to call it, I believe—the defective structure of their larynx. It takes a larynx like ours, he feels,

to articulate, and the other primates do not have such. I do not know if you have considered that as a possibility.

DR. THORPE: All one can say is that the vocal organs of birds are apparently much less appropriate for imitating human speech than those of the chimpanzee or gorilla. I think it would be true to say that if you showed a bird syrinx to a laryngologist who had never seen one and said, "How is it that the animal with this can talk?" he would say, "It is utterly impossible!"

DR. SCHEVILL: Very likely. As for mimicking by other animals, such as the cetaceans, which I study, I have no evidence for it. You have described animals which can for the most part be seen, so that you can know what they are doing. I cannot ordinarily see my subjects very well, since I am usually concerned with cetaceans at sea (not even captives).

It has impressed me that within these limitations we have no evidence that a wild cetacean ever imitates the calls of another species. They apparently do not do any imitating on their own. At least we have never been fooled when we have finally run down the calls of the few species we do know. We do not know the phonation of very many, rather less than two dozen. There are probably a hundred species in all.

CHAIRMAN MILLIKAN: Dr. Mason.

DR. WILLIAM A. MASON: Like Dr. Thorpe, my interest is chiefly in animal behavior. Discussions of animal language are always a little embarrassing, I think, to people in animal behavior because all of us recognize the many important differences between animal communication and human language.

My own research has been concerned with monkeys and apes, and the following remarks apply to them rather than to other animals with which I have had no personal acquaintance. Certainly we can say that communication plays a prominent part in the social activities of the nonhuman primates, and that many species have evolved fairly elaborate modes of communication. Until more information is available, we cannot offer any precise assessment of the limits of the nonhuman primates' communicative skills, but we do know that the signals of monkeys and apes are stereotyped and species-typical—the form of the signal, its structure, is more or less fixed, and is similar in different individuals of the same species, in spite of wide variations in experience or social history. (The response to the signal is, I suspect, more variable and more heavily dependent upon experience.) Furthermore, most of the postures, facial expressions, and vocalizations which comprise the basic "vocabularies" of the nonhuman primates occur under conditions of patent emotional arousal. These may be analogous or even homologous, to some forms of human communication, but human language obviously includes much more than this. For man, language is an integral part of learning and problem solving. It is one of the primary avenues of cognitive growth in the child, and in the adult, a major intellectual resource.

I have no intention of minimizing the potential importance of studies of natural forms of communication—studies which are primarily concerned with describing signals, and establishing the situation in which these signals occur, and the effects they produce in other animals—but, at the same time, there are other approaches which could prove at least as pertinent and fruitful. It might be profitable, for example, to review the extensive literature on primate intellectual performance—especially the many excellent studies of discrimination learning and brain function—with a view to establishing their relevance to language and communication. Thus far, little attention has been given to this question, either by specialists in language or by comparative psychologists.

The final point that I would like to consider concerns the kinds of changes that may have occurred in primate evolution that led toward or permitted the development of language. This problem has been widely discussed, of course, and it obviously is central to the question of what animal studies can contribute to the understanding of human language.

There are several aspects of primate behavior which seem to vary significantly with phyletic status among the living primates, and these may offer some clues as to the nature of possible evolutionary trends. Going from the prosimians, through monkeys and apes, to man one would probably find an increase in discriminative capacity, or the ability to detect slight variations in input or signal. This is probably accompanied by an increase in the capacity to respond to relationships between stimuli—to organize perceptions in new or unusual ways. On the response side, there is an increase in behavioral flexibility. The chimpanzee, as compared to the monkey, for example, probably produces a greater variety of sounds and in a larger number of combinations. The response units are, so to speak, smaller in the chimpanzee and more loosely bound together.

Such changes are of the kind that would help to make language possible. They do not, of course, suggest why language emerged. The selective pressures that led to the emergence of language must have been social, and among the more likely specific possibilities is the prolongation of social dependence which brought with it the need for more subtle social adjustments and more elaborate forms of cooperation.

CHAIRMAN MILLIKAN: Dr. Lilly, will you continue the discussion of animal vocalization?

Dolphin Vocalization

JOHN C. LILLY

Communication Research Institute
Miami, Florida

WE HAVE BEEN PURSUING some research with one of the cetaceans, *Tursiops truncatus*, the bottlenose dolphin, in captivity.[240] This animal has a brain approximately the size of ours. As he ages, his brain passes ours; as an adult he has about 10 to 20 per cent more cerebral cortex than we have. About 98 per cent of his brain surface is cortical, as compared to our 96 per cent. The density of the cells in corresponding areas of cortex is close to ours. The number and kind of major connections between cortical areas correspond to those that we have. There are some quantitative differences, however. For example, his visual inputs are about one-tenth those of ours, 120,000 fibers/eye, for our 1,200,000. However, on the ear side, he has $2\frac{1}{4}$ times the number of fibers we have. His hearing frequency spectrum is approximately five times ours. His usable spectrum, in terms of complex pattern hearing, is something of the order of five times ours in frequency.

If we compare his highest and lowest frequencies and their ratio, it comes out about the same as the ratio for our speech band. If we accept the telephone speech band as the one that carries the most essential meanings for us, that is, from 300 cycles to about 3,500, and you now multiply those frequencies by the ratio of the speed of sound in air to that in water,[5] you come out with the bands that the dolphins apparently use in their intraspecies communication (1500-17,500 cycles).

We have made several thousands of measurements of the ranges which they cover in exchanging whistles one with the other and have found that about 90 per cent of the lowest frequencies that they choose run around 6 kilocycles whereas the highest frequencies of the fundamental that they use run around 24 kilocycles. They can use higher intrinsic pulse frequencies (for sonar) than these (though not higher pulsing rates). The upper limits that we have worked with run around 300 kilocycles. However, most of the energy seems to peak between 40 and 120 kilocycles in this band.

The vocal versatility of a given individual is rather extreme. They can "mimic" simple tunes that are played to them, a few notes each. They can mimic the variations in the human voice (not all the variations but certain aspects of the human voice) extremely well, through rather long passages when newly played to them.

In a recent issue of *Science*[243] I published a paper dealing with two of the physically measurable aspects of this mimicry. If one makes up a set of "nonsense" syllables so as to avoid the problem set up by using "meaning" in the transmissions, one can then furnish the animal with a set of sonic human stimuli, voice given, including all the complexity of our speech, with very large numbers of variations in various parameters of the sounds.

We chose a set of seven vowels ($\bar{e}$/, $\breve{\text{i}}$/, $\bar{a}$/, $\breve{e}$/, $\ddot{a}$/, $\bar{o}$/, $\overline{oo}$/) and two diphthongs (a $\breve{\text{i}}$/ and o $\dot{\text{i}}$/). We chose eleven consonants: r/, l/, z/, v/, ch— or —tch/,

13

w/, m/, n/, t/, k/, and s/. We combined these in vowel-consonant and consonant-vowel pairs and randomized a set of these in the usual fashion with a set of random numbers. Then we divided them into groups, randomly ordered as to the number of nonsense syllables in each group, in groups from one to ten (see Table 1.).

This list was then read to the dolphin in air by the human operator standing by the tank in which the dolphin was resting (Fig. 11). Within a matter of 15 minutes, a dolphin who had been exposed to a number of kinds of different sonic emissions and who had some operant conditioning training in this area, picked up the rules of this particular experiment and proceeded to put out *matched numbers of bursts* of sound which matched the numbers that the human had just given. For example, if the human said, "ez, ot, ir," the dolphin came back with three corresponding bursts of sound. I do not attempt to mimic the dolphin mimicking the human. This is a very difficult thing for us to do; their usual pitch runs from about 500 to 1000 pulses/second, whereas the human operator's pitch is running from about 125 to 300.

Under very special conditions we have obtained direct mimicking of pitch down to as low as 250. This is not a usual performance.

Let us pay attention to the bursts of sound themselves and the inter-burst silences, their durations and the numbers in the bursts. In the first experiment the dolphin reproduced the number that the human put out in 206 different emissions; he mimicked the number within 91 per cent of the correct value. In the second experiment he was up to 92 per cent. In the third experiment he was running 98.5 per cent. In the fourth

TABLE 1.

Vowel or Diphthong		r	l	z	v	ch--tch	w	m	n	t	k	s
ē	ē	ēr	ēl	ēz	ēv	ētch		ēm	ēn	ēt	ēk	ēs
		rē	lē	zē	vē	chē	wē	mē	nē	tē	kē	sē
ĭ	ĭ	ĭr	ĭl	ĭz	ĭv	ĭtch	wĭ	ĭm	ĭn	ĭt	ĭk	ĭs
		rĭ	lĭ	zĭ	vĭ	chĭ		mĭ	nĭ	tĭ	kĭ	sĭ
ā	ā	ār	āl	āz		ātch		ām	ān	āt	āk	ās
		rā	lā	zā	vā	chā	wā	mā	nā	tā	kā	sā
ĕ	ĕ	ĕr	ĕl	ĕz	ĕv	ĕtch	wĕ	ĕm	ĕn	ĕt	ĕk	
		rĕ	lĕ	zĕ	vĕ	chĕ		mĕ	nĕ	tĕ	kĕ	sĕ
ä	ä	är̤	äl̤		äv̤	ätçh		äm̤	än̤	ät̤	äk̤	äs̤
		ra	la	za	va	cha	wa	ma	na	ta	ka	sa
ō	ō	ōr	ōl	ōz	ōv	ōtch		ōm	ōn	ōt	ōk	ōs
		rō	lō	zō	vō	chō	wō	mō	nō	tō	kō	sō
oo	oo	oor	ool	ooz	oov	ootch		oom	oon	oot	ook	oos
		roo	loo	zoo	voo	choo	woo	moo	noo	too	koo	soo
aī	aī	aīr	aīl	aīz	aīv	aītch		aīm	aīn	aīt	aīk	aīs
		raī	laī	zaī	vaī	chaī	waī	maī	naī	taī	kaī	saī
oi	oi	oir	oil	oiz	oiv	oitch		oim	oin	oit	oik	ois
		roi	loi	zoi	voi	choi	woi	moi	noi	toi	koi	soi

Randomized sets of vowel-consonant and consonant-vowel pairs used to test dolphin mimicry. (From Lilly.[243])

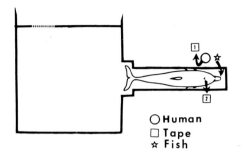

Fig. 11. Schema of experimental configuration. The Tursiops is in the recording position in the side-arm. The investigator (O) is standing beside the side-arm; his voice is recorded through microphone #1 and tape channel #1. The emissions from the blowhole of the Tursiops are recorded through microphone #2 and tape channel #2. When a food reward ("fish"*) is used, it is either manually given to *Tursiops* or by means of a mechanical feeder triggered outside the tank room. The fiberglass tank (2.5 x 2.5 meters) has a door (........) opening into other tanks. The transparent side-arm is approximately 2.5 meters long by 0.5 meters wide by 0.5 meters deep.

experiment it dropped to 93. By the fifth experiment he was down to 98, and by the sixth experiment he did 98.7 per cent. At the seventh session he failed to perform at all (Fig. 12).

The same list was used in each experiment; we started at a different point in the list each time and alternated in direction for the 198 different items. I do not know whether it was possible for the dolphin to memorize any portion of this list. We did our best to prevent this contingency. No portion of it was gone over any more than any other portion. The emissions, in duration, matched within plus or minus 50 per cent of the duration of the human in 96 per cent of the emissions (Fig. 13). The inter-burst silences matched similarly. Thus, we have a physically determinable series of events with high levels of interinvestigator agreement.

The usual experiment was terminated by the dolphin leaving the experimental situation. He could swim away to his home tank, rest, and then return. Usually he broke the

experiment at the end of 10 minutes; at this time the emissions were coming at a rate of about one per second. He then took a five minute break and came back for another ten minutes of work. Experiments varied in duration from 12 minutes to half an hour. We staged three or four such experiments a day when the human operator could stand the pace. The dolphin apparently would "loaf" through them very well. The novelty factor was absolutely essential to elicit this kind of performance. The dolphin stopped this kind of experiment and refused to go on. But if we changed the list to another set of sounds, he would start again with similar accuracies as he had in the first list.

Tursiops truncatus is an animal that varies

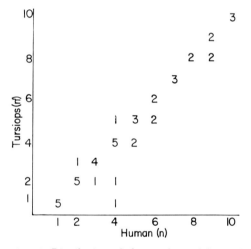

Fig. 12. Distribution of the numbers of bursts in each of 40 human emissions and in each immediately consequent dolphin emission. The number of bursts in each human emission (n) is on the abscissa; the number in the consequent dolphin emission (n') is on the ordinate. The instances of exact equality (n = n') are on a 45° line (starting at n = 1 with five instances and running up to n = 10 with three instances). The two instances in which the dolphin added one burst are at n = 2 and n = 4. In seven instances it deducted one; in one instance, deducted two; and once deducted three. In no instance did the dolphin fail to reply to the human emission. (From Lilly.[243]) Figs. 12-14 copyright 1965 by the American Association for the Advancement of Science.

from about 100 Kg. to about 200 Kg. in weight. The brain varies in the newborn from 685 Gm., in one case we have, to 1800 Gm. in the older animals, with all the variations in between. Brain weight increases linearly with body length from birth to full development.

These animals have a long beak ("bottlenose"). The true porpoises do not have this beak and also do not have this size brain. Their brain is comparable in size to that of the chimpanzee.

A usual dolphin's brain weighs 1600 Gm.; the usual man's brain weighs 1400, including the cerebellum in each case. With regard to

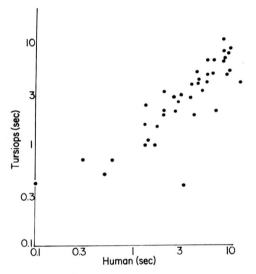

Fig. 13. Distribution of durations of human emissions and of each consequent emission by the dolphin. The duration of each human emission is on the abscissa; of each dolphin emission, on the ordinate: each is a log scale. Exact equality positions are on a line at 45°. Within each emission, the time from the beginning of one burst to the beginning of the next burst, averaged over the whole series, is 0.84 second for the human and 0.78 second for the dolphin's replies. Some longer emission times by the dolphin are accounted for by more bursts per emission (seven instances); in two instances of shorter emissions, the number of bursts was also reduced; in other instances, variations in duration of bursts and of silences between bursts accounted for the differences. (From Lilly.[243])

cortical weights, the dolphin's is approximately 15 per cent more than that of man. The gyri and sulci are more complex. This is true even in the newborns and also in the fetal brain, as we have seen recently.

Do not make the mistake of thinking that *Tursiops* brain is the largest of its kind. The brain of a killer whale is much larger and far more complex. One we collected weighed 4500 Gm. for a 17-foot female *Orcinus orca*.

We are developing an atlas of the dolphin, *Tursiops'*, brain, in collaboration with Yakovlev. This atlas is scheduled for publication in 1967 by Pergamon Press. There are now 2500 slides from which templates are being prepared. The basic portions of the brain, below cortex, are now in hand. For instance, the archeocortex recently has been gone over, and the findings agree with those of Filimonoff,[94] who recently looked at *Delphinus delphis'* brain. The temporal lobes in these animals are very much larger than ours. Currently we are estimating their area as being something of the order of $2\frac{1}{2}$ times the area of ours. However, their occipital poles are very much smaller than ours.

Those who have studied human cortices microscopically agree that the dolphin has the same number of layers of cells as does man, and the cellular density is the same, within a first approximation. The areas of differentiation of cortex are currently being done in our laboratory.

Practically the whole vocalization apparatus, except that portion in the larynx, is innervated by the seventh cranial nerve. They have an intranarial pair of vocalization apparatuses, one on each side. Each one is innervated by about 30,000 fibers. If we added up all the nerve fibers we have for our vocalization, we seem to come out with about the same order of magnitude numerically. On the output side, they come up to where we are, and on the input side somewhat better than we are, in terms of vocalization and the hearing side.

Figure 14 shows the results of one of the experiments in which the animal is mimicking certain aspects of our voices. Another portion of a record showed ten responses— ten nonsense syllables given by the human, immediately followed by the dolphin giving ten sounds in response to those ten. The performances are really remarkable to listen to.

These experiments demonstrate some rather dramatic differences between this species and the mimicking birds. The mimicking birds, as I understand it from those who have worked with them, and I have not, will mimic extremely well, probably pronouncing much better than the dolphin does, but they will not stick to the task nor use the degree of concentration that the dolphin has.

The diligence with which a dolphin will spend minutes working with you, at very high speed, in this kind of exchange is startling. The only other animal species I know

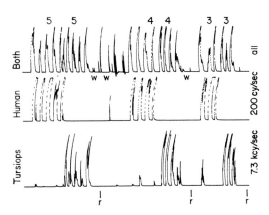

Fig. 14. Three typical vocal exchanges, man-dolphin. Analysis and graphic presentation of a portion of a magnetic tape recording without cutting or editing (real time, continuous). Five, four, and three bursts in each of three human presentations are matched exactly by those of the dolphin. In the middle and bottom traces the two voices are separated for graphic purposes by two narrow pass band filters (Spencer-Kennedy) and displayed separately. To cover the wide amplitude range (40 db) an automatic gain control circuit was applied to the combined signals, and the resulting signal is displayed in the uppermost trace. Food reinforcement was used at the times indicated by r; w indicates water splashes. The duration of this segment of record is 25 seconds. (From Lilly.[243])

of that will do this is the human species; I know that my four year old daughter can give a performance very similar to that of the *Tursiops*. However, she and I both flunk out at about five or six nonsense syllables on a new list, whereas the dolphin maintains his accuracy right up to ten in that list. (Additional references: [234-238,241,242,244-246.])

CHAIRMAN MILLIKAN: Dr. Geschwind.

DR. NORMAN GESCHWIND: Returning to Dr. Thorpe's presentation, I would like to comment on Konorski's theory about why human beings can repeat and why primates cannot. The structure of which Konorski spoke, the arcuate fasciculus, is one which runs from the postero-superior temporal lobe to the lower frontal lobe. The best evidence seems to indicate that this tract runs backward around the posterior end of the Sylvian fissure and then runs forward in the lower parietal region, eventually reaching the frontal lobe. I agree with Konorski about the particular type of aphasia which results from a lesion of this structure. He calls it "audio-verbal" but it has a more classical name, which is "conduction aphasia." It is a distinctive and not uncommon syndrome.

Konorski based his views on the failure of macaques to repeat on a diagram which was published by Bonin and Bailey.[40] In their diagram of the long corticocortical connections in the nonhuman primate, you do not see the arcuate fasciculus; that is, the posterosuperior temporal region and the lower frontal region are not connected by a pathway which runs back around the Sylvian fissure and then forward in the lower parietal lobe. However, as was pointed out by these same authors in a later publication, the reason for this was that the technic they were using for showing the connections was the technic of strychnine neuronography. With this method you know where the fiber begins and you know where it ends, but you have no way of knowing what pathway it follows since all you can pick up is the firing at the end of the fiber. In drawing their earlier diagram, instead of drawing the pathway to follow that of the known arcuate fasciculus, Bonin and Bailey had drawn a more or less straight line running through the temporal lobe and ending up in the frontal lobe. It is clear, however, from their diagram that the two regions mentioned by Konorski are connected in the macaque. Bonin and Bailey pointed out, furthermore, that it was quite likely that the pathway ran in the lower parietal lobe, but they could neither definitely confirm nor reject this on the basis of the technic that they were using. In conclusion, I agree that the arcuate fasciculus is very important in man for repetition, but I do not believe we can argue that a monkey fails to repeat because he lacks this pathway. I think it is clearly present in the nonhuman primate, and we must therefore seek another explanation for the failure of repetition in these animals.

DR. GIAN FRANCO ROSSI: A very simple question. I was impressed by the similarity between some of the expression of human language and parrot language. I wonder if you know of any evidence of the existence of brain dominance in birds. Has anybody tried to make lesions, on one side only, of the brain of the birds to see whether and in what way language was affected and, above all, to see whether the possible language impairment occurred only or chiefly following lesion of one side of the brain?

DR. THORPE: No, as far as I know, that has not been done.

DR. H. W. MAGOUN: With respect to Dr. Thorpe's remarks on vocalization in birds, experimental studies on a range of experimental animals, which include birds, carnivores, and subhuman primates, indicate that vocal and related mimetic responses involved in the expression of affective states are managed by a mechanism in the middle brain stem. This subcortical mechanism for faciovocal expression is present in man as well as in animals. Midbrain lesions in man may impair such behavior without impairment of his speech. Conversely, widespread bilateral cortical injury in man may be followed by a pathologic exaggeration of laughter and

crying, interpreted as release of lower functions from higher inhibition.[254]

It has sometimes been proposed that man's capacity for speech has developed from this subcortical mechanism for nonverbal communication, but no intimate relationship is known between this deep-lying mesencephalic mechanism, present widely through the animal kingdom, and the topographically distant cortical region for speech, which has only appeared with the relatively recent evolution of associational cortex in the human brain. In keeping with their phylogenetic differences, these two mechanisms for communication display widely differing maturation times in the ontogeny of the human infant. The older, more stereotyped, subcortical emotional mechanism is already functional at birth. By contrast, activity of the cortical mechanism in understandable speech only develops between one and two years after birth and its capacities in written language are not gained until the child is five or six years of age.

These observations seem to oppose the view that man's capacity for speech evolved from the abilities for emotional vocalization present in lower animals. On the contrary, man's communication by symbols, both vocal and written, appears to represent an entirely novel functional increment related to the acquisition of associational cortex in front of the face and hand parts of the motor area in the case of speaking and writing, and around the cortical sensory areas for audition and vision in the case of recognition of spoken and written language. Man's capacities for communicating by symbolic language are unique also in depending upon neural mechanisms which develop only in the dominant one of the two cerebral hemispheres, rather than bilaterally. One can conclude that there are two unrelated central neural mechanisms for vocal expression in vertebrates: one for nonverbal affective communication, widely present in the animal brain stem, and a second for verbal communication, present only in the lateral neocortex of the brain of man.

DR. THORPE: I think it is very important

to distinguish in birds those vocalizations which can be produced without any practice or training, which are not learned from those which can be modified by experience.

I did not speak about what we usually designate "call notes" because, in general, these do not require learning for their expression. You can rear birds in auditory isolation and they will come out with the perfectly normal call notes of their species, and there is no impairment.

Where I think you can say that a learned language does come in in bird communication is in the context of song. If you rear a bird such as the chaffinch in auditory isolation, it comes out with only an extremely simple sequence of notes, resembling the full song in only a few respects. If it is kept in isolation until it is about 14 months old, then it can never develop its song further. It retains the restricted kind of vocalization as its "song" for the rest of its life. So that all the fine structure of the song vocalization is the result of learning from conspecifics during the period from the time it leaves the nest through the first autumn but, particularly, again the following spring. Then it is that all the fine detail is put in, and then it is that the individual characteristics of the vocalization appear. This seems to me to be very similar to what we call language. In many species the songs are in fact signals acquired in such a way as to be characteristic of the individual. They are recognized by other individuals as characteristic, as identifying that particular individual.

Coming to the question of language, it seems to me that if you use these three characteristics I mentioned—propositional, syntactic, and purposive—it is difficult to find an animal in which we can say quite definitely that all three exist together, but you can find examples of these characteristics separately in a great variety of animals.

After all, the dance of the honeybee is propositional in that it does give precise information about direction and distance of a good supply. The songs of these shrikes I was describing to you are syntactic. There

is, it seems, careful organization of the different phrases in a particular order, as characteristic of the pair. And, as I said, there is a lot of evidence that much communication in animals is purposive. So it seems to me that we can find good examples of all these three characteristics of language, but we cannot at the moment say quite definitely that they are all present in one particular animal.

CHAIRMAN MILLIKAN: Are there other comments or questions? Does that conclude your commentary, Dr. Thorpe?

DR. THORPE: I would like to ask Dr. Lilly in regard to the imitative sounds of the porpoises, what the sound spectrograph shows. The very striking feature, of course, about the vocal imitations of a bird like the Indian mynah (*Gracula religiosa*) is the extraordinary precision of its imitations. The vocalization is so good that you can distinguish individual human voices and vocal inflections; the bird can imitate, say, the same thing in the voices of two or three different human beings it knows. When you look at the sound spectrograms, you find that the hubs of the vowels are present in almost exactly the same relation as they are in the voice of the model. In all respects, this is an extraordinarily precise imitation. I may give an anecdote to show how precise it is. I have had mynahs which can produce, I think one can say perfectly, every phoneme in the English language, and many other phonemes as well. It is easiest to train the mynahs by having them taught by a person. You can train them by tape, but they do not learn so quickly or so securely that way. I had one of my mynahs trained by a lady who was very keen on doing this. I asked her, in order to get some sounds which I had not had from a mynah before, to teach the bird to say, "I just saw a zebra."

She taped all the training sessions, so I could study the details of the learning process. The mynah came out saying this very well. "But," she said, "you know, it is curious that it says 'I just saw a *debra*.'" Actually the teacher is a Hungarian who came to England as a girl, a refugee, and now speaks absolutely perfect English, but she does occasionally mispronounce the "z." She noticed the mistake at once when the mynah said "debra" and not "zebra." That is just a little anecdote indicative of the extraordinary precision of their imitation. But one finds it again and again in one's training experiments.

Mynahs learn a very great deal which they do not often utter. Yet they have phrases which are particular favorites, which they will repeat constantly. They can store away a very great number of sounds but it is often difficult to get them to reproduce their full vocabulary.

I would like to know what the sound spectrogram shows in the case of the dolphin vocalizations, because that seems to me to be the real criterion for good imitation of the human voice. Also I would like to know is there anything known about the range of discrimination of the dolphin's hearing.

DR. LILLY: I think the answer to that is, as the speech people keep saying, that the spectrograph is a very poor measure, a very poor judge of how well anything is mimicked. One can pick up, of course, with the mynahs and the parrots, the basic pitch and various formants of things. Also one can do this to a certain extent with the dolphin, but we have many technical problems here; one is that the dolphin's voice goes to extremely high frequencies, and his hearing apparently falls off very rapidly in the very low frequencies but continues way beyond ours.

To get the best enunciation from a dolphin, we found that we had to chop off the fourth formant very sharply at about 80 db./octave, using very sharp filters, in order not to confuse him with the presence and absence of the fourth formant because apparently his receiving side has such a high amplitude that he tends to overemphasize it in what he puts back. When we cut off the fourth formant, we then find he will mimic very well our formants 2 and 3, as measured on the sound

spectrograph. He cannot do very well either with our basic pitch, formant 1 region; in other words, he cannot work down in that region well, except by changing his repetition rate which, of course, does not give you the resonances in that region. In other words, he is copying formants 2 and 3 but putting them at characteristic frequencies two to four times our characteristic frequencies.

This means that, with the ordinary speech spectrograph and with the filters used, you cannot see very well the resemblances. You must widen out the pass band of the analyzing filter, and you must do other things to the spectrograph before you can, as it were, make a one-to-one correlation between these two vastly different regions in frequency.

I do not feel that the dolphin is as good a mimic in our hearing and speech frequencies as are the mynah birds or the human being. This is obvious to anybody who listens to the tapes. As I said before, the pitch is way too high; practically everything is way too high.

All we are saying is that there are certain aspects in which he can mimic extremely accurately with new material over long periods of time, in very complex sequences, which the mynah bird or the parrot cannot do. The dolphin has abilities not matched by the bird, and the bird has abilities the dolphin cannot match. The two are very, very different animals and both very, very different from us. Can Dr. Thorpe's mynahs produce on first exposure without practice 10 nonsense syllables immediately after a human utterance of them, and then 9, 3, 7, 2, etc., at an average rate of 1 per second for stimuli and responses and latencies between human and bird of 0.5 second?

CHAIRMAN MILLIKAN: Dr. Thorpe, do you have any final comment?

DR. THORPE: No, I don't think so, except to say that some birds also can imitate long and complex new sequences.

CHAIRMAN MILLIKAN: Dr. Hirsh will now discuss "Information Processing in Input Channels for Speech and Language."

Information Processing in Input Channels for Speech and Language: The Significance of Serial Order of Stimuli

IRA J. HIRSH

Central Institute for the Deaf
St. Louis, Missouri

LET ME SAY, first, that I am astounded to see you all here, not only at this hour but also in such number. My remarks were planned for what was advertised as a small group of people gathered around a luncheon table and, thus, they are primarily notes intended to stir up discussion.

In Dr. Thorpe's terms, his remarks can be divided into two parts: first, a "territorial proclamation," and the second part will be the beginning of what I trust will be an "antiphonal chant."

This Conference is intended to be directed toward those brain mechanisms that underlie certain behavioral functions or processes that comprise speech communication. Thus, one of my roles appears to be that of pointing out certain characteristics of speech communication, particularly with reference to hearing and the reception of spoken language.

Though I know very little about the brain, I should confess to you initially that those very aspects of speech perception that appear to me best known are those that brain mechanisms do not appear to underlie. They concern transformations, codings, and processing in those physiological mechanisms disdainfully called "peripheral" by those whose interests are in "higher" centers.

The speaking and understanding of language probably represent the most elegant and complicated example of human perform-ance in dealing with sequential patterns. There are other, only slightly less complicated forms of sequential behavior, like walking, throwing a ball, returning a ball in tennis, and driving a car, but I am informed that these are no better understood, particularly with regard to underlying physiological mechanisms, than speech.

We know a fair amount about the speaking mechanism, especially if we ask about speech particles. We also know something about the processes involved in the perception of speech. But, again, that knowledge is most adequate when we are discussing individual speech sounds, syllables, and words.

There does appear to me to be something quite special about the auditory perception of speech. It takes two forms: one concerns auditory perception as such, and the other concerns language. The patterns that one distinguishes and recognizes in hearing are formed or articulated in time, and these temporal patterns are rather peculiar to hearing. Furthermore, language, as received by the ear and not by the eye, is similarly formed in time. Not only can we note that speech consists of elements and element combinations that are themselves temporal patterns, but also the structure of language involves, to an enormous extent, storage, perceptual stretching, and relation-making over rather long extents of time.

21

What I propose to discuss is really an attempt to elaborate and support two points. (1) Auditory perceptual theory requires the concepts of sequence and temporal pattern to play the same role that Gestalt or form or shape has played in visual perception; (2) the rules that govern temporal pattern perception in hearing must be combined with rather different sets of rules, still concerned with sequence and temporal relationships, but these second sets arise from the structural aspects of spoken language. We shall concentrate on only one input channel, the sensory modality of hearing and its associated systems.

Although the auditory sense receives information-bearing stimuli of all types, our present concern will be restricted further to the sounds of speech. I would emphasize, first, the *sounds* of speech, and here we find a fairly decent state of understanding of the bases of speech perception. In addition, this emphasis will point up the dearth of connections that have been made between speech-sound perception and the utilization of speech perception by language users.

Speech Perception

Our present understanding of speech perception results, I believe, from a marriage between clinical audiometry and electrical engineering, with linguistic phonetics, until recently, playing the role of the ignored lover. This speech perception most often means the perception of isolated words so far as the measurements in the literature are concerned. Inferences from word intelligibility have been extended in two directions, opposite directions in fact: on the basis of word intelligibility we attempt to predict what was the underlying phonemic discrimination on which the word recognition was based and, in the other direction, we have also attempted to predict a listener's capacity to perceive long strings of words as they occur in ordinary linguistic context. I should say, parenthetically, that neither prediction is working out very well.

Let us review a few items about *phonemic discrimination* where we focus attention on the way in which speech sounds are processed by the auditory system. According to Jakobson and Halle[185] there are about a dozen distinctive features on the basis of which listeners can distinguish one speech sound from other speech sounds. A trained phonetician using a broad transcription would probably encounter in his transcribing of my speech about 40 classes of sounds, each of which would be designated by a different symbol. Although we would then say that I used about 40 different phonemes, an acoustical analyzer would show that I have uttered many more than 40. The listener and the listening phonetician generalize across certain others. The listener gives different values to different phonemes but not to what are called allophonic variations. The acoustic spectra of the sound /s/ in my words "seat," "soon," and "saw" are different. The mouth is already formed for the following vowel when the /s/ is pronounced. So there are, physically, three different /s/ sounds but the listener each time hears the /s/.

So far as the physical or acoustical basis for speech-sound perception is concerned, let me review very quickly, in so roughshod a manner that it will surprise and disturb perhaps some of my audiological and phonetic colleagues, the evidence. In general, it appears that, in order to discriminate among vowel sounds, the listener must recognize spectral distribution. A spectral analysis of a vowel reveals a fundamental or vocal frequency and separate harmonics, peaking at three or four places, corresponding to what are called the formants or resonant peaks of the vocal tract. Thus, I say, one of the kinds of cues in speech perception is a spectral kind, where the identification of a speech sound depends upon either the recognition of a spectrum, spectral shape or spectral envelope, or the discrimination of that spectral envelope from others.[275]

Certain consonants are discriminated on the same basis, in particular groups of consonants that are made in the same manner. The unvoiced fricatives are distinguished from each other on the basis of spectrum, when they are sounded alone in isolation. The sounds of /s/ and /sh/ are noises with continuous spectra that also show peaks, but in two different frequency regions. These two fricative consonants are also distinguishable on the same general basis as are all vowels, namely, on the basis of spectrum.[179]

But there are many other kinds of discriminations that have to be made in the recognition of speech sounds, and these apparently involve, to a much lesser extent, recognition of spectra. For example, in order to distinguish a voiced consonant from a voiceless one, /z/ versus /s/, for example, one must distinguish a continuous noise spectrum from one with line or harmonic components.

The acoustical variables responsible for the distinction that corresponds to what the phoneticians call different manners of articulation, whether plosive or fricative, and so on, are much less clear. Some of these surely involve cues that depend upon change and rate of change of acoustic variables as a function of time. The /t/ versus /s/, for example, is not only short versus long as duration discrimination but also as rate discrimination. One builds up very rapidly, the other less so. The underlying, nonspeech psychophysical abilities are not clear.[168]

Most of these overgeneralized statements about phonemic discrimination come from studies in which the phonemes occur in the context of words. From the early 1930's onward, both engineers and clinicians have presented lists of words to listeners. The listeners were to identify the words. The chief purpose of such studies has been to know the effect of various features of a telephone or radio system on the transmission of speech, or the effect of different kinds and degrees of hearing disturbance or hearing impairment on such word intelligibility. The measured quantity of interest was, for a long time, just the total number or percentage of words that the listener identified correctly. More recently, workers following the pattern set by Miller and Nicely[276] have analyzed not only how many words were missed but the kinds of errors that were made, in order to know something about particular kinds of confusions that appeared between speech sounds.

From those studies we learned that errors in word identification, when a transmission system is degraded by a limited bandwidth or by noise, follow quite regular patterns. Errors with respect to voicing, for example, are rare as are errors with respect to the manner of articulating consonants. Confusions are much more frequent that concern the place of articulation. I am almost tempted to say that spectral cues to phonemic identification are more fragile and less resistant to distortion than the nonspectral ones, but the clear separation of these two classes of cues is not easy.

Still more recently the juxtaposition of multiple choice responses, where you do not ask the listener to dredge up a word from his memory but tell him what the alternatives might be, combined with certain formal restrictions in the set of possible responses, for example, the rhyme test of Fairbanks[112] or its adaptation by House[174] and his colleagues, have yielded test technics whereby these errors, or confusions, can be analyzed in greater detail. But the conclusions from applications so far are not so different from those based on older technics.

I feel a duty to remark on physiological considerations, in spite of my lack of knowledge in this area. We should be diverted momentarily to consider what information is available on the relations between such molecular speech perception as I have discussed and the integrity of the nervous system. Those of you concerned with the brain and complex language functions must feel that the processes that I have discussed so far are not quite the interesting ones, particularly in the context of clinical neurology. What little is known about the physiological substrates of speech perception comes also from clinical practice, but usually the practice of otologist or audiologist. What have we learned? Disease processes that affect hearing do indeed interfere with the patient's ability to understand speech.

In the case of most disorders of the sound-conducting system in the external or middle ears, the difficulty is brought about only because the mechanical waves entering the cochlea are now too weak. Speech perception is not usually otherwise deranged, as can be demonstrated when the levels are restored to more nearly normal values with surgery or with a hearing aid.

Other disease processes affecting the cochlear mechanism, or the nervous system immediately following, show complications in speech perception but not in a very orderly fashion. When the speech levels are raised through amplication sufficient to compensate for the change of sensitivity that is indicated by the pure-tone audiogram, these patients do not always discriminate speech sounds in a normal fashion. That is to say, they do not identify a normally high percentage of single words presented to them in lists.

We could conceive of even more possibilities than have been suggested in the literature to account for this faulty speech perception, like frequency distortion that is related to the shape of the audiogram, or amplitude distortion or compression that would follow from the reduced dynamic range that is shown by loudness recruitment, or even a sluggish response in either cochlear or nerve mechanisms—sluggish with respect to rapid changes in the stimulus in time. But, unfortunately, even when specific confusions between /s/ and /t/ and /o/ and /r/ are analyzed, according to open-set word lists in the study of Rosen,[333] or a restricted set as applied by Schultz,[346] there appear to be very few patterns of specific confusions that characterize different diagnostic categories. There

should be such, but we have not yet figured out how to find them.

LANGUAGE COMPETENCE

Let us agree that speech communication requires certain performance, both with respect to motor output and auditory input and that, for the moment, we have focused on the input side. Consider, also, the difference in interest between psychologists and linguists in language. The latter are interested in language as a system, code, rules, while the former are interested more in the behavior that exemplifies or reifies the language system. It has been suggested by others that perhaps these two interests correspond to the subjects of de Saussure's *la langue* and *la parole*.[86]

Again, holding to the input side, we can be certain that what I have summarized here about speech perception doesn't tell the whole story about the listener's ability, even in *la parole*. Even though we were interested in the atomic particles or phonemes of language, and though we tested with the molecular particles or words of language, yet we learned very little about the listener's use of such discrimination or particle identification in listening to the running speech of the talker. By isolating these components and forming them into arbitrary lists, we deprived ourselves of the knowledge of their contextual role in the very structure that is language.

This kind of formal shortcoming is not new to psychology. John Stuart Mill had to bring mental chemistry to explain certain emergent properties of combinations of unitary ideas, and von Ehrenfels and the Gestalt psychologists got us to think about these emergent whole properties as rather independent of their constituent parts. For language behavior, similar arguments have been inveighed against traditional conditioning theory as explanatory of speaking or listening behavior, because even sequential dependencies among elements in a string do not sufficiently tell about the structure of which the string is an example.

TIME AS A PERCEPTUAL DIMENSION

This part-versus-whole matter is familiar to all of you. My main reason for introducing it here is to show that there are two quite different aspects, both concerning time. A first Gestalt-like conclusion is that you cannot deal appropriately with the discrimination of acoustic elements and expect to understand their role in longer temporal patterns. That is not very profound. It is just that here, in the context of auditory perception, we must have a concept-like pattern or sequence to describe the complexities of auditory processing. But, in addition we must note that the hearing of either an elementary event or combinations of events cannot account for the remarkable performance that listeners show when they deal with spoken language. Here very long patterns, changeable in many respects, depend upon the listener having learned a complicated structure that determines which sequences are orderly in his system and which are not. These rules of grammar, particularly in English, concern unfolding, unidirectional time as well. I would like to deal briefly with these two roles of time, one having to do with its function as a dimension in auditory perception, and the other having to do with its background role for the ordering of events in language structure.

There have been lots of psychological treatises on time. Most of them, however, have dealt with the nature of the experiences past, present, and future, or apparent duration or rhythmic grouping or psychological and chemical clocks that respond to temperature, drugs, and so on.

My own notion about duration is that, if you are expected to make judgments of duration, it is best that you learn about time through your ears. But that is another story, based upon a very little study I did with Deatherage and Bilger[169] some years ago, in which we showed that you could modify a man's estimation of time by modifying his auditory background, but his estimation of time was very stable no matter how you modified his visual background. My present concern, however, is with time as a physical dimension along which, or within which, various stimulus values change to yield different perceptions.

It is true that visual perception also includes some time-dependent phenomena, like apparent movement, but it is auditory perception that requires time as the gridwork for its chief stimulus patterns. The referents for visual perception are often called objects, and they are defined by size and shape. The referents for auditory perception, on the other hand, might better be called events, whose qualities and cues for recognition depend upon what it is that changes, by how much, and how fast in time.

Temporal frameworks may operate at very different levels and for different purposes, as the following speculative outline will show. Here I go into some matters I wrote about in 1959,[167] and I think that my time is so short that I should just mention them briefly.

Time can play a role in determining the quality even of single events. Here I mean, for example, the difference in sound between a rapidly rising and a slowly rising note, say, in music, the difference between sforzando and legato sounds or chords, where the same frequencies may be involved, the same apparent pitch, the same loudness, even the same quality having been produced by the same musical instrument, but yet another quality is given by rise rate, namely, sharpness of attack or other kind of descriptions. In speech, such cues probably account for the distinction between /s/ and /ts/. Similarly, there is a whole range of times separating two very brief clicks that may be, at most, a millisecond apart, and therefore are fused as a single image, and yet the quality of that image, whether click or thud, depends upon how far apart within that millisecond those two are placed.

Similarly, we have examples in single speech sounds or syllables. Let me just take two from a long list of examples from the work of our colleagues at Haskins Laboratories[227] in New York. We find that the difference between the consonant sounds, /b/, /d/, and /g/, for example, are not only dependent upon the spectra characterizing those sounds but, when they are followed by vowels, depend upon the frequency region from which the transition is made to the spectrum characteristic of the following vowel.

Consider the syllables "ba" and "wa." The spectra for the isolated initial sounds /b/ and /w/ are very similar. If you set this spectrum just before one corresponding to the vowel /a/, whether the listener hears "ba" or "wa" is determined almost entirely by the rate at which one changes from one spectrum to the other.

Then there is another whole set of phenomena dealing with temporal fusion, the judgment of simultaneity and successiveness. This has been an interesting group, particularly for comparing the behavior of the visual and the auditory systems, where visual flicker frequencies are of the order of 50 interruptions/second and those in the auditory system are as high as 800 or 1000 interruptions/second. A characteristic figure is 500 with a corresponding reciprocal of 2 milliseconds to separate what can be judged as successive events.

The fact that auditory successiveness here can be given by intervals almost an order of magnitude lower than those that characterize the visual system suggest that this kind of judgment, of fusion or successiveness, is limited probably by the peripheral system (the two systems being quite different, visual and auditory) and not by more central processing.

We come finally to another aspect of temporal judgment, which is the judgment of serial order, the requirement that a listener be able to judge which of two successive stimuli came first. This is a question that I have asked subjects many times, to their

eventual nausea, in fact. There, some of you may recall,[167] we found a figure characteristic of trained observers of about 20 msec., an order of magnitude higher than for successiveness in hearing, but characteristic not only of the auditory system but also of events, one to one sense modality and one to another. This, it seems to us, is not characteristic of a particular sensory modality but, rather, of a more central processing stage.

It is also, incidentally, this judgment of temporal order in which we first begin to find some relation to brain. I won't tell you about Efron's experiments;[100] he is here and he can tell you about them himself. But he does find when there are lesions, primarily in the temporal lobe but some others, that this ability to judge temporal order is severely impaired.

I would remind you also that ordered sequences of pitch, as in melodies, is the first task in which Neff[87] with his colleagues demonstrated that brain function was clearly involved. For any lower-order performance, apparently, you can hack away on cortical tissue a lot before you interfere with that performance.

These were temporal orders of pairs of events. What we mean by sequences are much longer and much more complicated strings, rhythmic and melodic perception, if you like, for which we have much less quantitative information. As these sequential stimulus patterns become parts of speech, then rather special problems are introduced. I think it might be worth some minutes to take one example, again from the Haskins Laboratories,[229] because I think it is worth serious attention.

(Blackboard)—If I may use the musical notation Dr. Thorpe introduced, only call it a spectrogram, then I might show you one example having to do with the distinction between the words "slit" and "split." We have high-frequency friction corresponding to the /s/ sound followed by some formants corresponding to the /l/, which then change up to /I/, and then there is a pause and the /t/ explosion. This is the word "slit." Now the spectrogram for the word "split" is essentially the same form, but the interval between /s/ and /l/ has been prolonged. There is a silence introduced between the /s/ and the /l/ that corresponds to closing off the vocal tract when you close the lips to make "split." This interval in normal speech corresponds to the time for bilabial closure in speech behavior, and it is, if you like, either there or not in speech.

If you have a synthetic sound-making machine like the one at the Haskins Laboratories, you can take that interval between the /s/ and the /l/ and prolong it at will, setting any values in there that you like. This they did and found that there was a range of very small values where the listener always said "slit," and then there was a range of rather longer values in all cases of which the listener said "split." The critical duration that separated these two classes of response corresponded naturally to the duration that one finds in everyday speech.

They did something else which is of interest here. They abstracted out this pause between noise and a following phonation and asked the listeners whether these sound pairs were the same or different. These sounds could be different with respect to the duration of the silent period. What they found was that discrimination between different values of this duration was much better near those durations of the pause that corresponded to speech than at very long ones or very short ones that, if you like, the lips could not make in a bilateral closure gesture.

This is one of the observations on which the motor theory of speech perception[228] depends, and I do not want to talk about that. I would simply call to your attention either that we listen with our tongues or that those particular characteristics of auditory perception that are extremely sharp in listening to the sound of speech correspond to particular sound combinations that we have overlearned, having listened to them

many, many times, all the times that people have been talking to us.

We have talked about some of the sequential factors in speech and language perception. Some are imposed by habitual listening, by the mechanical limitations, as I have just indicated, of the speaking mechanism. But there are others where time is that part of language structure that gets imposed in a rather different way. This business is much clearer on the output side. If I could talk about speech output, then I think I could make the point better, but I know less about it, and I think that less is known.

Lashley's[223] treatment of this question of sequential patterning in motor output tells us that a successive S-R, S-R kind of conditioning just does not work; there is much too much variety in the specific behavior to allow for that kind of interpretation. One must put upon the talker or the singer or the web-spinner a knowledge, a plan that is known before the behavior gets set up.

I can do no better than read to you from an authority in this field who wrote some years ago. St. Augustine[342] wrote as follows:

"I am about to repeat a psalm that I know. Before I begin, my expectation alone reaches itself over the whole; but so soon as I shall have once begun, how much so ever of it I shall take off into the past, over so much my memory also reaches; thus, the life of this action of mine is extended both ways; into my memory so far as it concerns that part which I have repeated already, and into my expectation too, in respect of what I am about to repeat now; but all this while is my marking faculty (*attentio*) present at hand, through which, that which was future, is conveyed over, that it may become past; till the whole expectation be at length vanished quite away, when namely that whole action being ended, shall be absolutely passed into memory. What is now done in this psalm, this holds too throughout the whole course of man's life."

CHAIRMAN MILLIKAN: Dr. Hardy, will you open the discussion, please?

DR. WILLIAM G. HARDY: I suppose I have nothing to add to this very remarkable presentation. I would like to emphasize one or two aspects, however, that we have to deal with daily, clinically, always with the firm conviction that we know very little about what it is we are trying to study, let alone what to do with it. Specifically, in the many many complexities that our small children present to us, particularly the group—and it is a rapidly growing group these days—which seems not to have any clear or overt history of damage. You are all acquainted with the many kinds of perinatal and prenatal events that can damage children. Although I do not believe our clinical load is unique, it is peculiar in that we see many children with multiple kinds of interference, disturbances, disorders, that interfere with learning, particularly learning of language and speech, which seem not to be accountable in any traditional terms. This is the group which nowadays is often referred to as representing aplasias, developmental slowdowns, or anomalies or peculiarities that, in due time, one hopes may be traced out through physiologic or even structural variants. We do not know enough about structure or function, as yet, to do this.

Many of their specific problems have to do with what Dr. Hirsh has presented to you as his No. 2 concept of time, so aptly demonstrated from St. Augustine, in which one calls upon long- as well as short-term memory to try to bring about an orderly array into which and through which to fit an understanding of the events that are ongoing, particularly the incoming events, which are the topic of this discussion.

We find many of the multiply-involved children, however, who apparently have just as many kinds of integrative disturbances in temporal sequencing and in integrative pattern-making, relative to their uses of visual stimuli, as they do to auditory. I suspect if one were better constituted to study other kinds of modalities—I am talking about pre-schoolers now, two, three, and four year olds —if we knew enough to study the other modalities in detail, we probably would find evidence of disturbance or slow-down or distortion and incapacity there, too.

Dr. Hirsh has treated us to a very nice discussion of the capacity of allophones to convey much more meaning, perhaps, than is usually considered. I suspect he would agree that one of the reasons for our lack of information is that we have been so stimulus-bound with word lists which are themselves only scientific inferences or abstractions from the realities of the communicating act, that we are just beginning to pay some attention to the flow and the sequence, and the meaning of the sequence of flow.

You get into some perfectly horrendous word games if you want to consider what it is that a small child has to do. One of the group of 28 little preschoolers we have been studying very intensively for the past three years—a fascinating little fellow—did not seem to be able to know how to get to first base in terms of auditory sequencing and then to develop useful patterns that were immediate and relative to the communicating act pertinent to the situation.

One of the first phrases he learned was "Go get Ann." Mother typically stopped by to pick up little Jimmy in this preschool arrangement, and then, in the course of the orderly timing of the family, about midafternoon would swing a few blocks across town to get Ann, the elder sister, to whom little Jimmy was devoted. So "Go get Ann" became a signal and a directive fraught with a tremendous amount of emotional substance for him. It did not surprise us that this was the first three-word phrase he picked up. One day his mother reported a rather shocking interruption in sequence. This day the time schedule was changed, and mother stopped for Ann first. She was sitting in the back seat when little Jimmy bounced into the front seat, smiled at Ann, and turned to the mother and said, "Go get Ann." This is precisely the kind of disturbance we meet in these children. It is not automatic.

I think it was George Miller who first began to play an interesting kind of word game, which I heartily recommend to you. Dr. Hirsh referred to him. You take a simple series (and you may write this down if visual support is necessary)—you take a simple series like, "The good candy came anyways" —the last "s" is Brooklynese—and simply change time pattern No. 2 to make this read, "The good can decay many ways." You see where we are going in this whole sequence. This is a very troublesome thing for some of the small children we are talking about.

If you take another one—I was playing with it last evening—"Candor is best topped" and you convert that into another time form, "Can Doris be stopped?" we think of some other kinds of confusion.

It must have been about a year and a half ago that a 12 year old, who happens to be the youngest of a couple present here who shall not be further identified, began to play around with some of the possibilities of the Londonderry Air, as he converted it over to London Derrière. So, even 12 year olds fiddle with this kind of time patterning. I think this may seem facetious; I hope it is, but these are the kinds of things that present our very young children with most profound problems in learning.

Just in very broad terms relative to another remark that Dr. Hirsh made, Mr. Chairman, I think it might be profitable to call the attention of this group once again—this is not a new thought—to the fact that we tend to look to the brain for information about communication, when perhaps we might better spend more time looking at the details of the communicative acts and their resulting behavior for information about the brain.

CHAIRMAN MILLIKAN: Thank you, Dr. Hardy. Now open discussion, questions, and comments.

DR. RICHARD ALLEN CHASE: Dr. Hirsh has spoken at some length about the role of temporal parameters of acoustic signals and speech perception, but he also reminded us that the perceptual system that operates upon acoustic inputs can operate in more than one mode. It is this question I would like to comment on briefly.

Dr. Hirsh spoke about the discrimination of phonemes alone, the discrimination of phonemes in words, the discrimination of words, and the discrimination of words in strings that have linguistic integrity. It seems that one does not process a phonemic element in the same way when it is listened to alone as one does when it is embedded in words. One does not discriminate words in the same way when they are presented alone as one does when they are presented in linguistic strings. Once a sound is embedded in context, there is a scheme of probabilities that assists us in recognition, and it would seem to become less necessary to discriminate a lot of the fine structure of the stimulus under such circumstances.

In the case of phoneme recognition, Dr. Hirsh spoke about the acoustic cues underlying the "split-split" distinction. It has been demonstrated that a sufficient acoustic cue for this distinction is the duration of silence between the /s/ friction and the vocalic portion of the syllable.[17,230] It is quite clear that in this case the nervous system is discriminating a very small time interval, and it is on the basis of this discrimination that one distinguishes "slit" from "split." However, it has also been demonstrated that if the interval of silence between the /s/ friction and the vocalic portion of the syllable is continuously varied, subjects hear the continuously varying stimuli as either "slit" or "split."[17,230]

These observations suggest that perceptual accuracy and efficiency is also based on the ability to "fail to process" certain small time differences. I would think, as one moves up the line, embedding phonemes in words, words in linguistic chains, and linguistic chains in specific semantic spaces that, indeed, there would be dramatic shifts in modes of processing acoustic elements.

I would like to suggest that we turn our

attention to a consideration of how many modes of processing might be applied to the same acoustic stimuli. I would further like to suggest that some of the problems we are confronted with clinically may not be predicted upon the inability to process in a certain mode but upon the inability to shift modes when such a shift would be the appropriate strategy to follow.

DR. ROBERT EFRON: Dr. Hirsh has been focusing our attention on the issue of temporal sequence in speech. He is concerned with order of speech sounds and, in relation to this temporal order, the intelligibility of speech. Of course, a word *is* a temporal order, that is, a temporal sequence of sounds. The issue before us is how does the nervous system keep track of the input *order* of sounds and, finally, how do we recognize a specific order of sounds as a word? The experiments of mine on this subject which Dr. Hirsh has just mentioned are probably known to most of you. For those who do not know of them, I will describe them briefly.[99-102]

The experimental problem was to find out, in patients with temporal lobe lesions, the minimum interval between two rather simple but different sounds, at which the subject could indicate which sound came first. This is the classical temporal order experiment that Hirsh and Sherrick[170] did some years ago in normal trained subjects. Essentially I obtained similar kinds of results in neurologically normal but untrained hospitalized patients. For the visual as well as the auditory system, I found that, for inexperienced observers, the two stimuli have to be approximately 50-60 msec. apart before the subject can identify the correct order in which they occurred.

Now, the neurologist is faced with many patients who cannot understand speech. The question which we asked was, "Can there be a disturbance in this capacity to sequence a set of simple sounds which might account for the failure of these patients to understand speech?" The answer, very definitely, is "yes." We found that patients who had aphasia —I am using the term "aphasia" very broad-

ly at the moment—frequently require enormous intervals before they can separate and give a correct report of which sound occurred first. I have already given you the normal figure—60 msec. I have come across aphasics who have required as much as a second between two brief, 10 msec. sounds of very different frequencies before they could correctly identify the temporal order. We can, of course, show that their pitch discrimination was normal by routine audiometry. When the intervals between two sounds are made sufficiently long, these aphasic subjects achieve a 100 per cent correct score, proving that they understood the instructions and performed reliably. However, as the interval between stimuli was reduced, they failed miserably and their reports of the correct sequence of sounds became random.

This defect of sequencing of auditory stimuli in aphasics has now been replicated by Edwards[98] in California, by Holmes[173] in Boston and by Lowe and Campbell[248] in Atlanta. We can thus consider it to be definitely established that aphasics as a group do suffer from a profound defect of auditory sequencing. What is not established is the relationship of this clearly defined defect of auditory function to the understanding of spoken language. We now know that there is an *association* between aphasia and this type of sequencing defect. It has not been proved that the defect in temporal sequencing is the *primary cause* of the inability to understand speech.

There are some further data that have not been published which might interest you in relation to this problem. To the extent that the two sounds which the subject must sequence are closer together in pitch, to that extent the aphasic subject has even greater difficulty in identifying a temporal order. While some patients succeed in reaching near normal discriminability thresholds if the intervals are several seconds apart, the slope of the decay in function is much sharper if the sounds are more similar in pitch. If we used sounds of, let us say, 256 and 300 cycles/second, these patients have much greater difficulty in detecting the temporal order. They require much more time between the two sounds to identify the order correctly than they do if the sounds are, let us say, of 256 cycles and 3000 cycles.

The puzzling feature about these experiments, in understanding the possible role of this defect of sequencing in aphasia, is this: neither in my work nor in the work of Edwards or Holmes was a major or really significant correlation found between the severity of aphasia (as gauged by clinical criteria) and the degree of difficulty these patients have with sequencing. That is to say, you can have patients whose understanding of speech is quite reasonable (by clinical standards) who are virtually hopeless on this test; other patients who are profoundly aphasic sometimes get near normal results.

To try to clarify this problem, I have recently been doing some experiments on a patient of Dr. Geschwind's who would be clinically called a word-deaf patient. While this man clearly understands *some* spoken speech, his major difficulty is that of understanding spoken speech. His reading is virtually normal. This man's defect in temporal sequencing is extraordinarily profound, frequently requiring an interval of over 800 msec. between two tones that are very different in frequency. With tones more similar in frequency, he often needs an interval of more than one second to identify the temporal order correctly.

The question that has been concerning us, and to which we do not know the answer, is this: how much of the general language disturbance of these patients can be attributed to this defect in temporal sequencing capacity? One might look at patients with various different clinical types of aphasia and attempt to parcel out several different physiological disturbances which give rise to them. The type of defect which I have been studying may be only one of several different defects of temporal ordering which may be found among a large group of aphasics. Dr.

Hirsh has indicated other types which may exist, particularly the temporal intervals between *complex* patterns, rather than the simple pattern so far studied. The further suggestion by Dr. Chase that defects may be found in the temporal analysis of long chains of sounds and in the contextual relationships between sounds deserves further study. I think that we will have to examine many aphasics systematically using these technics and find out how much of their speech defect can be attributed to problems of temporal sequencing—on the input as well as the output side.

DR. ARTHUR L. BENTON: I have a couple of questions. Have you checked the identification of order in visual stimuli in your aphasics or with this word-deaf patient?

DR. EFRON: This word-deaf patient has no defect in the visual sequencing tasks. In fact, the patient was more accurate than I was on visual sequencing even without training. Edwards did not attempt to replicate my experiments on visual sequencing but Holmes did. She was unable to find a defect in the visual sequencing in her group of aphasics. This may have been due to the fact that my group had several patients with more posterior lesions. This point remains to be clarified.

DR. GESCHWIND: I would like to highlight one of the points that Dr. Efron made which illustrates some of the complexities of these problems. Some of the patients who, in his original study, had the worst defects in temporal ordering were people whose auditory comprehension was, by clinical standards, excellent. One might expect that if a disturbance in perception of temporal order was relevant to aphasia it would show up in comprehension disturbance.

We can also, conversely, be sure that certain types of comprehension disturbance could not be the result of difficulties in perceiving sequences. Thus, there are aphasic patients whose comprehension is grossly impaired but who yet show the ability to repeat perfectly. It is obvious that in this group the disturbance could not be due to a difficulty of temporal ordering at the auditory level since the intact repetition insures that the sounds were perceived in the correct order.

DR. HILDRED SCHUELL: We have a little information about the patients referred to as word-deaf, or partially word-deaf. I prefer Dr. Roberts' term, partial auditory imperception, which is more comprehensive as well as more accurate. I agree with Dr. Geschwind that patients who show this disability are not all alike but have more or less extended involvement of other cerebral systems.

We have found consistent impairment of phoneme discrimination in patients we have studied. One test we use requires subjects to discriminate between paired words, such as *mail* and *nail*, and *face* and *vase*, by pointing to an appropriate picture. We experimented with a good many paired words and eliminated those that were consistently missed by nonaphasic subjects, presumably because of high frequency hearing losses.

Twenty-six of 30 nonaphasic subjects from the same hospital population and with a similar age distribution to the aphasic subjects made no errors on the test, while four subjects made one error each. The median error was zero for both aphasic and nonaphasic subjects. For 31 aphasic subjects, the mean error was 1.23, with a standard deviation of 2.11. Thus, four errors was almost one standard deviation from the mean, while six errors was two standard deviations away. So far every patient we have tested who has made four or more errors on this test has been classified, on the basis of overall test pattern, in the group characterized by partial auditory imperception. This test appears to pick them out.

As we have worked with patients with auditory imperception in the clinic, it has become clear that they have more persistent difficulty discriminating phonemes than other aphasic patients. Study of error patterns shows that they usually can hear no difference between short vowels in isolation or in syllables and reveals a tendency to confuse phonemes with similar loci of articulation or

similar movement patterns, such as /p/, /b/, /m/; /t/, /d/, /n/, /l/; /f/, /v/; and /k/, /g/. Substitutions rarely cross these boundaries. Discrimination does improve, however, and percentage of errors on relevant tasks gradually decreases.

A striking phenomenon is the on-off effect of auditory imperception. I have been working for more than a year with an extremely intelligent man, a writer and news analyst, who presented severe aphasia with auditory imperception following a cerebral hemorrhage. Now he follows most ordinary conversations and usually responds with appropriate, although limited, language which frequently sounds very normal. He is writing a little, although this has been difficult. For more than six months he has been writing his name, address, and the date spontaneously every day, then reading it back. After he has done this, I may say, "What year is this?" and sometimes he has no idea what I have asked. He may repeat the word, "Year —year—year," and add, "It doesn't get in." Although he uses a very literate vocabulary now, a word as simple as "year," "name," "street," or "city" on some occasions evokes no response while on other occasions the response is prompt and accurate. The random on-off effect is very puzzling. I would be happy if anyone could throw some light on it.

CHAIRMAN MILLIKAN: Before we go on, Dr. Rosenblith, would you care to make any comments about the relationship of sequencing and temporal patterns as they influence the ability of an electronic machine to set and store information?

DR. WALTER A. ROSENBLITH: Frankly, I would not.

CHAIRMAN MILLIKAN: Dr. Rich, does a computer have difficulty in the matter of sequencing of temporal patterns?

DR. ROBERT P. RICH: I think I must not understand your question. The machine accepts the pattern, through any of its modalities, in the sequence in which it is given, or else it is busted and we fix it. Machines are different from people in this regard.

DR. ERIC H. LENNEBERG: Regarding Holmes'[173] data to which Dr. Efron referred, the patient simply had to say whether the high-pitched tone came first or the low-pitched tone came first. Normal subjects were compared with patients with aphasia and with other brain-damaged subjects. All the aphasic patients were extremely light cases; approximately half of them had predominantly expressive disturbances and half receptive.

It is interesting that for the normal patients the interval can be extremely short, certainly much less than 100 msec., usually from 20 to 40 msec. The aphasics differ very dramatically, making a much higher percentage of errors.

Similar tasks for visual material (involving colors) and cross-modal material does not bring out a difference between aphasic patients, brain-damaged patients, and normal subjects. It is just the auditory material that brings out this very dramatic difference.

I think this is suggestive that Dr. Geschwind's point is well taken, that generalizing from these artificial, somewhat contrived experiments may not be entirely appropriate, but I do think that here we have some indications that language is peculiarly involved in auditory temporal processing.

DR. RAYMOND CARHART: This has been a very interesting discussion, but it has moved from the realm of the sound spectrogram to that of the cerebral cortex without much attention to the processes that occur between these two end points.

Dr. Hardy made a remark which offers one way of increasing our understanding of these intermediate processes. He stresses that we should use speech tests to get information about the brain. Now I want to stress that clinical patients can be very useful as research subjects when we follow such a plan. These individuals present different kinds of clinical problems leading to different types of auditory breakdown in the central processing of speech information. By analyzing these distinctions insightfully we can acquire a great deal of knowledge regarding the functions and activities of the structures that lie be-

tween the peripheral sensory system and the cerebral system. In other words, we can learn much about the roles of the several levels of the auditory nervous system through appropriate testing of patients with neurological lesions. Let me clarify this thought by brief mention of three topics that illustrate the kind of information which auditory testing can make available when applied in clinical research.

The first example is found in the pure tone audiogram which typifies hearing loss due either to kernicterus neonatorum or to birth anoxia. Such an audiogram ordinarily shows a very mild loss for low frequency tones with substantial impairment of thresholds for high frequency tones. Remembering that the lesions in this type of case are probably in the cochlear nuclei, the hearing pattern just described may be taken as evidence that within the cochlear nuclei there are two mechanisms for coding and transmitting information on the frequency of the stimulus. The rationale for this statement goes back to Wever's volley-place theory.[409]

This theory, you will recall, holds that low frequency sounds are discriminated on the basis of volleys of nerve impulses. These volleys have the same frequency as that of the incoming stimulus. By contrast, high frequencies are mediated on the basis of information as to the place along the organ of corti where maximum stimulation occurs. People have not given too much thought in recent years to the clinical implications of this theory. However, one may interpret the audiogram typifying kernicterus neonatorum and birth anoxia as the result of a particular type of lesion which disturbs the capacity of the cochlear nuclei to pass on information as to the place of maximum cochlear stimulation much more than it disturbs the capacity to transmit volley information to higher centers. Here is an instance where a clinical entity supports the speculation that identification of place and identification of volley-rate involve two different activities at the first way-station in the auditory nervous system. Exploration of this hypothesis will add importantly to the understanding of auditory neurophysiology.

Another clinical observation has interesting implications. It is well known that unilateral lesions within the central auditory system, provided these are beyond the cochlear nuclei, interfere with the understanding of speech coming through the contralateral ear. Jerger,[187] among others, has shown this phenomenon to occur whether the damage is in the brain stem or the temporal lobe. Such observations lead to the opinion that the particular array of neural coding which is essential to the understanding of speech (and, hence, the input code which is essential to language acquisition) is transmitted from one ear through a crossed pathway to the opposite hemisphere. Said in another way, we do not have balanced bilateral representation of the neural code for unilaterally heard speech. Thus, it may be that meaningful sound complexes, as exemplified by speech, have a more restricted course through the auditory system than do at least some of the elementary attributes of these same stimuli.

Turning to the third topic, there are fascinating implications in the observations by Cherry,[65] by Kimura,[198] and by others[53,89] that two independent trains of speech material are completely separable when the two trains are received unilaterally but in opposite ears. There is ample proof that the ordinary listener can attend to one of these trains of speech and completely disregard the other. This fact, which actually is commonplace knowledge, raises the question as to how the two trains of speech information are kept separate within the cortical complex. More specifically, since each ear transmits speech information to the contralateral temporal lobe, one cannot help wondering whether substantial amounts of speech information are retained separately in the two cerebral hemispheres. It is worth remembering, for example, that studies such as Kimura's and Dirks' demonstrate cerebral dominance for received speech on the basis of the proportion of errors made via each ear when conflicting test materials are presented to opposite ears. Much of the material that is being received

under these circumstances by the nondominant hemisphere is being understood. One must, therefore, conclude that the advantage which the dominant hemisphere exhibits over the nondominant one is a modest statistical one. Both trains of incoming material are here kept sufficiently separate so that either may be subsequently reproduced with substantial success.

In summary, I suggest to you that we may learn a great deal about the ways in which the central auditory system processes the various types of auditory information if we will but study the disruptions and peculiarities of auditory behavior manifest by clinical patients with various types of neurological lesions.

DR. MAGOUN: With respect to altering input signals so as to modify what happens in the central machinery of the brain, may I ask whether these fascinating studies of phonemic differentiation, which are seeking to promote auditory comprehension and discrimination in aphasic subjects, are being extended to include other modifications of auditory signals in a way that would tend to aggrandize their impact upon the brain?

The simplest method known to the physiologist to amplify central responses to input signals is to increase the intensity of the stimulus, in this case its loudness. Next, whenever input signals possess the quality of novelty, they evoke an orienting reflex, a centrifugal influence of which upon the involved receptor increases its sensitivity, while a centripetal influence upon the cortex promotes an attentive state and increases the amplitude of the evoked cortical response. Orientation to the evocative signal is promoted also by contrast-enhancement, through central inhibition of all competing neural activity related to inputs from the peripheral surround. By contrast, when stereotyped signals are presented with monotonous repetition, a process called habituation ensues, which actively reduces central transmission of such signals in a manner preventing orientation and attention to them.

Third, a pronounced generalization and

amplification of central responses to afferent signals follows their associated reinforcement, irrespective of whether this is of a rewarding or an aversive type. This central facilitation of input signals is more persistent than that of the orienting reflex and does not attenuate upon repetition. Indeed, when a novel afferent signal, initially facilitated by the orienting reflex, is monotonously repeated until habituation occurs, the introduction of reinforcement immediately overcomes habituation and augments central responses far beyond their original amplitude and central distribution.

Do any of these means of magnifying the central impact of input signals, by augmenting transmission or by reflex or learned facilitation, promote auditory perception, comprehension, and discrimination in aphasia?

CHAIRMAN MILLIKAN: Dr. Hirsh, can you comment about that?

DR. HIRSH: Certainly not about normals and certainly not about aphasic patients.

CHAIRMAN MILLIKAN: Dr. Efron!

DR. EFRON: Changing the intensity does not significantly alter the performance, provided that the stimuli are above threshold. On the issue of novelty, Dr. Magoun, there is an observation which might be germane to your thoughts. If you give the patient two tones, separated by a fixed interval, and then just merely change the temporal order, the high and the low, the patient develops a "set" for that particular individual interval; he achieves a certain kind of performance. If, however, we deliver random intervals as well as a random order (this would be the feature of novelty to which you may be referring) the subject's performance is distinctly worse. He takes more time, on the average, to identify the correct order, if both interval and order are randomized. Whether this is what you have in mind, or whether this information helps you, is for you to decide.

DR. SCHUELL: We have found that there seems to be some optimal level of stimulus intensity that varies from patient to patient.

Particularly at the beginning of treatment, patients become disturbed if intensity is too great and respond in a disorganized fashion. However, below the level of disruption, increasing intensity sometimes produces a higher percentage of correct responses.

Slowing down the rate of speech also seems to increase ability to respond. This appears to be a transient effect, however. Most patients with impaired auditory perception cannot use the Language Master at first, because the taped words come too fast for them. One patient damaged the instrument by holding on to the card to try to slow it down forcibly as the tape passed the electrodes. After two or three weeks of training, however, there seems to be no difference between responses to normal and to slowed speech.

If you slow down speech too much, I think you probably produce enough pattern distortion to impede recognition. I do not know what these limits are, and I do not think they are the same for all patients nor for the same patient in all periods of recovery. I am sure, however, that there is an effect of intensity, of rate of presentation, and of stimulus duration. I am not sure about stimulus novelty. We have found transient effects from presenting a series of stimuli, for example, in a new way. As far as I have been able to observe, this merely serves as a temporary distraction, without resulting in any permanent gain.

DR. BRENDA MILNER: I would like to elaborate a little on Dr. Hirsh's reference to Doreen Kimura's experiments on dichotic listening. When different sets of digits are presented simultaneously to the two ears by means of a dual-channel tape recorder and stereophonic earphones, more digits are reported accurately for the right than for the left ear, this result being reversed for subjects known to have speech representation in the right hemisphere.[199] Thus, the channel contralateral to the dominant temporal lobe is favored for this verbal material. Dirks[89] has extended these findings to filtered, phonetically balanced words, different words being presented to the left and right ears. With such simultaneously conflicting verbal input, accuracy of report is again greater for the right ear in normal, right-handed subjects.

What I wanted to add is that Dr. Kimura then went on to devise a dichotic melodies task, in which different snatches of music (solo passages from baroque concertos) are presented simultaneously, one to each ear, and the subject must then select from a series of four items played successively, the two which had been presented previously. For this nonverbal, melodic material, normal subjects obtain better recognition scores for the left than the right ear, the same subjects showing the expected right-ear superiority for reproducing dichotically presented digits. Since Broadbent and Gregory[55] have shown right-ear superiority for digit recognition and not merely for digit recall, the different results obtained by Kimura for melodies and digits are clearly due to differences in the stimulus material and not to differences in testing technic. Hence, the relative efficiency of the two ears can be reversed by switching from words to music, reflecting the greater involvement of the left hemisphere in verbal and of the right in nonverbal functions.

CHAIRMAN MILLIKAN: Dr. Rosenblith.

DR. ROSENBLITH: I will still not rise on behalf of machines but on behalf of pink boxes instead of black ones. The point that Professor Magoun has raised on speech processing and the relation of what might be happening in terms of orienting reflexes, I think is one that deserves a good deal more discussion.

It seems to me that the time scale of phenomena at the level of orienting reflexes is a good deal more related, in this domain of speech communication, not to the questions of immediate chaining of sound but to the problems of the grammatical structure of a sentence—the intonation patterns that, in some sense, set the processing at a higher level. What we must be talking about, when we talk about processing of speech, is not precisely a question of what we do with word lists, but rather of the chaining of events. In a way, the grammatical structure provides the continuing orienting reflex towards the process. But, again, we do not really have very much evidence about that. The gap between the kind of phenomena that we can examine neurophysiologically, let us say, occurs because the level of evolution at which we are operating is not quite the level of evolution of the species that deals with language. But if we address ourselves to this question that seems to have been in the foreground of some, namely, this question of serial order, we have, certainly on a very different time scale (a microtime scale), the problem of the effect of the two ears. That is probably the best investigated problem of this type, as far as the nervous system is concerned.

If one deals with the problem of binaural effect, one finds, as have a variety of workers have who worked on it—Rosenzweig, Galambos, and perhaps most quantitatively, Joseph Hall—that there are in the superior olive a lot of units whose particular job is precisely to weigh the information, depending upon from which ear it comes in first. You have the single units that operate there at a spontaneous level of activity. If the right ear should come ahead 10 microseconds, then this unit might, for instance, exhibit strong excitation, while if the left ear should come in 10 microseconds ahead, the unit will show inhibition. Out of this model of a population of neurons in the superior olive you can predict quite well the upper limit of performance that a psychophysical experiment will give you in a trained observer—how he will judge lateralization or which side the stimulus comes from.

This happens at a level that Ray Carhart would like to address himself to, namely, between the cochlea and the cortex. The cortex is not just a mimicker of what the superior olive does, as we all know. The problem that does arise here is, with this information now available, that these units seem to be highly specific in this respect. But perhaps the more important thing to say is that the output of these units seems to have effect not only in terms of getting later copies, albeit abstracted copies of this message, but that, to a very large extent, in various regions at higher levels of the nervous system, sequencing influences the way in which a variety of sounds that come in a chain are being processed.

I think we must distinguish three kinds of problems: (1) the type of problem that deals with this trivial kind of priority allocation, as to which ear came first; (2) the problem that information of this type influences processing at various levels of the nervous system; and (3) the type of problem that in my opinion is most directly related to the kind of language behavior that we seem to be fixing our attention on, namely, the one that has to do with the kind of grammatical structure, translated into physiological mechanisms, which Dr. Magoun has mentioned in speaking of the orienting reflex.

DR. W. GREY WALTER: I feel that we are really confused in discussing the peripheral mechanisms and just the cortex. The question I want to raise is, "Which cortex and where?" In relation to what Dr. Magoun said and to revert to his discovery of the diffuse projection systems to the frontal cortex, there are three cortical regions involved. There is the specific projection area, the adjacent specific association areas, and the enormous mass of gray matter in the frontal cortex. It is in this region that we may find the answer to some of these puzzles. A good deal of confusion is caused in the clinic by what one might call "specific dysphasics" who think and understand quite well. The answer to this puzzle may be quite straightforward.

In the frontal lobes we have a part of the sensory system. All sensory information is relayed to the frontal cortex, and in this region a new effect appears during semantic conditioning, a slow potential change which we have called the *expectancy wave*. If the frontal cortex is intact, it develops an expectancy wave in relation to semantic signals, however weak, whether novel or not, provided they have some degree of redundancy, and in this condition the person will understand the communication, whether it is a single event, word, or sentence. But if the frontal cortex is damaged in some way, either by disease or trauma or developmental anomaly, then the person may have perfect pitch discrimination and be able to repeat and echo all that is said to him, yet be quite incapable of comprehending or using this information.

The frontal cortex of man provides a system for almost doing without the specific signals from the specific receiving areas. For example, we have seen patients in whom there are no evoked responses to auditory stimuli. The degree of damage is so great that the specific regions in the association areas, and even the nonspecific pathways to the frontal lobes, provide no evoked responses, and yet these people can produce an expectancy wave in response to a semantic stimulus.

So the frontal cortex, particularly the superior and medial frontal cortex in man, can fulfill the role of signal discrimination, even when the primary data are only just redundant enough to provide the essential information. Our language is usually at least 50 per cent redundant, and the brain is very well adapted to deal with this type of language, having created it in the first place. You only have to try a foreign language, where every syllable may be significant, to see how pathetic your response could be when the redundancy is reduced to zero. I think this may provide a clue to the distinction between specific and nonspecific disabilities in speech disorders.

CHAIRMAN MILLIKAN: Dr. Hirsh, will you close?

DR. HIRSH: I did not know things were that simple! (Laughter) That is marvelous. When people like Broadbent put a model of the receiving system on the blackboard, or on a slide, I sometimes catch myself thinking that that is the nervous system that is being displayed. I am not sure it really is.

There are a couple of points that were brought up in the discussion that I think bear a little further discussion, if not just a summary. I would like to go back to Dr. Hardy's advice that we concentrate our attention on the communicative behavior. I think this is because I feel more comfortable there than I do talking about which part of the nervous system might be related to which kind of function.

The kind of time that I did not talk about, because I had very little to say about it and because the time was short, we might call syntactic time. That has been implicated in several of the remarks that have followed. There are a couple of problems, the most important of which, I suspect, is the one that Dr. Hardy touched on.

When we write words on the blackboard, or when we pronounce words in lists, we have already performed for the listener or the viewer a segmentation. We have broken up the stimulus pattern into parts that correspond to categories in the linguistic system. This is a very difficult problem that has not been dealt with adequately. That is, the acoustic signal that comes to the listener in running speech is an essentially continuous wave form, and he must impose, first, segmentation in order to have events that can be ordered in time. If the segmentation is not performed, then he has a continuous time function where the concept of order is much more difficult to deal with.

The evidence appears, based on psychological experiments, where you have competing signals, where it is clear that not all the information that comes to the ear goes to the mind, that the information must be collected in baskets or categories of some kind before decision-making takes place. Think of the task, for example, of the German listener who must listen to 12 or 14 words before he gets to the verb and then must let the information given by the verb act back on all those signals that have been received up to that time.

I outlined, before Grey Walter started speaking, three different ranges of time, on which I would like to focus three different kinds of interest. The first one I called microtime. Just to set some limits, I think microtime, at least so far as auditory perception is concerned, extends upwards to about 2 msec. Then there is a range from about 2 to 200 msec., where we are dealing with a kind of macrotime, which determines the nature of individual auditory events—individual acoustic patterns or temporal patterns, if you will. And then the time that is related to grammar probably involves intervals longer than about 100 msec.

I am using as a base here a syllabic rate in talking. I am sure this is what I mean also by syntactic time. Dr. Rosenblith has spoken about the strings being organized according to the linguistic structure that the listener has learned up to that time. It seems to me that on these long-time intervals one operates on at least three features of the spoken language.

(Blackboard) I write this sequence of words (I write it in order to make it ambiguous from the acoustic point of view): "Had he not gone." One of these three features is intonation. One form of intonation would follow this with a question mark. Another intonation would follow this with a comma, and go on with a clause. This is a kind of clue. Another kind, a morphological clue, still dealing in macrotime, less than the syntactic time, has to do, for example, with the fact there is a "had" here rather than "has."

Finally, the other aspect of grammar, namely, word order, involves rather larger chunks of time. You can see that with this word order we know it is not a simple declarative sentence. With this intonation pattern, we know something else must follow, and so on. I do not think that we can subsume all these roles that time plays in the understanding of spoken language, even in the context of structure, in one basket. I think they are quite separate. Whether they involve separate parts of the nervous system or not, I am not sure, but I think our further treatment of them will benefit from this separation.

CHAIRMAN MILLIKAN: Thank you, Dr. Hirsh. Dr. Evarts will now discuss "The Output Side of Information Processing."

The Output Side of Information Processing

EDWARD V. EVARTS

National Institute of Mental Health
Bethesda, Maryland

ONE HUNDRED YEARS AGO Broca[56] published a paper entitled "Sur la faculté du langage articulé" and the neurological world entered an exciting period of investigation of the central representation of speech. It is indeed fitting to have a meeting such as the present one on the one hundredth anniversary of Broca's paper. Having made this opening remark, I must immediately apologize for the fact that the experimental results I will present do not deal with speech mechanisms *per se*. Because of this lack of direct relevance, I thought it might be worthwhile, in introducing my topic, to go over some of the ideas that neurologists have had about the cerebral organization of the movements essential for speech, since their ideas may suggest some slight relevance of my own data to the topic of this Conference.

As I have already mentioned, it was one century ago that Broca published his well-known series of papers. However, even before Broca, some very interesting ideas about the cerebral organization of the movements underlying speech were developed by Bouillaud,[43] who in 1825 pointed out: "Since certain movements of the tongue, such as those of prehension, mastication, deglutition, *et cetera*, persist, although those necessary for the articulation of sounds are abolished by lesion of the anterior lobes of the brain, it follows that the tongue has in the nerve-centre several sources of distinct action."

Bouillaud clearly recognized that the occurrence of speech in man and its absence in lower animals was not primarily the result of a difference in the lower motor apparatus but that speech was related to the organization of the higher centers. Thus, again in 1825[43] he said, "If we are asked why animals do not speak we should not reply with many naturalists that they have no suitable external organs but we should add that this lack of speech arose from a more potent cause, to wit the absence of the internal organ, the cerebral centre, which dictates, so to say, and coordinates the complicated movements by means of which man expresses the operations of his understanding."

Thus, Bouillaud made a distinction between the lower motor mechanisms necessary for the occurrence of speech and the higher nervous activity essential for the control of these lower mechanisms.

With Broca's series of papers from 1861 to 1865, emphasis shifted from the question of the general organization of motor mechanisms of speech to the problem of the precise cerebral localization of the centers for speech. Since my concern at this meeting is not one of cortical localization, I will not discuss Broca's contributions further. Rather, in this introduction, I will shift attention to Hughlings Jackson, in whose work analysis of the cerebral organization of movement reached its highest point of development. I believe that physiological analysis of cerebral mechanisms in movement can very well take as a point of departure the overall principles which Jackson put forward.

In considering speech, Jackson distinguished between intellectual and emotional language, a distinction which is similar to

39

the one proposed by Dr. Thorpe: propositional versus emotive sounds. It is the former
type, the propositional type of communication, which is particularly affected by cerebral lesions. Jackson described cases of
speech defect in which the patient could not
protrude his tongue on being commanded to
do so, but could use it perfectly well in all
automatic movement, as licking his lips. In
describing this differential effect of cerebral
lesions on movement, Jackson pointed out
that the magnitude of the effect depended
upon the context in which the movement took
place. This could be seen not only in the
case of speech disorder but also in cases of
other disorders of movement—of hand movement, for instance. Head[148, Vol. 1, p. 197] makes
the same point as Jackson. He states, "Speechless patients are not necessarily wordless, for
they can swear or even ejaculate appropriate
expressions. A man, usually speechless, may
at times produce a complete phrase." In describing a particular case, Head says, "No.
21 could reply 'yes' and 'no' correctly but
could not repeat these words at will. Asked
to say 'yes' he answered 'No. No, I can't
repeat this.' When told to say 'no' he would
shake his head, and once replied 'No, I don't
know how to do it.'"

The relation of these clinical observations
to modern neurophysiological studies has
been extensively and critically considered by
Walshe.[398] In his analysis of this subject,
Walshe devoted particular attention to Jackson's hypothesis concerning the representation of *movements* rather than *muscles* in the
motor cortex. In considering the alternative
hypotheses of muscle versus movement representation, Walshe stated: "That muscles
are not therein represented in the cortex is
illustrated daily by every case of residual
hemiparesis, where we may see the extensors
of the wrist paralyzed as prime movers in an
attempted voluntary extension of the wrist
but powerfully active as synergists in every
forceful grasping movement of the fist. Were
a direct representation of muscles in question,
this familiar, clinical phenomenon could not

occur." At the present time there is still much
controversy between the proponents of the
notions of Jackson, as dealt with further by
Walshe, and the ideas based on certain
physiological studies, best exemplified by
those of Chang, Ruch, and Ward,[59] on a
punctate muscle localization in the cortex.

Until recently it has been impossible to
study the activity of the cerebral neurons in
association with movement occurring under
physiological conditions; the reason has been
largely a technical one. The neurophysiologist
who investigates cerebral mechanisms in
movement has in the past employed the technics of electrical stimulation of the brain
or ablation of cerebral tissue. While very
useful for certain problems, these technics are
clearly limited in the elucidation of the
process underlying normal movement.

Recently it has become possible to add a
third technic to the two previously employed
methods. This technic involves the recording
of discharge patterns of individual cerebral
neurons during normal movement. Of course,
the technic of single unit recording is an
old one. But because the recording of individual neurons requires that the electrode
remain very close to the individual cell, it
was long thought that recording of single
neuron activity in moving animals would not
be possible. Now, however, the technical
obstacles have been overcome by the work of
Hubel,[176] who worked out a system for fixing
a microelectrode to a chamber attached to
the head, such that when the head moved,
the recording system went right along with
it, there being no net displacement between
the recording electrode and the neuron from
which activity was being recorded. The report
which I am going to give will present the
results of studies in which the activity of
neurons in the motor cortex of the monkey
has been observed during a variety of physiological movements.

METHODS

In the monkey the classical motor cortex
is located in the precentral gyrus. Though

this particular region is one of special significance in the control of movement, widespread additional regions also have an important role in movement. But, in preliminary studies, it seemed that the classical precentral motor cortex would be a reasonable region in which to begin recording. Furthermore, it seemed that rather than recording from *all* neurons whose action potentials the microelectrode succeeded in isolating, it might be good to select a certain subclass of these neurons. The subclass selected was that consisting of pyramidal tract neurons (PTNs). The cell bodies of these neurons lie in the cerebral cortex and their axons descend to the spinal cord via the medullary pyramid. I am going to talk about what happens to the activity of PTNs when the monkey moves. The movements which will be dealt with are hand movements, and the region of the precentral gyrus from which PTNs were picked up was the hand area.

Before going on to describe the actual experimental results, I will say a few words about how the PTNs in the hand area of the precentral gyrus were distinguished from the much more numerous neurons which do *not* send axons to the spinal cord via the medullary pyramid. This identification of PTNs is made possible by the fact that PTNs (whose axons pass through the medullary pyramid) respond antidromically to brief electric shocks applied to the medullary pyramid; cortical neurons whose axons do not descend via the pyramid will not have such antidromic responses.

In the actual recording sessions, a movable microelectrode is lowered into the precentral gyrus several days after stimulating electrodes have been permanently implanted in the medullary pyramid. As the microelectrode is lowered into the precentral gyrus, the ipsilateral medullary pyramid is stimulated once a second, and occasionally the microelectrode will pick up the action potential of a neuron which responds antidromically to the pyramidal shock. The occurrence of the antidromic response identifies

this neuron as a PTN and the electric stimulus to the medullary pyramid may be terminated. Now the activity of the PTN may be studied in association with movement of the hand.

In addition to identifying PTNs, the antidromic response provides information about axonal conduction velocity. The distance between the point of stimulation in the medullary pyramid and the point of microelectrode recording in the precentral gyrus is about 70 mm. Thus, for a PTN whose axon has a conduction velocity of 70 meters/second there will be a delay of 1 msec. between stimulation of the PTN axon in the pyramid and occurrence of the antidromic response in the PTN cell body in the motor cortex. This delay between stimulus and antidromic response is called antidromic latency (ADL) and is inversely proportional to the axonal conduction velocity. The information gained about axonal conduction velocity allows inferences to be made concerning the axonal size, since conduction velocity is directly proportional to axonal diameter: the conduction velocity of an axon in meters/second is about six times its diameter in microns. Thus, an axon with a conduction velocity of 60 meters/second has a diameter of about 10 microns.

RESULTS

In presenting the results, I am going to divide the material according to several points. The first will deal with the relation of axonal conduction velocity (ACV) to the pattern of output which the PTN has in association with movement. In a number of other neuronal systems any wide variation in ACV within a population of neurons has important functional correlates. It thus seemed reasonable to look for the functional correlates of ACV in PTNs.

The pyramidal tract contains axons which vary in diameter from about 20 microns to 1 micron, with ACVs from 120 to 6 meters/second—an enormous spectrum. The very largest axons arise predominantly from the

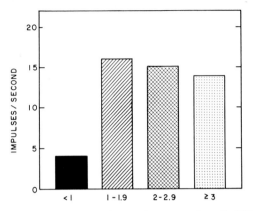

Fig. 15. Mean discharge frequency for 62 PT units divided into four groups according to latency. It may be seen that the mean discharge frequency of the shortest latency group is considerably less than that of any of the three groups with longer antidromic response latencies. (Reprinted from Evarts.[110])

precentral gyrus and, in particular, from the cells which have been referred to as Betz cells. The pyramidal tract was once thought to arise entirely from Betz cells, but it has since been learned that the pyramidal tract arises from small cells as well as large, with only about 2 per cent of PTNs being Betz cells.

Figure 15 illustrates the relation of discharge frequency of PTNs to ADL when the monkey is awake and just sitting in his primate chair. Remember that the less the ADL of a neuron, the more rapid its conduction velocity. Thus, in Figure 15 units in the group with ADL less than 1 msec. have very rapidly conducting axons. Figure 15 shows that the group of PTNs with the most rapidly conducting axons (shortest ADLs) is rather inactive when the monkey is awake but not moving, whereas the remaining tract neurons with longer ADLs have tonic discharge even in the absence of movement.

Figure 16 shows the change in discharge frequency of these groups of PTNs with movement. The movements here are spontaneous—the monkey is given a banana or

grape which he may squeeze, manipulate, etc. (he is not allowed to eat it). It may be seen that the neurons with the larger axons and the highest conduction velocities (shortest ADLs) show the greatest increase in activity in association with these spontaneous movements, whereas the neurons with the smaller axons and lower conduction velocities (remember that they were tonically active when the monkey was not moving) may actually show a net decrease in discharge.

Figure 17 illustrates this relation of discharge frequency and ADL in two PTNs recorded simultaneously with the same microelectrode. During absence of movement one of the neuron's discharged tonically; the other neuron, which has a shorter ADL, has very little activity when the contralateral arm was at rest. When the monkey moved his contralateral arm, the neuron with the shorter ADL which had been silent went into action, and the neuron with the longer ADL, which

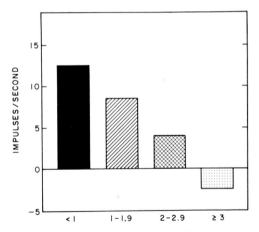

Fig. 16. As in Figure 15, the 62 PT units have been divided into four groups according to latency of antidromic response. For each of these four groups, mean discharge frequency during waking without movement has been subtracted from mean discharge frequency during contralateral arm movement. This difference, the increase in discharge frequency with movement, is greatest for the shortest latency units. The longest latency group of units shows a slight average decrease in discharge frequency with movement. (Reprinted from Evarts.[110])

was tonically active even in the absence of movement, had a modulation of this discharge frequency—the modulation being both up and down.

In general, then, it was found that the PTNs with larger axons have *phasic* discharge properties: they are inactive in the absence of movement but become very active with movement. In contrast, PTNs with smaller axons have *tonic* discharge properties. In terms of the processing of output information, one sees that those PTNs which conduct most rapidly transmit information related to transient phenomena, and tend to become inactive in the steady state.

The movements referred to above were spontaneous and uncontrolled and for this reason allowed detection of only the grossest types of correlations between PTN activity and movement. The determination of information concerning the latency between the "command" to move and the occurrence of discharge in the pyramidal tract was the next goal of these studies, and this determination required a more reliable movement. To this end, monkeys were trained to extend the wrist in response to the onset of a light. In what follows I will present data obtained in relation to this learned movement. Information on this point seemed of interest because, in fact, it had not previously been shown that pyramidal tract discharge

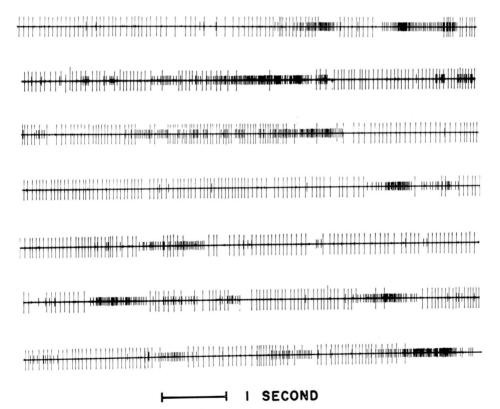

├──────────┤ I SECOND

Fig. 17. Discharge patterns of a pair of PT neurons. The larger spike responded antidromically with a latency of 1.5 msec., and the smaller spike had a latency of 0.8 msec. The shorter latency unit (small spike) was relatively inactive in the absence of movement but discharged during contralateral arm movement. The longer latency unit had regular discharge in the absence of movement and showed both speeding and slowing when movement took place. (Reprinted from Evarts.[110])

actually *precedes* the occurrence of voluntary movement.

Monkeys were trained to depress a telegraph key (closing a contact) until a light came on and to release the telegraph key promptly following the onset of a light. Figure 18 shows an electromyographic correlate of the hand movement which the monkey was trained to make. Wrist flexion was necessary for production of contact closure and, as would be expected, the EMG showed a predominance of activity in the wrist flexors during contact closure; contact opening involved a reduction in the activity of wrist flexors and an increase in the activity of wrist extensors. Within a short time (usually less than a second) after the monkey had opened the contact following light onset, she usually closed it again, beginning a new sequence. The period of time for which the

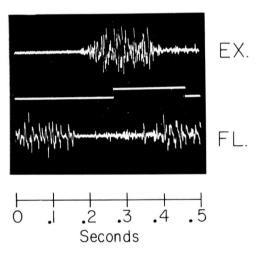

EX.

FL.

0	.1	.2	.3	.4	.5

Seconds

Fig. 18. This figure illustrates the reciprocal activity of extensors (top) and flexors (bottom) during the wrist movement which monkeys were trained to perform. Sweeps start at the onset of the light, at a time of wrist flexion. At about 150 msec. following light onset there was a reduction in flexor activity and a reciprocal increase of extensor activity. This EMG response was followed by opening of the contact, as indicated in the center line. The term "reaction time" as it is used in this paper is the interval from light onset to contact opening. (Reprinted from Evarts.[109])

monkey was required to flex (maintaining contact closure) prior to light onset was varied from trial to trial over a range of 1 to 5 seconds so as to prevent the monkey from predicting the time at which the light would appear. A premature release by the monkey (that is, a release prior to light onset) did not result in reward, and following such a premature release the press had to restart from time zero. Thus, when the monkey released prior to light onset, she reduced the overall frequency of reward. As a result of these contingencies, the monkey maintained steady wrist flexion until light onset, extended her wrist for a fraction of a second following light onset, and then started steady wrist flexion again. During training, two of the five monkeys were required to alternate right and left hands rather frequently—the aim being to have them gain equal proficiency in the use of both hands. The remaining three monkeys were trained on only one hand. In the present experiments it was desirable that performance become highly stable prior to single unit recording and to this end monkeys were given 100,000 trials or more before unit recording was begun.

The detailed results obtained in this study will not be described in the published report of this conference, since some have already appeared and others will be published in complete form in the *Journal of Neurophysiology.*[109-111] Rather, I will here summarize the major findings. In summary form then, the studies provided answers to four questions of pyramidal tract physiology. These questions and their answers follow.

1. At what point in the interval between conditioned stimulus (light onset) and conditioned response (wrist extension) does modification of discharge in PTNs occur?

It was found that even in cases of minimum (180 msec.) reaction times by the monkey, the latency of the antecedent modification of pyramidal tract discharge does not fall below 100 msec. This 100 msec. latency stands in sharp contrast to the 30 msec. latency with which PTNs in the motor cortex discharge in response to a photic stimulus in animals anesthetized with chloralose.[397] It is clear, then, that for this conditioned movement, the latency of response in PTNs is delayed at least 70 msec. beyond the minimum latency demanded by the anatomical connections between the retina and motor cortex. What sequence of neuronal events takes place during this 70 msec. delay? An answer to this question would provide useful clues as to mechanisms of sensorimotor integration.

2. Is the occurrence of the wrist movement temporally locked to the PTN response?

There was a strong positive correlation between the reaction time of the monkey and the latency of response in PTNs. Thus, in the most proficient monkeys PTN discharge might begin 100 msec. after the conditioned stimulus; the arm muscles might begin to show electromyographic responses about 140 msec. following the conditioned stimulus; and the final response (opening the contact) might occur in 180 msec. For longer latencies of PTN response there were longer reaction times. Thus, it was found that not only did PTN activity precede the behavioral response, but also that lengthening of response latencies in PTNs was associated with lengthening of behavioral response latencies, that is, reaction times.

3. What is the relation of axonal conduction velocity of a PTN and the response which it shows in association with movement?

In a previous section of this report it was pointed out that PTNs with high axonal conduction velocities tend to be silent in the absence of movement but to become extremely active during movement. PTNs with lower axonal conduction velocities are ton-

ically active even in the absence of movement. The present study of a conditioned movement revealed an analogous relationship between axonal conduction velocity and discharge properties in PTNs. Thus, units which were silent while the monkey was maintaining wrist flexion but sprang into intense activity prior to wrist extension had high axonal conduction velocities. Units with low axonal conduction velocities did not show sharp transient responses and when their discharge patterns were modified in relation to the wrist extension, they showed either a reduction in discharge frequency or an increase of what had been tonic discharge persisting throughout wrist flexion.

4. Is activity of PTNs related only to contralateral movements, or are there some PTNs whose discharge is related to ipsilateral movements as well?

The great majority of PTNs examined were related to movements of the contralateral wrist and were relatively inactive in relation to ipsilateral wrist movements. Some units were found, however, for which the reverse was true, and this finding provides additional evidence for the role of the pyramidal tract in control of ipsilateral movement.

Before closing, I wish to make one final point concerning the reciprocal patterning of discharge which adjacent PTNs (simultaneously recorded with the same microelectrode) may show during normal movement. Figures 19 and 20 illustrate a record of the activity of a pair of PTNs in association with movement of the contralateral arm and hand. One of the neurons (ADL = 0.7 msec.) was inactive when the monkey was alert and not moving, whereas the other member of the pair (ADL = 1.3 msec.) showed continual regular discharge under these circumstances. When the monkey moved his contralateral arm (the onset of movement is indicated by the EMG), there was a modification of activity of both of the PTNs: the neuron which had been inactive showed bursts of activity and the neuron which had been tonically active showed modulation of its resting discharge pattern, at times having high frequency discharges and at other times showing transient cessation of activity. The re- sults pictured in Figures 19 and 20 are quite typical: units with higher conduction velocities tend to be phasically active in relation to movement, whereas units with lower conduction velocities tend to be tonically active in the absence of movement and to show

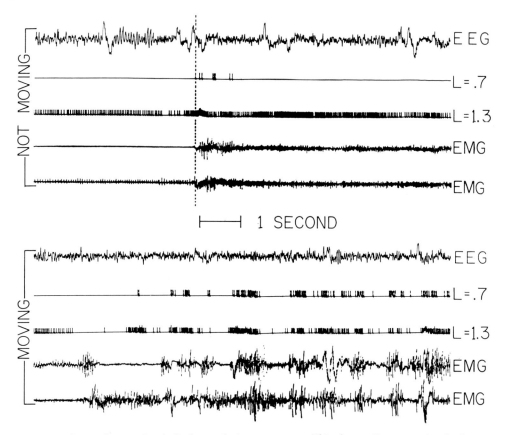

Fig. 19. Positively correlated discharge during movement. This figure illustrates the discharge patterns of two simultaneously recorded PTNs whose spikes were separated electronically and used to deflect the pens of an ink-writing oscillograph. The units had latencies of 0.7 msec. and 1.3 msec. During the period marked "not moving" the monkey was relatively quiet, though he shifted his arm position and appeared to become more alert at the point indicated by the dotted line. Prior to this shift in position the EMG records showed relatively little tonic muscle activity. Following the shift of position the EMG records showed considerable increase in activity. At the time of the shift the tonic unit (L = 1.3) had a marked increase in discharge frequency and the phasic unit (L = .7) had several discharges. Following the shift the tonic unit slowed somewhat, but its discharge frequency remained higher than it had been prior to the shift. In the lower section of the figure (marked "moving") is shown what occurred when the monkey was picking at hairs with his contralateral hand. Note that during movement both units discharged with relatively high frequency and that bursts in the two tend to occur at about the same time. The electromyographic recordings were obtained from muscles of the contralateral arm and serve to indicate the occurrence of movement. (Reprinted from Evarts.[110])

both upward and downward deviations of this tonic discharge during movement.

The relation between adjacent PTNs during movement was observed in 13 pairs of units. The correlation between discharge frequencies of adjacent PTNs varied depending upon the particular movement which the monkey was making. For a particular pair of neurons it was sometimes possible to discover a movement which was associated with a striking reciprocal discharge pattern; for other movements the reciprocal relation was not clearly present or the discharges of the two neurons were positively rather than negatively correlated. Figures 19 and 20 show the same pair of units having synchronous discharge at one stage of movement and reciprocally related discharge dur-

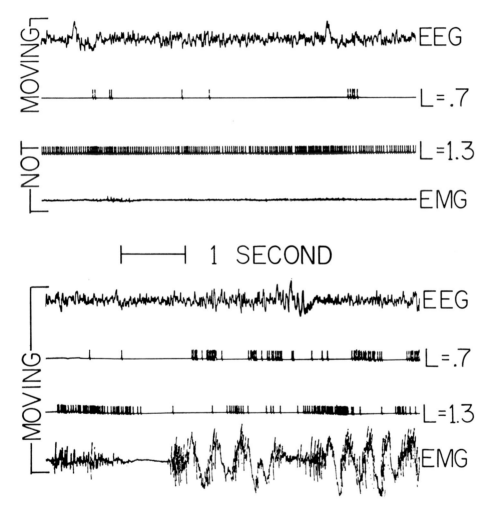

Fig. 20. Negatively correlated discharge during movement. This illustrates the activity of the same pair of PTNs shown in Figure 19. In the upper section (marked "not moving") the monkey was alert but inactive; the unit with latency of 1.3 discharged regularly, whereas the shorter latency unit was relatively inactive. In the lower section (marked "moving") the monkey was scratching himself. In this series of movements the discharges of the two units were negatively correlated, discharges in one of the pair being associated with relative silence of the other. (Reprinted from Evarts.[110])

ing a different movement. Pairs of units whose discharge was positively correlated during movement sometimes showed phase differences: the change of discharge frequency of one of the units preceded the change of discharge frequency of the other, so that as a movement progressed, one neuron started discharging slightly before the other and also stopped before the other.

These findings concerning the reciprocal relations of adjacent PTNs during movement may cast some light on a problem with which neurophysiologists have been concerned for many decades. Sherrington[361] observed that lesions in the arm area of the motor cortex are followed by degeneration of axons which extend to the sacral as well as to the cervical segments of the spinal cord. This observation made it clear that neurons of the cortical arm area project to the region of leg as well as of arm motoneurons. In contrast, the experiments of Chang, Ruch, and Ward[59] on electrical stimulation of the motor cortex indicated a rather punctate muscle representation within the motor cortex. In interpreting the results of electrical stimulation of the cortex, one must bear in mind that this unphysiological stimulus causes large groups of neighboring PTNs to discharge synchronously. If adjacent PTNs were to have predominantly positive relations during normal movement, then the pyramidal volleys elicited by electrical stimulation might be said to mimic normal discharge. In view of the prevalence of reciprocal patterns of activity during normal movement, however, it is not surprising that ideas of motor cortex organization based on the results of electrical stimulation have occasionally been at variance with theories of Jackson[183] and Walshe[298] based on studies of motor function and its modification by disease of the nervous system in man.

CHAIRMAN MILLIKAN: Dr. Silverman, will you open the discussion?

DR. S. RICHARD SILVERMAN: If I were one of Dr. Thorpe's shrikes, I would have used the skill and the ability which those shrikes have, in reverse. Instead of declaring territorial proclamation, I would have declared territorial abdication. (Laughter.)

I am as aware of the need for interdisciplinary enterprises but—if I may borrow from the activities directed at Christian unity—it is carrying the scientific ecumenical movement a bit too far to ask a teacher of deaf children to discuss the technical advances that result from recording discharge patterns from significant cortical neurons during movement. I simply am not able to do that, particularly since I heard the presentation for the first time this morning. Nevertheless, I should like to raise some questions, if I may, which may be quite remote from recording from single neurons but still may, in some way, be related to them.

As I said, my daily work has to do with teaching deaf children, some of whom may have some hearing. To go back to perception for a moment, Dr. Hirsh's delineation is useful. For the deaf person speech is a spatial display, the moving of the lips in time or of the fingers in the use of the manual alphabet. Here we are dealing with something very complex—the effect of that kind of perception on the use of the motor system in producing articulatory movements and other features of speech.

I would like to share some experiences with you that lead to some questions in another form. For example, Dr. Hirsh alluded to the Haskins' view of the motor theory of speech perception; to use their language, they ask, "What are the neuromotor commands to the articulators?" Dr. Evarts has given us some form that these commands may take, but my own experience, of course, has been with the gross behavior. Both at the phonologic level of articulation and the more complex one repeatedly alluded to this morning the capacity for language, the errors that deaf children make in their speech, are interesting. We can categorize them in a number of groups, most of which have to do, I believe, with some feature of motor performance. I find, in my experience, that one source of error is the poor motor feedback, whatever the sources may be—proprioceptive, tactile, and movement. It is interesting, for example, that in articulating the front vowels, they will tend to be off target by enough to confuse a listener. One can see that the slightest overshoot here confuses the listener.

In some studies we have made we have found that 90 per cent of the errors in listening to vowels have to do with these particular vowels and, also, kind of one place away in this continuum of downward movement. So we have the motor system again producing information for the talker and affecting his articulation.

A second source of error is the ambiguity of what it is that is presented. Here we have the familiar /m/, /p/, /b/ confusions, and the feedback here is not much of a problem.

Another difficulty results from movements being invisible. So, those who must teach these children articulation tend to want to give the child a little more information than is necessary to produce the sound, because he cannot see it. We find, for example, in the case of the articulation of the /k/, which can be either a linguavelar or a linguapalatal sound depending upon the phonetic context in which it is imbedded, that the sound is not visible. The teacher, opening the mouth wide and showing a rather posterior articulation, literally induces a lot of bad speech by the model that is given to the child. The child then seems to fix this image for this sound and finds it very difficult to make some of the movements that context requires.

So the motor system is an exceedingly critical item in articulation in the speech of a child who does not have the perceptions that Dr. Hirsh spoke about. The only other comment that I can make, that I would like to address to the linguists and the psycholinguists among us, is the question of the so-called innate capacity for language that has been cited in some of the more recent work of people like McNeill[270] and others, in the absence of any kind of auditory input.

What is the situation here? What are some of the questions we can raise which would give us some insight into that situation? Most of my comments have had to do with the relation of that input to the formulation and the capacity for language.

CHAIRMAN MILLIKAN: Dr. Purpura.

DR. DOMINICK P. PURPURA: Dr. Evarts has presented some very important findings which require further discussion. There are several ways of interpreting these data. Dr. Evarts is telling us that neurons of the motor cortex are being controlled by some subcortical systems which impress distinctly different patterns of activity on different elements of a cortical network. His data also tell us that these circuits do not altogether involve simple collateral feedback relations as indicated by the remarkable differences in unit discharges observed in adjacent elements.

In regard to the subcortical systems which are regulating or influencing the behavior of motor cortex units, I think there is little doubt that these must arise for the most part in specific and nonspecific thalamic nuclear organizations. One tends to think about the specific projection system from the ventrolateral nuclear complex as being exclusively involved in somatic motor activities. However, recent studies from several laboratories have now shown that stimulation of these ventrolateral nuclear groups of the thalamus as well as some related basal ganglia structures may severely disturb the ordering and motivational factors of speech. Many of these data have been summarized in a recent symposium on the thalamic mechanisms regulating sensory and motor cortex activities.[328]

It is likely that some of the patterns of discharge which Dr. Evarts described are related to differences in membrane properties of cortical pyramidal neurons. This has now been quite nicely demonstrated in recent studies by Takahashi.[375]

Thus tonically active cells appear to be smaller, have a larger membrane resistance, and have different after potentials than phasically active neurons. The same seems to hold for spinal motoneurons, which suggests the operation of common principles in the regulation of "upper" as well as "lower" motoneurons controlling movement. These are but a few of the problems which Dr. Evarts' data have touched upon. They are, of course, of basic importance for the understanding of cerebral mechanisms in speech.

DR. FRANK MORRELL: I just would like to comment briefly on the other side of what Dr. Evarts said, that is, to emphasize the nonplasticity side. What was really of concern to me to hear, as he described it, was the clear relationship between axonal size and discharge patterns in relation to movement pattern. A lot of work has been done and a lot of words have been written about the randomness of the relationship between unit activity and behavior on several levels. For example, workers using histological and histochemical methods have found, with various staining technics supposedly designed to assess the level of activity of cortical cells, that sections show random differences in staining properties throughout the cortical laminae. These have been interpreted to indicate that no particular pattern exists in the organization of activity at any particular time. Other kinds of recording have also been interpreted as showing a relatively random relationship between unit discharge and motor activity. It seems to me Dr. Evart's work goes far toward showing that the organization is really not random but that it is quite specifically organized.

CHAIRMAN MILLIKAN: Other comments, questions, or discussion?

DR. CHASE: When we think about the organization of motor activity, we must again consider the question of how many modes the system can operate in. Dr. Evarts spoke to this point toward the end of his presentation when he discussed his interest in looking at the monkey performing the same pattern of movement but with different loads.

We should be mindful of the fact that the speech motor system can undoubtedly also operate in different modes. If I am imitating another person's speech, without any concern about transmitting information but simply doing an acoustic matching job, the neurophysiology underlying the organization of my speech motor activity is probably quite different from the neurophysiology underlying the organization of the same patterns of sounds when I am spontaneously piecing these sounds together in an effort to transmit information. Our laboratory experiences have taught us that the disorganization of speech motor activity that results from delayed auditory feedback of speech is less marked if the subject is reading a passage than if the subject is engaged in spontaneous propositional speech.

Dr. Evarts' comments also call attention to the relationship between the peripheral receptor apparatus and central organization of motor activity. This general question suggests two more specific questions that deserve our attention. One is, "What is the role of the peripheral receptor apparatus during the course of learning movements?" The other is, "What is the role of the peripheral receptor apparatus with respect to the organization and control of movement during different modes of operation of the motor system?"[62a, 63]

With respect to the first question, we must be mindful of the fact that speech motor gestures are acquired patterns of movement. It is very important that an infant be able to acquire a system of phonology that conforms to that of the adult's in his culture. We know that under normal circumstances, he gets a great deal of his information about what his phonological system should be like through acoustic representation of adult speech patterns. However, we also know that if there is a deficit of sensation involving oral area structures in a patient with normal hearing, such a patient does not acquire a normal phonological system.

While I was working at the National Institutes of Health, Dr. James F. Bosma called my attention to a patient on his service who had a congenital sensory syndrome, which I will not describe fully here, that involved a failure to appreciate the position of lips and tongue. This patient had normal hearing acuity and normal intellectual function. However, her speech was barely intelligible.[62]

Dr. MacNeilage has used electromyographic technics to define the organization of speech movements used by this patient.[331] He found that muscle groups that normally function in relative independence during the speech of normal subjects were closely interrelated during the speech of our patient. Our patient demonstrated simpler speech motor gestures than normal English-speaking adults, but her speech motor gestures were stable, suggesting that her problem was not one of monitoring speech motor activity but rather represented aberrant initial construction of a finite set of speech motor gestures, resulting in a lack of conformity between her speech motor gesture system and that of the adult culture.

I cite this material to focus our attention on the fact that learned motor activity involves incorporation of sensory information that must serve as a substrate for the organization of movement. Whenever we scrutinize patterns of activity in the nervous system underlying the organization and control of learned motor activity, we must be mindful of the fact that there has been a past history to this, and that some elucidation of this past history will undoubtedly constitute a very important chapter in our understanding of the organization of movement.

DR. JAMES F. BOSMA: I shall comment on a comparison between the afferent experience we have from our speech effector apparatus and those described by Dr. Evarts. As we compare the limbs and the mouth, in particular, we note that the mouth differs in important ways.[42] The limbs are comparatively simple in anatomy and have few and simple functions. The oral area, however, is without the segmental design of the limbs and also without the skeletal joints that define and limit their potential directions and the extent of their motions.

In oral actions the tongue and lips, the soft palate, the mandible, and the hyoid bone are moved in coincidence. As in the limbs, the oral motions are immediately guided by sensations which the motions evoke. The principal afferent resource of the mouth is its large and continuous mucosal surface, with varied possibilities of apposition, with or without the interposition of solid masses. This is, in some sense, analogous to the guidance of the mature human upper extremity by cutaneous sensation of the hand.

Within the hand, sensation is remarkably more discriminate at the finger tips. Thus, the fine manual coordinations may be guided by this apically oriented surface tactile system. We apparently have a comparable arrangement in the mature human mouth. During object manipulation and exploration, the tongue, plus the mandible and the hyoid, follows the probings of the exquisitely sensitive tongue tip. These tongue motions occur within the receptor-rich walls of the mouth, which is, to our perspective, sort of a chambered sensorium, like the eye or the inner ear. Within this chamber the tongue performs as a spatial caliper and a manipulator, employing a dimensional system which is unique in the spatial parameters which it uses. Its information is supplied to the nervous system in terms of the oral anatomical relationships. This is quite different from the hand, because our hand shares with the eye the external world's geometric relationship and conveys the information in those terms.

The sensory differences between the mouth and limbs are further describable in degree. The sensitivity of the tongue tip to tactile and to two-point discrimination is greater than that of other body areas, even greater than that of the finger tips, as Sherrington[360] pointed out to us many years ago. The oral area of the mucosa of the mouth is large compared to the surface of the hand. The sensory guidance of oral area motor functions is from a remarkably large area input, and the inputs are compounded by the two contacting surfaces as, for instance, between tongue and lip and tongue and hard or soft palate: the uniquely compounded tactile experience of the mouth.

In further developmental perspective, I would like to point out that the human infant has a mouth which is essentially similar to that of the mammalia in general. The mouth of the human child, in development, differentially expands in comparison with the mobile tongue within it. This expansion of cavity, compared to the contained manipulator, is similar to that which occurs in the human pharynx. Because of this differential expansion our soft palate has an area in which to achieve its extensive displacements.

In coincidence of development, the human mouth acquires the sensory resource needed for guidance of this mobile tongue in its discriminate displacements in speech articulation.

CHAIRMAN MILLIKAN: Dr. Evarts, do you have a final comment you wish to make?

DR. EVARTS: I would just like to make one final remark on some thoughts that the information on latency I mentioned brings up in terms of the organization of this output system.

I mentioned that, when a stimulus is delivered, and the monkey is highly motivated to make a very rapid movement and learns to do it as quickly as highly motivated man can do it, it still takes a long period (100 msec.) from the arrival of the stimulus until the volleys begin leaving the motor cortex. It is interesting to note that this delay is in no way inherent anatomically in the system.

Wall et al.[397] have found that under chloralose anesthesia, volleys descend in the pyramidal tract 30 msec. after the occurrence of a flash of light to which the animal has never been conditioned at all. Thus, there exists an anatomical pathway which could save 70 msec. over the 100 msec. minimum latency with which PTNs responded in my monkeys. The waking and normally functioning brain seems to hold and delay input information which makes it hyperexcitable, or with chloralose anesthesia, one can see that the delay imposed by this holding mechanism has disappeared. One of the major challenges now facing the neurophysiologist is the riddle of what happens in this 70 msec. delay.

CHAIRMAN MILLIKAN: Thank you very much. Dr. Ettlinger will now discuss "Analysis of Cross-Modal Effects and Their Relationship to Language."

Analysis of Cross-Modal Effects and Their Relationship to Language

GEORGE ETTLINGER

Institute of Psychiatry
London, England

MAN'S CONCEPTUAL THINKING may be more or less abstract. He may indulge in flights of higher mathematics or merely in a leisurely contemplation of the fruits of the earth. Even in this event, he recognizes one such fruit as a particular source of calories and flavor, whether it confronts him in roasted, baked, boiled, mashed, or french-fried form. He has acquired an object-concept of the potato. This merely means that he recognizes and treats a potato as a potato, irrespective of its momentary shape, color, culinary disguise, or other variable characteristics. (I am not now concerned with generic concepts.)

Man has also learned to apply a particular label to this object, the name "potato." There are distinctions between the object-concept and the name. For one thing, the object-concept may remain intact in cases of neurological disease, when the name is lost (for example, in dysphasia). Also, the name may have greater generality than the object-concept and bring together concepts that might, without the name, be regarded as separate. I am thinking here of names such as "black currant" and "red currant," and, in a different way, of "plum" and "prune" (both are plums) and "grape" and "raisin" (both are grapes). The name can at present be regarded as a supra-modal symbol of the object. This is so because only a single neural mechanism is thought to be involved in the designation of the object by its name, irrespective of the sensory channel through which the object is perceived. (The supra-modal status of names remains acceptable at least until such time as systematic evidence of modality-specific nominal dysphasia may become available.)

Returning to the object-concept, we do not know for certain whether a single process of recognition takes place in one and the same neural system irrespective of the modality of the sensory inflow. Instead, recognition may occur in one neural system when the potato is seen, in another neural system when it is tasted or felt. This would imply the existence of individual object-concepts for the recognition of any one particular object through each separate sensory modality.

Classical neurology, with its acceptance of the occurrence of modality-specific agnosia, has adopted such a scheme. A patient with visual agnosia was said to be able to recognize an object by touch but not by vision, suggesting loss of the visual but not of the tactile object-concept. However, the clinical evidence for the occurrence of such selective recognition defects is not compelling. So it is wise to look elsewhere than to clinical neurology to determine whether the object-concept is supra- or uni-modal. (A distinction is made at a later stage between supra- and cross-modal concepts.)

Our subhuman relatives also acquire object-concepts. The dog recognizes a bone although its characteristics vary. However, it is not easy to make use of objects in experiments because we cannot gain control over the animal's prior experience with the object.

53

Fortunately there is a simple remedy. We can train an animal to distinguish by vision between two unfamiliar shapes (or forms), say a triangle and a disc. If, then, we alter the properties of the triangle (its configuration, orientation, size, color, and so forth) the animal may continue to treat the triangle as if it were possessed of the original properties. We can then say that it has acquired the concept of a triangle, a shape- (or form-) concept. (Such shape-concepts are analogous but not identical to object-concepts.) From now on I assume that animals having learned to make a discrimination have thereby acquired a concept and that in both cases we are dealing with classical or associative learning.

There are now two possible ways of proceeding, the former involving experimental brain lesions, the other not. We can train monkeys, say, to discriminate between the same two shapes by vision and also by touch. After this we can remove inferior temporal cortex, and we find impaired performance on the visual (but not the tactile) version of the discrimination task. Similarly, we can

remove posterior parietal cortex in other monkeys, and we find impaired performance on the tactile (but not visual) version of the task. Such an experiment was reported by Bates and myself,[18] although there was some confounding between measures of learning and re-learning.

The figures in Table 2 represent learning scores, that is, trials required to reach a standard level of performance, namely 90 per cent correct responses in 100 successive trials. The final 100 trials have been excluded as representing a constant which serves to dilute differences between the animals. Parietal animals, when compared with unoperated control animals, are impaired on tactile learning but not on visual retention. Similarly, they are impaired on tactile relearning or retention but not on visual learning. The temporal animals show the converse effect. Insofar as the selective impairments we found can be shown to have been independent of sensory defect (that is, amblyopia and loss of tactile sensitivity) and both reflect an equivalent defect, we can conclude that separate neural systems are

TABLE 2.

Animal	Test 3 Hexagon and Disc			Test 4 L and T		
	Preop. Learning	Postop. Learning	Postop. Retention	Preop. Learning	Postop. Learning	Postop. Retention
	Light (1)	Dark (2)	Light (3)	Dark (4)	Light (5)	Dark (6)
P1	330	1,150 F (53)	0	--	240	--
P2	30	1,150 F (49)	0	--	130	--
P3	--	1,150 F (54)	--	320	130	680 F (57)
P4	--	1,150 F (56)	--	680	140	450
T1	80	730	330 F (58)	--	500 F (59)	--
T2	130	Died	Died	--	Died	--
T3	--	310	--	310	500 F (71)	50
T4	--	1,150 F (56)	--	160	500 F (59)	130
C1	160	440	0	--	90	--
C2	80	1,120	0	--	170	--
C3	--	230	--	120	120	0
C4	--	670	--	180	140	10

The effect of parietal and temporal ablations on the performance by monkeys of visual and tactile tasks: the parietal lesion impairs tactile but not visual performance; the temporal lesion impairs visual but not tactile performance. Diareses (—) indicate that the animal was not tested at this stage of training (From Bates and Ettlinger.[18]) Reprinted by permission of the American Medical Association.

concerned when the monkey learns through two sense modalities to perform a single shape discrimination task. Such findings support the notion of uni-modal object-concepts. However, we need not depend on findings based upon the behavior of brain-damaged subjects. A more direct behavioral test of the supra- or uni-modal nature of concepts is available.

We train monkeys to distinguish by vision between a triangle and a disc. Then we retain all the original properties of the triangle (its configuration, orientation, and so forth) but exclude vision. (We already know that monkeys can learn to distinguish between a solid triangle and a solid disc by touch or palpation in the dark.) If monkeys trained to make this particular discrimination in the light (but having no previous experience with these shapes in the dark) are now confronted with the triangle and disc in the dark, how will they respond? Will the animal respond to the triangle it feels in the same way as it has learned to respond to the triangle it sees, a result implying supra-modal shape-concepts? Or will it treat the triangle it feels as totally unfamiliar, a result implying that shape-

TABLE 3.

Experimental design used in a study of cross-modal transfer of training with unoperated monkeys. Design eliminates confounding effect of nonspecific improvement between successive tasks. Animals C–1 and C–2 belong to Group I, animals C–3 and C–4 to Group II. Tests A and C are shape discriminations; Test B is a size discrimination. The sequence of training, from first to last test, is represented by successive lines, from top to bottom. The modality of training is the same for both groups of animals on their first, second, and all subsequent tests, although the differing sequences of the individual tests are balanced for the two groups. (From Ettlinger.[106]) Tables 3-6 reprinted by permission.

TABLE 4.

Animal	Group I		Group II	
	C 1	C 2	C 3	C 4
Visual	159	75	—	—
Somatic Visual	432	1112	230	661
	0	0	—	—

Transfer from visual to somatic modality. Scores represent the number of trials (in excess of 100) required by each of four unoperated monkeys to reach the standard level of performance on the visual or somatic form of Test A (shape discrimination) at various stages of training. Animals C–3 and C–4 (Group II) were not trained on the visual form of this test. The first line of results refers to the stage of learning, the second line to the stage of transfer testing, and the lowest line to the stage of retention testing of the original habit. (From Ettlinger.[106])

concepts are uni-modal? Obviously, intermediate results can also occur.

Let us now look at some experimental investigations. The design of this kind of experiment has been described in an earlier paper.[106] The design is complicated because, when we are dealing with specific habit formation we wish to exclude the nonspecific effects of learning set, which I shall deal with later on. We have in Table 3, first, the stage of learning. Next, we can assess transfer from vision to touch and from touch to vision. Then we wish to ensure, if there is no transfer, that the animals have not for-

TABLE 5.

Animal	Group I		Group II	
	C 1	C 2	C 3	C 4
Somatic	—	—	111	176
Visual Somatic	86	166	112	135
	—	—	0	1

Transfer from somatic to visual modality. Scores represent the number of trials (in excess of 100) required by each of four unoperated monkeys to reach the standard level of performance on the visual or somatic form of Test C (shape discrimination) at various stages of training. Animals C–1 and C–2 (Group I) were not trained on the somatic form of this test. The first line of results refers to the stage of learning, the second line to the stage of transfer testing, and the lowest line to the stage of retention testing of the original habit. (From Ettlinger.[106])

TABLE 6.

MEAN NUMBER OF TRIALS TO CRITERION

Training condition	N	Visual discrimination	Auditory discrimination
Negative	20	219	531
Positive	19	295	747
Matched-negative	11	260	469
Matched-positive	11	260	819

Transfer from visual to auditory modality in monkeys. (From Wegener.[399])

gotten what they were taught in the first modality. So finally, there is a stage of retention testing.

The results are consistently negative. There is no evidence of positive cross-modal effects, or of transfer of training as we say, from vision to touch (in Table 4) or from touch to vision (in Table 5).

We[57] have also asked the following question: Will monkeys that have been trained to discriminate between two rates of interruption of a light maintain their accuracy of discrimination when a sound is interrupted at the same two rates? Our results provided no evidence that accuracy was maintained across modalities.

Wegener[399] has been examining similar questions. Monkeys were trained to discriminate between two levels of illumination, presented one after the other. They then learned to perform an equivalent auditory discrimination task, when sounds of different intensity were presented. Half of the animals

were trained to respond in a certain way both to the high intensity light and high intensity sound, a condition which Dr. Wegener calls "positive." The others were trained to respond in the same way to the high intensity light and *low* intensity sound. The first group of animals did not learn the auditory task more rapidly than the others (Table 6), even when matched for learning ability on the visual task.

Wilson and Shaffer[414] have conducted two relevant series of experiments. In the former, there were 11 pairs of three-dimensional forms which the monkeys learned to discriminate by vision, in the light, and by touch, in the dark. The odd-numbered discrimination tasks were learned first by vision and then by touch, while the even-numbered tasks were learned first by touch and then by vision. There was no evidence of significant cross-modal transfer effects in either direction. However, in the second experiment care was taken to ensure that the animal "felt" the same part of the stimulus that it "saw." Using errors as the measure in Table 7, there was a significant cross-modal transfer effect in the first, but not in the second part of this experiment; using learning scores (trials), the effect failed to reach significance in either part. I am informed by Dr. M. Wilson that on replication, the same trend as before was observed but no significant effect was found, even though eight animals were now used.

The same kind of experimental investiga-

TABLE 7.

Group	Tactual (1) Positive stimulus	Visual Positive stimulus	Visual Errors in first 30 trials	Tactual (2) Positive stimulus	Tactual (2) Errors in first 30 trials
I	Short	Short	9	Long	28
	Short	Short	13	Long	24
	Short	Short	14	Long	16
II	Long	Short	16	Short	16
	Long	Short	18	Short	20
	Long	Short	21	Short	27
			$P < 0.05$		$P > 0.05$

Transfer between somatic and visual modalities in monkeys. (From Wilson and Shaffer.[414])

tion can be made with human instead of animal subjects. Cole, Chorover, and I[70] sought to determine whether learning of a rhythm discrimination in one sense modality (audition) leads to more rapid learning of the same rhythm discrimination in a second modality (vision). Table 8 shows that our experimental design gave us two separate measures of the presence of cross-modal transfer effects. One was the learning score of the experimental group on the visual task when compared with the mean learning score of the two control groups, neither of which had experience with the relevant auditory task before learning to make the visual discrimination. The second measure we used was the "difference" score for the experimental subjects, which reflects how many additional trials each subject required to learn the visual discrimination after learning to make the auditory discrimination. We failed to find evidence for cross-modal transfer effects with either measure in our adult subjects.

Blank and Bridger[33] have reported a similar experiment, involving discrimination

TABLE 8.

Group I (N = 6)	Group II (N = 6)	Group III (N = 12)	Group IV (N = 12)
VISUAL	Auditory	Alternating	Matching auditory vs. visual
• – – vs. – –• (+) (–)	······ vs. ··· (+) (–)	VISUAL and auditory	• – – vs. – –• • – – vs.• – –
followed by	followed by	• – – vs. – –•	– –•vs. – –• – –•vs.• – –
auditory • – – vs. – –• (+) (–)	VISUAL • – – vs. – –• (+) (–)	(+) (–)	

Transfer between auditory and visual modalities in man using different learning sequences with four groups of subjects. In the rhythm discriminations temporal parameters were as follows: duration of short components, 148 msec.; duration of long components, 504 msec.; duration of intervals between components, 110 msec.; duration of intervals between rhythm cycles, 990 msec. In the rate discrimination the sound was interrupted 10 times/sec. for the positive stimulus and 4 times/sec. for the negative stimulus. (From Cole, Chorover, and Ettlinger.[70]) Reprinted by permission of *Nature*.

first between a single and a double flash of light and then between a single and a double sound. There were three kinds of instruction and procedure adopted with their subjects, children of different ages. One group of children, aged four to five years, showed significant cross-modal transfer effects if there was verbalization during training; two other groups of the same age but tested with different instructions and procedure gave no evidence of significant cross-modal transfer. No other study with human subjects and specific habit formation is known to me.

(Rudel and Teuber[338] have reported significant transfer across sense modalities of the decrement in the Müller-Lyer illusion. However, it is not known what kind of behavioral process gives rise to the decrement of the illusion within a modality. It is unlikely to be an effect of associative learning, as no knowledge of results is given to the subject after each trial. By contrast, the formation of object-concepts and discrimination habits takes place largely as a consequence of associative learning. So, a positive cross-modal effect with the Müller-Lyer illusion cannot be held to contradict the negative results obtained with specific discrimination habits.)

I shall now consider cross-modal effects of two different kinds: first, cross-modal transfer of learned principles and, second, cross-modal matching or comparison.

It has been known for many years that animals, for example, monkeys, improve their performance over a series of 100 or 200 discrimination problems, even when nothing specific about the stimuli in one problem can be transferred to succeeding ones. This improvement between problems is termed the formation of a "learning set." In the present terminology, the animals can be said to have learned a principle. Wilson and Wilson[412] and Wilson[410] have demonstrated a small but consistent transfer effect across modalities of this improvement at learning discrimination tasks. Their most recent results show that the size of this cross-modal effect is about 3.5 per cent (mean of the effect in two directions). Wilson[411] has also shown that the basis for this nonspecific transfer across modalities may be the utilization, during performance in the second sense modality, of certain hypotheses or response tendencies acquired by the animal during training in the first modality.

Blakemore and I[108] have recently investigated the possibility that there is cross-modal transfer of another kind of principle in the monkey. We have trained animals to select by touch the cylinder of a pair having the smaller diameter, when both cylinders are tall; and the cylinder of larger diameter when both are short, or conversely. With such tactile conditional training the animal does not learn merely to make a specific stimulus-reward association: because on some trials it learns to select the thin rod, on others the fat rod, depending upon whether both rods are tall or short. The same test-objects were subsequently made available for visual selection and then again for tactile discrimination, with the reward contingencies being reversed for half of the eight animals on each change of sensory modality. We found no clear evidence of cross-modal transfer effects for any one of three measures.

There have been a few investigations of cross-modal transfer of principles in man. Positive effects were reported as long ago as 1954 by Semmes et al.[350]

Finally, we come to the cross-modal matching or comparison of equivalent stimuli in two sense modalities. The experimental conditions here differ in at least three ways from those of the transfer experiment. First, when tested in the second modality of a transfer experiment, the subject is not usually made aware by any experimental procedure that there is an equivalence between the original and concurrent discrimination tasks. By contrast, in matching experiments the procedure is designed to make the subject explicitly aware that equivalent stimuli are made available in the two modalities. A human subject may be instructed to palpate

an object in the hand and to indicate which of the five objects presented for visual inspection is the same: "Is this it? Is this the one you felt?" So the subject is given an attitude (or set, as we say) by the experimenter, that identities or equivalences exist between the stimuli presented in different modalities. Second, in the transfer experiment some alteration in performance, usually learning, takes place during training in the first modality. It is this *change* of performance that may or may not become manifest in the second modality. However, change in performance within a single modality does not form any essential part of the matching experiment. Third, an interval of days or weeks may occur in a transfer experiment between the last presentation of the stimuli in the first modality and the subsequent exposure of equivalent stimuli in another modality. So in transfer experiments we are dealing with persistent cross-modal effects. In the matching experiment the longest interval of this kind rarely exceeds a few seconds, while the stimuli may, indeed, be presented concurrently in the two sense modalities.

Apart from these differences in procedure, it seems to me on theoretical grounds that the ability to transfer across modalities (whether this be transfer of a specific habit or of a principle) presupposes an ability to match (either stimuli or principles of response) across modalities; whereas cross-modal matching performance does not presuppose an ability to show transfer across modalities.

It is important to emphasize the differences between the transfer and matching experiments because certain authors (for example, Birch and Lefford[30] and Rudel and Teuber[338]) have used positive findings derived from cross-modal matching experiments in support of their claim for the occurrence of specific cross-modal transfer. On the present argument, positive findings in matching experiments cannot be adduced to support or contraindicate the occurrence of cross-modal transfer (though negative findings would contraindicate the relevant kind of transfer). And I should emphasize that *transfer* is chiefly relevant to the neural organization of object-concepts since the basic process is the recognition of *familiar* stimuli (whereas matching can occur with unfamiliar stimuli).

The results of experiments concerned with cross-modal matching have been variable. In the majority, there has been evidence of significant but not perfect cross-modal matching (see, for example, Hermelin and O'Connor[163]; Blank and Bridger[33]; in a few, only weak (if any) cross-modal matching ability was detected.[70,196] The only attempt to observe cross-modal matching between equivalent stimuli in animals which is known to me is that of Wilson.[413] Significant but weak effects were found. Blakemore and I are currently seeking to train monkeys to match across sensory modalities. Although we suppose we are using near-optimal conditions, we have so far been remarkably unsuccessful.

Let me try to summarize the experimental findings and then briefly revert to the problem of language.

1. *Cross-modal transfer of a specific discrimination habit* has not been demonstrated in man or animals except under conditions where (a) verbalization (by human subjects) was possible and was reported by the experimenter to have played an essential role; (b) animals were trained to respond to the onset of a single stimulus, so that a principle ("respond to a change") may have been learned; or (c) animals were trained to a low criterion in the first modality so that, instead of showing genuine transfer of specific training, they may have shown faulty differentiation or confusion between two different test conditions. Studies in animals to which these last two statements apply, that is, (b) and (c), have been reviewed by Dr. J. G. Wegener (unpublished). The single demonstration that specific cross-modal transfer can occur without verbalization and not under conditions discussed in (b) and (c) above is the experiment of Wilson and Shaffer,[414] and here only one of two measures

was significant in one of two transfer tests. This critical experiment gave no significant effects on replication.

2. *Cross-modal transfer of a principle* has been shown to occur in the majority of experiments. However, the effect is usually weak. In some studies, transfer of a principle has been reported in only one direction (for example, by Stepien and Cordeau[372] from audition to vision) without a relevant control group, so that transfer effects are confounded with rapid learning of the easier task in the second modality.

3. *Cross-modal matching* of equivalent stimuli has also been shown to occur in the majority of relevant experiments with human subjects. More information is needed on cross-modal matching ability in the monkey. It has already been argued in this paper that the same kind of behavior is not being tested in transfer and matching experiments.

I would suggest, then, that cross-modal transfer of a specific discrimination habit may occur only with the aid of language, whereas cross-modal transfer of a principle and cross-modal matching may occur with or without the aid of verbalization.

What bearing does this analysis of cross-modal effects have upon our knowledge of neural mechanisms in language? Any formulation must at present be hazardous and impermanent.

First, we can tentatively suggest that object, shape and other similar concepts may be uni-modal. This implies that names may act as "bridges" between specific discriminations learned in different sense modalities but having common elements (as suggested by Burton and Ettlinger[57]). The suggestion leads to the prediction: given experimental conditions under which specific cross-modal transfer is known to occur (presumably through verbalization) in man, there should be a reduction in the degree of such transfer in dysphasic patients. In neural terms, the suggestion of uni-modal object-concepts implies that a separate neural system is concerned in the recognition of a particular object through each sensory modality; and that each of these systems is connected to a single further system (presumably in the speech areas) concerned with the evocation of the name of the object.

Next, we can tentatively suggest that certain learned principles may, at least in part, be supra-modal or, more strictly, cross-modal. This implies that verbalization may, but need not, act as a "bridge" in the behavioral implementation of the principle when sensory inflow is changed from one to another modality. It leads to the prediction: given experimental conditions under which cross-modal transfer of a principle is known to occur without verbalization (for example, in monkeys), there should not be a reduction in the degree of such transfer in dysphasic patients. In neural terms, the suggestion of supra-modal principles implies that a single neural system is concerned in behavior which exemplifies the implementation of a principle, irrespective of the modality of the sensory inflow. (This scheme leads to other predictions: for example, monkeys trained to acquire visual learning sets and then receiving infero-temporal removals might postoperatively show positive transfer effects when tested for tactile learning sets provided any cross-modal system is not situated in the region concerned with visual learning.)

Finally, we can tentatively suggest that cross-modal matching may take place at a perceptual level (without verbalization) or through the mediation of a verbal "bridge." It has been known for many years that cross-modal associations between nonequivalent stimuli may, perhaps, be formed in animals (from the results of experiments on cross-modal conditional learning). However, the learning of associations between nonequivalent stimuli and the matching of equivalent stimuli are quite different processes. When presented with equivalent stimuli, the human subject can reach a decision of "same" or "different" without learning and whether the stimuli are familiar or unfamiliar. Verbal labels will be assigned to the familiar stimuli more readily than to the unfamiliar, but even with unfamiliar stimuli the same label assigned to stimuli in different modalities could act as a cross-modal "bridge." However, when verbalization is precluded (as in the monkey) or when it is unlikely to occur (as when small differences in rate of intermittence or length are to be matched by human subjects), the matching process is likely to take place at a level prior to that at which associative learning takes place, that is, at the perceptual level. Little is known about the nature of such a process in neural terms. However, we can conclude that, although recognition of a potato as a potato when seen and when felt may involve two separate neural systems, recognition merely of the similarity or dissimilarity of two objects, the one seen and the other felt, may involve only a single system communal, in part, to vision and touch.

CHAIRMAN MILLIKAN: Dr. Myers, will you continue with "Cerebral Connectionism and Brain Function."

Cerebral Connectionism and Brain Function

RONALD E. MYERS

Laboratory of Perinatal Physiology
National Institute of Neurological Diseases and Blindness
San Juan, Puerto Rico

THE PRESENT PAPER deals with the processes and substrata involved in information handling and data transmission in the nervous system. Classic teachings on brain organization have emphasized the presence of rich associative linkages which serve to interrelate widespread areas of the cerebrum. Dependence is placed upon these presumed fiber systems in explanations of the functional interrelations and interactions of various cortical mechanisms. However, studies on connectionism in monkey brains after removal of the various lobes contradict such conceptions of brain organization. The present paper presents and discusses these new studies and also reviews recent functional studies relating to cerebral associationism. These new findings yield increased insights into the general problem of information handling within the brain.

The fiber projections extending from occipital lobe to other brain areas have been defined in the monkey by serial study of the brain using the Nauta technique after total occipital lobectomy. A heavy fiber system passes from occipital lobe down into the posterior half of the inferior temporal convolution with spillover into the depths of the adjacent superior temporal sulcus (Fig. 21). Another fiber system projects to the frontal eyefield. Only a few fibers pass from occipital lobe to the immediately adjacent posterior parietal lobe. Thus, the occipital lobe projections are limited to restricted regions leaving the major extent of the hemisphere free of fibers from occipital lobe.

The pattern of connections from occipital lobe to the contralateral hemisphere has been described in detail.[292,293] The occipital lobe sends commissural fibers only to the opposite

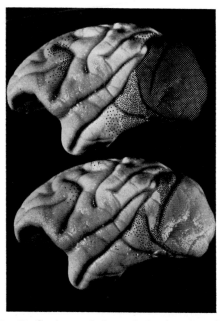

Fig. 21. Cortico-cortical associational systems from occipital lobe extending into ipsilateral and contralateral hemisphere as revealed by the Nauta technic. Density of dotting reflects density of termination of degenerating fibers within the cortical mantle. Shaded area represents the area of the lesion. (From Black and Myers.)

61

juxtastriate area 18 and area 18 proper with lesser numbers of such fibers to the posterior third of the inferior temporal convolution, the floor of the superior temporal sulcus, and still lesser numbers to the frontal eyefields. Thus, the regions of the opposite hemisphere receiving commissural fibers are the same as the regions of the ipsilateral hemisphere receiving the direct association fibers from occipital lobe. Note that the striate area, striate-receptive area 19, and area 19 proper all remain free of occipital lobe commissural fibers.

Study of serial sections of the monkey brain after temporal lobectomy reveals projection of fibers posteriorly into the occipital lobe as it borders on the lesion (Fig. 22). Small numbers of fibers pass from the area of the lesion into parietal lobe while virtually no fibers pass into precentral gyrus. There are, however, heavy projections from temporal lobe into prefrontal and orbital-frontal cortex and into cortex of the frontal eyefields. Contralaterally, commissural connections through corpus callosum and anterior com-

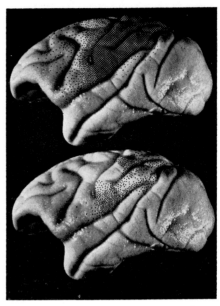

Fig. 23. Cortico-cortical connections from the parietal lobe to ipsilateral and contralateral hemispheres. (Unpublished, Ebner and Myers.)

missure from the temporal lobe are entirely confined to the opposite temporal lobe, a region closely corresponding to the extent of removal. Within contralateral temporal lobe the commissural fibers confine themselves mainly to its posterior half in accordance with earlier studies.[294]

The association fibers from the parietal lobe project massively forward into the precentral gyrus, particularly in its posterior half, as shown in Figure 23. Association fibers from parietal lobe also appear to enter the region of the frontal eyefields. These latter fibers, however, likely do not originate from parietal lobe but more likely represent fibers from the occipital and temporal lobes interrupted in their course within the parietal lobe white matter. The regions of anterior prefrontal and orbito-frontal cortex remain almost entirely free of connections from parietal lobe as do the regions of the occipital and temporal lobes, except in immediate relation to the lesion. Contralaterally, the commissural projections are restricted almost entirely

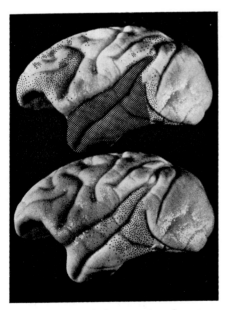

Fig. 22. Cortico-cortical connections from temporal lobe to ipsilateral and contralateral hemispheres. (Unpublished, Yamaguchi and Myers.)

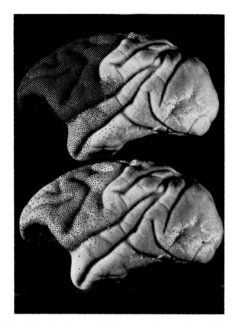

Fig. 24. Cortico-cortical connections from frontal lobe to the ipsilateral and contralateral hemispheres. (Unpublished, Myers.)

to the parietal lobe, a region homologous to the area of removal.

The associative connections from the frontal lobe may be seen from Figure 24. The frontal lobe sends fibers into restricted areas of the parietal lobe superiorly and inferiorly. These limited projections to parietal lobe likely originate from small zones of cortex cyto-architecturally extensions of the parietal lobe but located anterior to the central fissure as extended in these regions and, therefore, included in the frontal lobe removal. The major zone of fiber projection from frontal lobe is through the uncinate fasciculus into the anterior tip of the temporal lobe. There is a remarkable restriction of the commissural fibers from frontal lobe to the zone of the opposite frontal lobe.

It should be borne in mind that the above lesions are made in relation to gross lobar rather than to functional boundaries. Such is required since, in our present state of knowledge, only uncertain boundaries may be drawn in relation to the functional regions of

the cortex. For the sake of further analysis and discussion, however, an attempt is made to develop a functional map of the monkey's cortex. The map depicted in Figure 25 must be considered tentative in many of its parts though based upon diverse data taken from both physiology and anatomy. The following discussion relates to the derivation of this map and the map's relation to the anatomical findings following lobectomies in the monkey.

The visual functional sector of the cortex is considered to consist of the occipital lobe including the occipital operculum, the prelunate gyrus and, in addition, the posterior half of the inferior temporal gyrus along with the hidden cortex of the floor of the superior temporal sulcus. Also included as a part of the visual functional sector are the frontal eyefields. The justification for including the posterior portion of the inferior temporal gyrus and the cortex of the superior temporal sulcus within the visual sector are as follows:

(1) After occipital lobectomy there are massive fiber projections from occipital lobe to this sector of the temporal lobe.

(2) Lesions of this portion of the cortex in the monkey lead to deficits in visual discrimination performances.[287,69]

(3) The anterior commissure which interconnects these self-same regions of the two hemispheres functions in the interocular transfer of visual learning in chiasma-sectioned chimpanzees and monkeys.[32]

The frontal eyefields are included as a por-

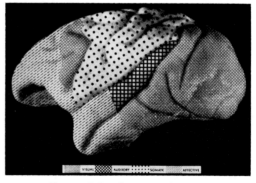

Fig. 25. Regional distribution of the functional sectors of the cortex in monkey.

tion of the visual functional sector because:

(1) The frontal eyefields receive heavy projections from the other portions of the visual functional sector including the occipital lobe and the posterior portion of the inferior temporal gyrus.

(2) The frontal eyefields are concerned in conjugate movements of the eyes in the opposite direction and may be considered as one of the motor mechanisms of the visual functional sector of cortex.[363]

The auditory functional sector of the cortex may consist of the posterior portion of the superior temporal gyrus along with a portion of the small angular gyrus of the monkey. This sector of the cortex, least studied in the monkey, has the least well-substantiated boundaries with other sectors.

The precentral gyrus and the parietal lobe are considered to be but parts of a single system subserving somatic sensory-motor functions. The motor mechanism of the precentral gyrus is considered the efferent mechanism of the somatic sensory system. The flow of impulses from somatic sensory receptors is through the parietal lobe anteriorly onto the precentral gyrus. Evidence for a flow from precentral gyrus back into parietal lobe is lacking.

There remains unaccounted for only the anterior half of the temporal lobe and the prefrontal-orbitofrontal cortex lying anterior to the frontal eyefields. These two regions of cortex are considered to be parts of a single functional unit for the following reasons:

(1) There are strong reciprocal anatomical interconnections between these two regions of cortex through the uncinate fasciculus.

(2) Epileptic discharges originating in both these zones in the human sometimes give rise to altered affective states associated with anxiety, fear, or pleasure.

(3) Both cortical zones are interconnected with the dorsomedial nucleus of the thalamus.

(4) Lesions of other cortical areas produce deficits either in sensory or motor functions. Lesions in the prefrontal or anterior temporal zones do not lead to such deficits but rather to deficits in social or emotional behavior.

The exposed surface of cortex then may be considered as consisting of four overall functional sectors or regions including those supporting vision, audition, touch, and emotion along with their respective behaviors. If the patterns of fiber association extending between the several lobes be reconsidered and interpreted in relation to the above functional map of the cortex, an interesting and far-reaching conclusion seems justified: *In almost all instances, passage of association pathways occurs between zones of cortex lying within specific functional sectors. Conversely, in no instance are significant fiber pathways found passing between one functional sector of cortex and another.* Only in fringe areas as one sector borders upon another can the possibility of cortico-cortical association occur between functional sectors.

The various functional sectors of cortex have been studied using the technic of ablation in relation to perceptual learning in the monkey. Similar interpretations of the lack of significant interactions or cross-assistance between the various functional regions of the cortical surface have emerged from these studies. For example, as may be seen from Figure 26, ablations of any or all regions of cortex outside of the parietal lobe and precentral gyrus leaves intact the memories of and the capability for performance of the most difficult tactual discrimination responses through the opposite hand. On the other hand, lesions which encompass the entire parietal lobe but leave intact other cortical areas permanently destroy the animal's capabilities for the recall or performance of even the most simple tactual discrimination responses. It is inferred that cortical regions outside the parietal lobe make no contribution to touch functions. Further, it appears that the parietal lobe alone constitutes the neural mechanism underlying touch perception and touch memory in the monkey. Similar findings may be described with relation to vision and lesions of the occipital-posterior temporal region. Thus, studies of

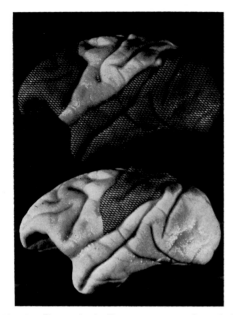

Fig. 26. Removal of all cortex except that of the parietal lobe and precentral gyrus as in the upper schema results in no measurable disturbance of tactual discrimination responses as tested through the opposite hand. Complete removal of parietal lobe leaving undisturbed other cortical areas as in the lower schema results in a complete loss of ability to discriminate between the most simple tactual stimuli through the opposite hand. (Unpublished, Myers.)

ablation and its effects on perception and memory in the different sense modalities generate interpretations of cortical organization similar to those derived from connectionism. From functional studies the cortical surface may be divided into several strictly defined sectors each relating to a specific function. One cortical sector appears not to contribute to the activities carried out by another. Lesions within a sector produce deficits confined to functions subsumed by that sector. Ablation studies suggest an absence of cross assistance or interaction between sectors of cortex.

Data derived from another type of functional study also tend to deny associative relationships between different functional sectors. Ettlinger has carefully investigated cross-sensory generalization of learning in the monkey and human. These studies fail to give evidence for generalization of learning from one sense modality to another. For example, the learning of a "largeness versus smallness" discrimination through the touch modality fails to assist or retard the subsequent learning of a "largeness versus smallness" discrimination through the visual modality or contrary-wise. For a fuller discussion of these experiments and conclusions, see Ettlinger, this volume.

A rich and long-time experience with the classical conditioned reflex has been achieved by Konorski in Warsaw. Konorski indicates that the learning of a conditional response through one sense modality neither aids nor hinders learning of a similar conditioned response through another sense modality (personal communication, 1964). Thus, studies utilizing a second quite different experimental psychological approach similarly fail to provide evidence for the cross-sensory generalization of the lessons of experience.

Still a fourth type of study yields evidence denying association between the various sensory neural mechanisms. Rats taught a conditioned emotional response to presentation of an auditory signal fail to give evidence of the conditioned emotional response on first presentation of a visual signal. The subsequent learning of a conditioned emotional response to presentation of the visual stimuli by these animals is indistinguishable from such learning by completely naive animals and is neither aided nor hindered by the prior learning experience with auditory stimuli (personal communication from L. J. Kamin, 1965). Thus, evidence for carryover of learning from one sense modality to another is absent in still another psychological test context.

Another problem of data transmission in the nervous system is the definition of the pathways through which sensory inputs of various sorts regulate the motor response system. For example, through what pathways and centers does the visual mechanism guide the hand in motor responding in reaching out to pick up an object seen? Many tasks are performed under visual control or visual guidance in this fashion. The presence of such eye-hand coordination suggests a transmission of data or information of some order from the visual functional sector of cortex to the somatic sensory-motor sector. Again, such data communication from the visual to the motor mechanisms may be ascribed to a rich associational network between these two cortical regions. However, in earlier work investigating this problem it was found that bilateral transverse wedge resections interrupting all possible association systems running between the occipito-temporal and the fronto-parietal regions of cortex does not interrupt the performance of eye-hand coordinations.[295] Similarly, transsection of corpus callosum and anterior commissure does not interrupt eye-hand coordinations of a crossed type in which the visual input to one hemisphere guides the motor response coordinated through the other hemisphere.[31] Hence, cortico-cortical association systems which might run from the occipital lobe to sensory-motor cortex of either hemisphere are not crucial to the carrying out of coordinations of the hand with the eye. These findings fit with the demonstrated absence of association fiber systems running from the occipital and temporal lobes to precentral gyrus or, in general, to parietal lobe. Rather, preservation of eye-hand coordinations in monkeys with transverse wedge resections or with commissure transections indicates that the transmission of visual information from occipito-temporal region onto the motor mechanism is through vertically oriented projection systems passing from the visual sector of cortex to thalamus or brain stem.

The utilization of downward projecting fiber systems from the visual sector of cortex for the visual control of movement suggests that other functional sectors may also exert their guiding influences over the motor mechanism through vertically projecting systems. Several lines of evidence give support to this supposition:

1. Lilly developed technics for implanting numerous electrodes over the cortical surface of the monkey.[236] In this way he was able to stimulate the cortex surface over wide expanses in completely alert animals. Movements were elicitable from stimulations over almost all points of the exposed surface. Thus, widespread areas of cortex have more or less direct access to motor mechanisms.

2. Tower,[390] working with lightly anesthetized cats, also could elicit motor responses on stimulation of widespread areas of cortex. She demonstrated the existence of areas of cortex in relation to each of the sense modalities which gave rise to motor responses on stimulation. The motor responses could be elicited from these loci even after removal of the definitive motor cortex at the anterior pole of the cat brain. Further, by removing the cortical grey tissue and stimulating white matter directly she was able to follow the several pathways which produced movements through the white matter directly to the pons of the brain stem. This study demonstrated fiber projections passing from diverse cortical foci directly to brain stem producing motor responses.

However, major differences occur in the types of responses elicitable on electrical stimulation of the different regions of cortex. Stimulations of the central somatic sensory-motor areas yield movements of the extremities or of the face. These movements are frequently discrete in nature especially with lower current intensities. Stimulations of loci in other functional cortical sectors tend to yield only conjugate deviations of the eyes and head to the opposite side with sometimes super-added related mass movements of trunk and extremities.

The controversial movements of eyes and head typical of electrical stimulation within the visual sector of cortex represents quite different phenomena from the detailed guidance of hands described above in relation to physiologically received visual stimulations. It is likely that these two movement types are expressions of two quite different motor mechanisms incorporated within the matrix of the visual functional circuitry. That mechanism producing movements of regard likely subserves the fixation reflexes and likely projects to neural systems having functional proximity to the primary motor neurons involved with head and eye movements. That mechanism having to do with eye-hand coordinations likely projects to portions of the motor mechanism removed from the primary motor neurons since direct cortical stimulations in the visual sector fail to produce or effect discrete motor responses in the extremities.

Are there still other types of motor responding brought about or influenced by the visual sector of cortex? The guidance of the hand toward an object at rest or moving within a three-dimensional field represents a type of tracking behavior. The carrying out of a tracking function also does not presuppose or encompass the motor skills required in dealing with the object once seized. May there, then, be another type of visual guidance of the motor response of a practic nature implying a visual direction or guidance of the hands in the proper manipulation of objects seen?

Chimpanzee studies deny practic functions for the visual sector of cortex. Chimpanzees which have learned simple latchbox problems while using only one hand are immediately able to solve the problems on first testing using the other hand. However, if the region of the corpus callosum which interconnects the parietal lobes is transected, the chimpanzees no longer are able to solve using one hand even simple latchbox problems learned using the other hand (R. E. Myers and P. Black, unpublished work, 1966). Remarkably, this outcome is not altered by the animal's observation of the proceedings with both eyes during the acquisition of the skill with one hand and subsequently during the testing with the other hand. Thus, completely informed eyes are unable to direct the uninformed of the two hands in the solution of simple motor tasks. Solution of problems of motor praxis seems to be a function, purely and simply, of the somatic

sensory system of the parietal lobes. Though in conflict with intuitive expectations, this conclusion conforms with the near absence of association fiber systems passing between the visual and the somatic sensory-motor sectors of cortex.

In summary, the cortical convexity may be divided into four functional sectors relating to vision, audition, touch, and emotional and social behavior. Anatomic studies have shown a surprising deficiency of association fiber systems running between the various functional sectors. Psychological studies of generalization of training from one sense modality to another have also failed to give evidence for functional association between the several sensory systems. Ablation studies have tended to support the concept of strictly demarcated and separate functional regions of cortex for the several sensory functional systems. Just as the above studies demonstrate an absence of cortico-cortical fiber systems passing between the functional sectors, so other studies reveal an absence of cortico-cortical fiber systems passing from other functional sectors to the somatic precentral motor mechanism. Hence, cortico-cortical systems do not account for the hegemony exercised by the sensory sectors over the motor response mechanism. Instead, the concept is developed whereby vertically oriented efferent fiber systems passing to thalamus and brain stem account for the guidance of motor response by the several sensory functional systems. Finally, the execution of learned motor skills with the hands is uniquely a function of the parietal lobes. Surprisingly, the visual system makes no contribution toward the direction of the hands in the solution of skilled motor tasks but does execute a tracking function to bring the hands to target.

It is appropriate at this symposium to question the significance of these findings to the neural organization of speech and language. Of course, in animal studies speech and language functions cannot be studied as such. However, speech may be thought of as a special instance of volitional somatic activity which has arisen late in evolution. If this is the case, it is interesting to conjecture that:

(1) Each of the several functional sectors of cortex may make its own contribution to speech and language functions just as each separately contributes to volitional motor responding in general.

(2) There are not likely to be significant association systems running between the several language repositories or speech mechanisms of the several sectors of the cortex.

(3) The several language mechanisms of the several sectors of cortex are not likely to be associatively tied to the precentral somatic motor cortex.

(4) Rather, the expression of language as organized within the several sectors of cortex is likely to occur through vertically oriented projection systems extending down to brain stem centers for speech production.

These deductions regarding speech organization are remarkably similar in many regards to the interpretations of Penfield based on the effects of surgical lesions in man.[309]

Recent studies have tended to highlight the importance of the corpus callosum to speech functions.[123] However, evaluations of the basis for this interpretation yield some doubt in several aspects. The conclusions are based upon observations on only three or four patients. Importantly the procedure of commissure section on these critical patients was associated with evidence for variable concomitant damage to the brain, particularly to the nondominant hemisphere. The neurosurgeons performing the procedure have given a detailed description of the status of the most critical patient in the series both pre- and postoperatively.[36] Preoperatively there were considerable deficits in the functioning of the right parietal lobe with hypesthesia in the contralateral extremities. After surgery the patient exhibited considerable further difficulties of a neurological nature. The patient was an akinetic mute for over a week's time. For a period of time, he exhibited a flaccid left hemiparesis. As the

hemiparesis lessened, he exhibited grasp reflexes at first bilaterally and then only on the left. For a period there were bilateral Babinski responses. After the period of depressed consciousness the patient exhibited a confusional state. The neurosurgeons suggested that these difficulties were directly due to the commissure section itself. However, a personal experience with commissurotomy in large numbers of monkeys and chimpanzees has failed to support the conception that the commissure lesions alone may produce such alterations in consciousness or in mental state or that it may produce alterations in motor status. In fact, in all instances where the procedure is properly carried out, experimental animals exhibit no mental or neurological changes of any kind on recovery from anesthesia. Conclusions based on a few human cases showing such widespread evidence of brain damage both before and after commissure section should be accepted only with considerable qualifications.

The conclusions based upon these several human cases are also in conflict with the results of studies carried out by Akelaitis, K. U. Smith, and others working in the 1940's.[4-7,362] Sixteen commissure-sectioned human subjects were carefully studied in a wide variety of ways. It was found that extensive commissure section did not result in definable deficiencies in the motor, sensory, mnemonic, interpretive, or linguistic spheres. More specifically, the capability for recognition and object naming in both homonymous visual fields was well preserved in these patients. The utilization of the two hands in practic functions either independently or together was not affected by the commissurotomy. Speech disturbances were not seen in these patients except in instances where there had been evidence for damage to one or the other hemisphere demonstrable in terms of new neurological findings postsurgery. Maspes has studied a single patient who sustained transection of the posterior portion of corpus callosum.[261] In this instance, once again, there was a remarkable preservation of the capability of recognition and naming of objects presented in both visual half-fields. In order to demonstrate deficits in the naming and recognition of objects it was necessary to resort to tachistoscopic presentation of stimuli. Then it was possible to demonstrate some slight differences in stimulus recognition in the two half-fields. Also here the field exhibiting deficit was related to the nondominant hemisphere, which was the hemisphere receiving retraction and manipulation during the brain surgery.

Thus, the importance of the corpus callosum to object naming and language function must remain uncertain. In studies of commissure function all individuals, whether animal or human, that exhibit demonstrable postoperative neurological disturbances, whether of consciousness, mental state, or motor performance, must be eliminated from consideration inasmuch as such deficits clearly are indicative of damage sustained by one or the other hemisphere and should not be considered as part of a "syndrome of the corpus callosum."

CHAIRMAN MILLIKAN: Dr. Purpura, will you open the discussion?

DR. ROSENBLITH: Will somebody tell us what the Akelaitis series is? A certain amount of mystery is nice, but not too much.

DR. MYERS: The Akelaitis series is a series of patients who were studied and described in the literature in the early '40's. There were about 20 patients in that series, all patients with intractable seizures of one type or another, usually with longstanding brain damage. The surgeon, Van Wagenen, was hoping to restrict the number and the severity of seizures by commissure section. There was some reason to believe that this might be helpful. There were one or two neurologists, one of them by the name of Akelaitis, who with two or three psychologists studied these carefully, pre- and postoperatively.

DR. ROSENBLITH: From what viewpoint?

DR. MYERS: From the viewpoint of laterality functions, capability of doing various types of tasks with one or the other hand, capability of recognition in the two visual half fields, or recognition in the two hands, etc. If one would summarize their results as a whole, almost without exception the story from that series was that the patients did not exhibit deficits.

CHAIRMAN MILLIKAN: Dr. Purpura!

DR. PURPURA: I am thankful to Dr. Myers for at least mentioning the word "brain" in his presentation. Obviously he did not talk about speech and I do not think I was invited to this meeting to talk about "speech" either.

It might be of interest to mention briefly some of the recent lines of investigation which have contributed to a better understanding of the control mechanisms involved in regulation of cortical activities that both Dr. Myers and Dr. Evarts have reported on earlier.

A major question that has been of considerable concern to us in recent years is, "What kinds of influences are exerted on motor cortex neurons by pathways arising in the thalamus?" To answer this question it has been necessary to look inside cells with intracellularly located microelectrodes and attempt to define differences in synaptic drives during specific and nonspecific evoked responses. It seems to be well established now that when one stimulates the specific ventrolateral relay nucleus of the thalamus, one records a series of repetitive discharges in pyramidal tract neurons. These discharges are effected by synaptic pathways which terminate on or very close to the site of impulse initiation in these cells. One consequence of this is a powerful burst of impulses which is usually succeeded by a phase of inhibition. In contrast to this, stimulation of a nonspecific nucleus produces a relatively low level of excitatory activity and sometimes very little in the way of cell discharge. Typically a slowly developing depolarizing excitatory postsynaptic potential (EPSP) is observed inside Betz cells during repetitive stimulation of a nonspecific thalamic nucleus. It is inferred from several lines of evidence that these synaptic events are generated at sites remote from the soma, presumably in dendrites.[326]

The data on specific and nonspecific thalamic effects on motor cortex neurons serve to emphasize the existence of a wide variety of afferent systems capable of influencing motor cortex elements. For example, it has also been shown that under conditions of barbiturate anesthesia, stimulation of a peripheral nerve may elicit a very long latency discharge in cortex that is generalized in distribution (Forbes' response). We have shown that the same type of very long latency response can be evoked by stimulation of the hippocampus. Both types of responses are associated with activation of pyramidal neurons of the motor cortex.[323] The fact that these responses exhibit mutual facilitatory and inhibitory interactions strongly suggests that pyramidal and hippocampal stimulation activates a common projection system probably arising in the ponto-mesencephalic reticular system.[321]

Although the subcortical systems controlling sensorimotor cortex activities have been well defined in recent years, it has also been of great interest to analyze the mechanisms regulating the activities of these subcortical organizations. Particular attention has been directed to studies of the manner in which nonspecific thalamic stimulation affects other thalamic neurons and leads to generalized synchronization of thalamo-cortical activity. Intracellular studies of this synchronization process at the thalamic level have disclosed the operation of powerful excitatory and inhibitory pathways which may be activated in a unique temporal sequence to produce alternating excitation and inhibition of many cells synaptically linked by complex networks to elements in nonspecific thalamic nuclei.[322] One synaptic pattern is typically encountered during thalamo-cortical synchronization whereas quite another pattern is observed during the desynchronizing action of high-frequency stimulation of a non-specific thalamic nucleus.[325] It is also of interest to point out that the effects which superimposed reticular stimulation exert on thalamic synchronizing mechanisms may be clearly related to changes in the patterns of inhibitory synaptic drives which characterize the synchronizing process.[324] You may recall that quite a few years ago Dr. Magoun together with Dr. Moruzzi from Pisa first demonstrated that high-frequency stimulation of brain stem reticular regions produced a generalized EEG-activation pattern associated with blockade of thalamo-cortical synchronization.[290] This work has, of course, greatly altered our views on the brain mechanisms controlling many types of complex behavioral activities. What has been accomplished in recent years is a better understanding of the cellular mechanisms underlying the effects of reticular stimulation on thalamic and cortical activities.

It would be presumptuous of me to continue outlining the several areas of investigation which have brought us closer to an understanding of cortical function at the cellular level. However, I cannot help mentioning a few more problems which are also of great current interest to neurophysiologists. There is, for example, the question, "What do dendrites do?"—and "How do the functions of cortical neurons change during ontogenesis?" Undoubtedly when we talk about the development of speech behavior or indeed any behavior, somewhere we will have to come to grips with the problem of the relationship of behavioral changes to morphogenetic changes in neurons and synaptic organizations. It has been suggested recently that the properties of neocortical neurons in immature animals are quite different from those in adult animals of the same species.[327] This appears to be particularly true in respect to the "plastic" responsiveness of dendritic elements of immature neocortical neurons. Much work is also in progress in attempts to disclose conditions for demonstrating similar "plastic" responsiveness of dendrites in neurons of mature cerebral cortex and other locations. These problems may appear to be trivial to many of the participants here engaged in the every-day activity of speech and language studies. But I doubt that we will ever be able to satis-factorily cope with the neurophysiological basis of these complex activities without a thorough understanding of the complex func-tions of single neurons and populations of neurons at different developmental stages.

CHAIRMAN MILLIKAN: Dr. Magoun, from your position in "antiquity" in which you have been referred to, have you any com-ments?

DR. MAGOUN: Simply to congratulate my little "grandson." (Laughter)

CHAIRMAN MILLIKAN: Dr. Sperry, do you have comments?

DR. SPERRY: Frankly, no.

DR. GESCHWIND: I would agree strongly with most of what Dr. Myers said about cortico-cortical connections. The pattern of connections which he has so elegantly dem-onstrated is certainly compatible with the patterns that have been found by strychnine neuronography and by the Marchi technic.

I am not prepared to accept the notion that the transcortical connections to the frontal lobe are of no importance. Downer[90] believes that there were disturbances of crossed visual reaching after commissure sec-tion. I think his results and those of Dr. Myers are somewhat discrepant.

Dr. Myers stressed that each functional sec-tor is independent. The one way, however, in which these sensory regions tend not to be independent, as shown by Dr. Myer's slides, is in fact that each of these does indeed pro-ject to the frontal lobe. He showed this to be true for visual, auditory, and somesthetic sectors. He was a little doubtful about the somesthetic, but the results obtained by strychnine neuronography show projections from this region to the frontal lobe. There is certainly a great deal of evidence that the animal can at times use the efferent pathways running directly to the brain stem, about which Dr. Myers spoke. I don't agree, how-ever, that the transcortical connections to the frontal lobe are of no importance. Thus

Glickstein, Arora, and Sperry[141] showed that while separation of the occipital and frontal regions did not indeed produce a failure in simple visual-motor tasks, delayed response tasks were permanently impaired. This would suggest that, for certain types of tasks, the occipital-frontal connection is indeed im-portant.

There is still another factor to consider in dealing with the transcortical connections to the frontal lobe. It is true that in many experiments the animal carries out motor acts despite the loss of those connections and must, therefore, be presumed to be using the direct subcortical connections. The possibility must be entertained that the animal normally uses the transcortical connections and starts to use the direct subcortical connections only when the normal transcortical pathway is no longer available. Thus Kennard[197] and later on Welch and Stuteville [402] showed that after small frontal ablations monkeys develop a dramatic syndrome in which they show no motor responses to sensory stimuli from the opposite side. This syndrome disappears in about two weeks. It is my feeling that the original ablation removes the region to which the three cortical sensory association cor-texes project, and that this area of the frontal lobe is the one normally used for carrying out motor responses to sensory stimuli. Fol-lowing ablation of this region the animal is able after a period of time to bring into use the direct descending pathways from these regions of sensory association cortex. We have evidence for similar phenomena in man. Thus, after acute unilateral frontal lesions in the appropriate location, humans may de-velop a disturbance of conjugate eye move-ments which is nearly always gone by two weeks, again suggesting that other pathways can substitute for the normally used trans-cortical connections to the damaged area. Although in this case man compensates read-ily, it is my guess that, in general, humans are more dependent than monkeys on their transcortical connections in the sense that they compensate less readily for damage to these pathways.

I find it difficult to accept the evidence cited by Dr. Myers for subcortical mechanisms in aphasia. Thus, Penfield and Roberts[309] cite one case with a thalamic lesion who was aphasic. This patient, however, had a large thalamic glioma. Just as patients with such tumors often have gross hemiplegia which we attribute to edema affecting structures outside the thalamus, we cannot accept the aphasia in this case as being the result of the thalamic lesion itself, but rather the sequel of pressure and edema elsewhere. There is to my knowledge no case of a well-studied stable aphasic patient who turned out at post-mortem to have an isolated thalamic infarct.

Dr. Myers spoke about the studies of Akelaitis. His studies are important and interesting. There is, however, excellent evidence in contradiction to his results. Thus among Akelaitis's cases there were six who had the splenium cut and did not develop alexia in the left visual fields. But the case of Trescher and Ford[391] and the two cases of Maspes[261] and the cases recently described by Gazzaniga, Bogen, and Sperry[123] did show alexia in the left visual field.

How can we account for these differences? I cannot believe that stormy postoperative courses explain the differences since it is hard to believe that none of Van Wagenen's cases had a stormy postoperative course while all the cases of the other surgeons did.

I cannot discuss all the reasons for the differences which I have discussed elsewhere,[130] but can outline some of the possibilities. One important difference is that most of the patients in the Akelaitis series had epilepsy dating from childhood. We know that following early lesions to the left hemisphere language is acquired by the right hemisphere. Therefore, patients with early lesions, such as those in the Akelaitis series, might well have more bilateral representation of language than would the usual adult cases. Since, however, many of the tests used to demonstrate callosal disconnection are based on language, we could in such a group of patients less readily find evidence of disconnection. The long-standing epilepsy of these cases is the second factor. Thus Erickson[105] showed that seizures will, after lesions in their usual pathways of spread, find roundabout routes to other brain regions. Long-standing seizures might facilitate the opening of pathways not normally used and thus account for some of the phenomena in the Akelaitis series. I would certainly hope that someone working with animals will take the opportunity to do commissural sections in animals with a long-standing history of seizures.

As a final comment on Dr. Myer's paper, I find myself a little hard put to accept the notion that we cannot use any patient who has a stormy postoperative course. Thus Geschwind and Kaplan[133] predicted, while their patient was still alive, that he was suffering from a callosal infarct. The patient came to postmortem while the paper was in press and had the predicted lesion. It would seem most odd that only in a patient with a callosal lesion should a stormy postoperative course have led to the effects we observed. This would be too much of a coincidence. Since that time we have examined over 100 postoperative cases and despite the most stormy of postoperative courses in some of them, we have yet to find another patient who showed such a syndrome.

I certainly would agree that caution is necessary in accepting the results of clinical studies. Thus, if a patient dies within a few days of the onset of his lesion, we would all agree that it would be unreasonable to accept readily the conclusions based on observations of his deficits. But we are not talking here of such cases, and it is clearly outside the range of chance that the only patients, with or without stormy postoperative courses, who have shown interhemispheric disconnection syndromes have been those who were subsequently proved to have callosal lesions.

CHAIRMAN MILLIKAN: Professor Chomsky will discuss "The General Properties of Language."

The General Properties of Language*

NOAM CHOMSKY

Research Laboratory of Electronics
Massachusetts Institute of Technology
Cambridge, Massachusetts

I WOULD LIKE TO make some rather informal remarks about certain aspects of language which I think will ultimately have to be taken account of if the study of brain mechanisms and the study of language are to have any real connection.

The straightforward way to approach this question would be actually to sketch what seem to be well substantiated properties of language. However, I don't know if I can do this in comprehensible fashion within the time limitations. Therefore, I will try to do it informally, using examples and rather metaphorical remarks to try to give some indication of the kinds of properties that must ultimately be accounted for by any neurological theory which hopes to get to the root of the matter.

I think it might be useful to begin the discussion by referring to several points that have already been raised in the last few days. In particular, I was interested in the question about whether it makes any sense to study, or whether there is any useful purpose served in studying, animal communication systems within the same framework as human language. Some skepticism was raised about this, and I must say that I myself rather share this skepticism. It seems to me there is no striking similarity between animal communication systems and human language. If we rise to the level of abstraction at which human language and animal communication systems fall together, then we find plenty of other things

incorporated under the same generalizations which no one would have regarded as being continuous with language or particularly relevant to the mechanisms of language. This is clear, if we consider the properties which, as was pointed out last night, are shared by animal communication systems and human language: specifically, the properties of purposiveness, of having syntactic organization, and of being propositional, in a sense, informative.

I think it is perfectly true that both systems are propositional, syntactic, and purposive, in the sense in which these terms were used in this discussion. So are many other things. For example, consider walking. Walking certainly is purposive. It is certainly syntactic, that is, it has some global organization. It is also informative; for example, the rate of speed with which someone is walking suggests to us how interested he is in his goal. In fact, it is perfectly conceivable that one could use rate of walking to give information about precisely that.

Or, to take something which one might think is, perhaps, a little bit closer to language, consider the common gestures one uses in helping someone park a car. When you indicate to him by the distance between your two hands how far he is from the car behind, your actions are purposive, integrated, and propositional. But, it is unlikely that any significant purpose would be served by studying such gestures and human language within the

*This work was supported by the Joint Services Electronics Program (Contract DA 36-039-AMC-03200 [EL]), NSF Grant GK-835, NIH Grant 2PO1 MH-04737-06, U.S.A.F. Contract AF 19 (628)-2487.

same framework. In fact, if you consider how these various systems are purposive, informative, and structured, then very striking differences appear between human language, on the one hand, and all the other systems (that is, animal communication, gesturing, and walking), on the other.

Consider first the matter of informativeness. As I understand it, animal communication systems are informative in one of two ways. Either they consist of a finite number, a finite population of available signals, or else, in the case where they have an infinite number of possibilities, there is a finite number of dimensions in the "language," each of which is correlated to some physical, nonlinguistic dimension in such a way that by picking a point along the linguistic dimension, you uniquely specify a point along the correlated nonlinguistic dimension.

If I understood Dr. Thorpe's remarks last night concerning birds that use alternations of pitch, the "linguistic" dimension is the number of alternations in high and low pitch; the nonlinguistic dimension is the intensity with which the territory will be defended, or something of this type; and these two dimensions are associated. Furthermore, there is a point-by-point correlation between them so that the bird specifies a point along the nonlinguistic dimension by selecting a point along the linguistic dimension. The same is true of the bee dances and the other examples mentioned. My example of walking has just this property. Rate of walking is informative about desire to get somewhere in just this sense, and the same is true of the gesture system that I mentioned.

But the devices used by human language are of an entirely different kind. If I say that there is a bird in the tree outside, or that I wish I could go to New York to see a movie tonight, or anything else, it is quite senseless to ask the question: "What are the dimensions of this utterance that correlate with some dimensions in the outside world, such that picking a point along the linguistic dimension selects a correlated point along the

dimension in the nonlinguistic system?" It is obvious that there is no sense in asking that question.

In short, if we rise to the level of generality at which animal communication and human language fall together, we find such other systems as, for example, walking. If we try to analyze these kinds of behavior into natural classes, we find that human language separates out as rather different in its fundamental properties from other types of behavior that fall together at this level of generality, for example, walking and animal communication.

It was remarked that there is some similarity between human language and animal communication systems in another sense, namely, that the ordinary use of language, like the ordinary use of animal communication systems, is to change behavior, to modify thoughts, or something of this type. I rather doubt that this is true. As a matter of fact, I think there is little reason to believe that the primary use of language is to modify behavior or modify thought.

Language can be used for all kinds of other purposes. It can be used to inform or to mislead, to clarify one's thoughts or to show how clever one is; or, in fact, it can be used for play in a very general sense, that is, to utilize intellectual capacities and maintain some feeling of relationship with others, or something of this kind. I am not using language any less, if I do not care whether I convince anyone or change anyone's behavior or change his thoughts—I am not using it any less under those circumstances than if I say exactly the same things, and I do care whether I convince him or change his behavior or change his thoughts. In either case, I may be using language in a perfectly normal way.

If one wants to find out something significant about the nature of language, I think it is important to look not at its uses, which may be almost any imaginable, but, rather, at its structure—to ask what it is, not what is done with it.

Language can be used for a huge variety

of purposes. On the other hand, almost any system that contains discriminable stimuli can be used to modify behavior or to provide information. It is a mistake, a bad habit, to approach the study of language by considering its "characteristic" uses. For one thing, the general assumptions about what are "characteristic uses" are highly suspect. Second, even if correct, these statistical guesses would suggest very little about the nature of language. The same kind of comment can be made about various attempts to "extrapolate" from experimental work with animals to conclusions about human language.

It has been brought out in the discussion in the last few sessions that "linguistic concepts" are rather different in important respects from concepts that are taught by so-called "associative learning," concepts specified in terms of some set of physical properties, such as the concept of round object with green spots in it, and so on. A good deal of evidence was provided concerning the failure of cross-modal transfer in the case of concepts developed in this fashion. Then it was observed that linguistic concepts do exhibit cross-modal transfer and are thus rather different from the concepts taught by associative learning. It was concluded that it is the verbal tag that mediates the cross-modal transfer.

There is another interpretation of such data, namely, that the linguistic concepts have nothing to do with "associative learning," that linguistic concepts are not characterized in terms of a network of physical properties. Then, instead of attributing cross-modal transfer to the verbal tag, we might assume simply that linguistic concepts (which, in fact, have verbal tags) differ in a fundamental way from these artificial concepts characterized in terms of some network of physical properties. Actually, I think there is good reason to accept that latter interpretation; on independent grounds, it is clear that the concepts normally assigned "verbal tags" are not, in general, characterized in terms of physical properties, as are the artificial concepts of

the concept-formation experiments. Concepts such as "knife" or "house" are not characterized in terms of some set of physical properties but are, rather, defined in functional terms, as has long been known. Ordinary human concepts simply do not have the property of being characterizable in terms of some collection of physical properties. They are concepts of a different type. There is no reason to expect the very different, arbitrary, and artificial concepts taught by "associative learning" to share the properties of concepts of the normal type, which are probably not "taught," in any interesting sense of this term.

Again, to call all these things "concepts" may be as misleading as to call animal communication systems and human language "languages." That is, although at some level of abstraction the word applies to both, there may be fundamental differences between them. One has to be careful about jumping to the conclusion that because such a thing as associative learning does exist, because you can demonstrate it, it therefore has anything to do with something else that exists, namely, human concepts.

In fact, there are many specific human concepts, such as the one I want to talk about more specifically, namely, the concept of a sentence (of English or of any other language) which certainly cannot be characterized in terms of some arrangement of physical properties or association or anything else of this kind. It is totally out of range of any of these notions.

With these introductory remarks, let me try to say a few things about what seem to be general properties of human language, more specifically, what it means to have command of a language. When a person has command of a language, when a person has command of English, what kind of things does he know? What kind of information is in some fashion represented in his nervous system? We may assume that a language is a specific sound-meaning correspondence, and that when a person has command of the language, he knows, in some sense, the intrinsic meaning of a variety of signals. Command of the language involves knowing that correspondence and involves the ability to select, when one of the signals is presented, the correlated semantic content; also the ability, given some idea in mind, to find the appropriate signal to express it. This connection between sound and meaning is not a connection at the level of words but at the level of sentences. That is, command of English involves an understanding of each sentence of English, a knowledge of what that sentence of English means. The most obvious and most important and most neglected fact about language is that this knowledge of the intrinsic connection between signal and semantic interpretation, between sound and meaning, is a correlation that extends over an infinite range of objects. This is no logician's quibble, or anything of this sort. Actually, the most obvious aspect of normal use of language is that it is unbounded, that it rarely involves repetition, even repetition of items of the "same pattern" as those that have occurred before. Repetition of utterances certainly is the exception in normal linguistic behavior. There are certain clichés, or idioms, like "Good morning," which may have empirically detectable probabilities of occurrence. Characteristically these clichés do not have the ordinary structure of the sentences of the language. But normal linguistic behavior, one's normal behavior, as speaker or reader or hearer, is quite generally with novel utterances, with utterances that have no physical or formal similarity to any of the utterances that have ever been produced in the past experience of the hearer or, for that matter, in the history of the language, as far as anyone knows.

If you want to convince yourself of the truth of this remark, the easiest way to do so is to take an arbitrary sentence and wait until you hear it, or read the New York Times until you find it; or take the first sentence in the first book in the Library of Congress and keep reading until you find a repetition of it; or any other such test you wish to try.

It is rather obvious, without trying the "experiment," that you are unlikely to find a repetition, or even an utterance which is similar, point by point, in category; or anything of this kind. Normal use of language has this property of unboundedness. It is not a matter of matching certain stimuli or forms of stimuli against associated meanings or kinds of meanings, or anything of this type; but, rather, there is some abstract system of rules which, in some manner, characterize an unbounded meaning-sound correspondence. The grammar of the language, which is somehow represented in the brain, must have this property of determining a sound-meaning correspondence over an infinite range. One normally encounters these absolutely new signals or produces them on the appropriate occasion without any feeling of strangeness or feeling of novelty. This is the basic, most elementary fact that has to be accounted for by anyone who is interested in dealing with the phenomenon of human language in a serious way. It might be thought that "animal language" also has this property. As I pointed out before, however, it provides for novelty and innovation in a very different manner.

Let me turn briefly to the question of the correspondence between sound and meaning. What is the nature of the grammar that determines this relation? Instead of trying to outline the structure of grammar and the general properties of grammatical structure that seem to be universal, what I would like to do is to give a few examples which illustrate the kind of property these grammatical rules seem to have, that must somehow be accounted for. I think I can probably illustrate this with only two or three examples.

I think someone mentioned earlier that the "integrity of the sentence," what makes it "hang together," is determined by relations among successive items. It is quite clear that that cannot be the case. The fact that it cannot be the case can be seen if you look at some very simple examples of sentences. Let me give you a couple to illustrate.

Consider the sentence: "What disturbed John was being disregarded by everyone." Consider the sound-meaning correspondence. First, we must ask how the signal is determined. I won't try to argue this here, but will simply assert that the form of the signal is determined by two factors: one, by the choice of words, for example, by the choice of "John" instead of "Bill"; and second, by the phrasing, in the normal sense of grammar school. It is clearly true that this sentence can be bracketed into a subject part "What disturbed John" and the predicate "was being disregarded by everyone." Furthermore, the subject part can be identified as a category of a particular type, a nominal category. Furthermore, the phrases "John" and "everyone" are also categories of this nominal type. I won't bother with details, but it is clear that a labeled bracketing of the sentence is an appropriate description of it at some level— I will call it level of "surface structure." This is a psychologically real level of structure in the sense that the rules determining the phonetic form make explicit and essential reference to this level of structure. That is, knowing the intrinsic, ideal form of each lexical item, one can determine from this labeled bracketing the ideal physical form of the signal.

I think this fact plays a role in perception as well as in production of speech. However, let me put this question aside and turn to another point, namely, how the semantic content of the utterance is represented.

A very significant fact about semantic content is that it is not in general represented by the system of labeled bracketing that constitutes surface structure. This is quite obvious if you think about this sentence, or almost any other you pick. Look more carefully at this sentence. Notice, first, that it is ambiguous; that is, it might mean that John is disturbed by the fact that everyone disregards him. That is one sense: "What disturbed John was the fact that everyone disregards him, John." But the sentence has another interpretation, namely, that everyone is disregarding

the thing which disturbs John. There is no physical difference between these two interpretations. This is easy to demonstrate. If you put this same signal in two different contexts, you force one or the other interpretation.

The basis for difference of interpretation, again, to use traditional and familiar terms, is the difference in the network of grammatical relations one finds in the sentence. For example, in the paranoid sense, in which what it means is that John is disturbed by the fact that everyone disregards him, it is clear there is a certain grammatical relation called traditionally the "verb-object relation," which holds between "disregard" and "John"; whereas in the other interpretation, where we mean that everyone disregards whatever it is that disturbs John—under that interpretation there is no grammatical relation between "disregard" and "John." Rather, this same verb-object relation holds between "disregard" and, perhaps, "what." Furthermore, the verb-object relation which holds in these two different ways also holds in other parts of the sentence between "disturbed" and "John," and so on.

Furthermore, if I add the word "our" to the sentence, giving "what disturbed John is our being disregarded by everyone," then the ambiguity disappears.

One could go on to show various other complexities in this network of relationships in a sentence. The important point to observe is that the structural properties of the sentence that determine its meaning are not represented in surface structure. So, there is some other aspect of linguistic structure— let me call it "deep structure"—which involves some rather abstract network of grammatical relations. It is this network of grammatical relations, not represented in the signal or in the organization of the signal, that determines the semantic content.

There are many other examples that illustrate the same point. Let me mention two more and say a word about each of them. I have just given an example of an ambiguous sentence. One can draw the same conclusion by looking at the opposite extreme, that is, at two sentences which are essentially synonymous. Compare the following two sentences: "I expected the doctor to examine John" and "I expected John to be examined by the doctor."

There is relationship of paraphrase between the two. That is, although the surface structure of the two sentences is clearly quite different—the signals are entirely different in labeled bracketing—nevertheless, there is something in common which determines the same interpretation.

One might be inclined to say that what makes them the same in meaning is that the embedded sentences, "The doctor examined John" or "John was examined by the doctor," have a very simple relation, namely, the active-passive relation. But matters are not that simple.

Consider the very analogous sentences formed by replacing the word "expect" by "persuade": "I persuaded the doctor to examine John" and "I persuaded John to be examined by the doctor." Although "persuade" and "expect" play the same surface role, it seems this change has made a fundamental difference in the deep structure. Though the two sentences with "expect" are paraphrases, the two sentences with "persuade" are definitely not paraphrases. It is not true if I persuaded the doctor to examine John, then I persuaded John to be examined by the doctor. But it is true that if I expected the doctor to examine John, then, in fact, I expected John to be examined by the doctor, and conversely. There is a much more abstract feature of the grammatical structure of these sentences which somehow determines their semantic content and does it in an entirely nontransparent fashion.

The two significant facts that I want to draw from this discussion are these. First, surface structure of any type, any type of labeled bracketing of the sentence, any attempt to account for the structure of the sentence in terms of contiguity of parts or association between successive parts or anything of this type is certainly going to fail, as you can see by examples of this type, by the fact that whatever it is that determines the structure of the sentence completely transcends any such representation. Whatever it is about the sentence that determines its semantic interpretation, whatever determines that aspect of the sound-meaning correspondence, is very different from the organization of the utterance into grouped parts, even if you categorize the grouped parts.

The second point is that observations of this very elementary kind illustrate the point I made before, namely, that one's knowledge of a language goes well beyond any experience and well beyond any possible teaching. It is entirely out of the question that everyone in this room was taught these facts about "persuade" and "expect"; in fact, nobody even knew them consciously, until a couple of years ago; at least, there is apparently no grammar of English which observes that "persuade" and "expect" differ in this respect. Certainly no one was taught the fact, yet everyone knows it, and knows it without having had experience with these sentences or anything like that. It is extremely unlikely that any of you has ever seen sentences like these or been presented with some kind of indication, by teachers or parents, that these sentences differ in this fashion. The same is true in the case of the first example.

So, somehow, one has represented in one's brain a set of rules which differentiate sharply between surface structure and deep structure in such a way that that aspect of the sentence structure which determines semantic content is extremely abstract and not represented in the physical form or in the arrangement. That is, I think, a crucial point.

Let me give one further example and make a final comment about it and then summarize briefly. Consider the following, again, ambiguous sentence: "Mary saw the boy walking to the railroad station." It is clearly ambiguous. It can mean either that the boy was seen walking toward the railroad station by

Mary or that the boy walking toward the railroad station was seen by Mary. So there are at least those two interpretations, and, in fact, others.

Furthermore, we can resolve the ambiguity very simply by replacing "walking" by, say, "walk," giving "Mary saw the boy walk to the railroad station," which has only one interpretation; or by inserting the words "who was," giving "Mary saw the boy who was walking toward the railroad station," which resolves the ambiguity the other way. These are facts that everybody knows and that are somehow determined by the grammatical structure of the sentences. But this is not the point I want to illustrate. The point I want to illustrate relates to the information that every speaker of the language has about the kind of operations that can be performed on these sentences, to assign new interpretations to them.

Although I cannot give details, let me try to illustrate in informal fashion. Consider the problem of how to form questions and relative clauses in English. Given the sentence "John saw Bill," we can form such questions as "Who saw Bill?" and "Whom did Bill see?" We do this by two operations: first, by an operation that we may call "*wh* placement*," in which we identify a certain noun phrase and assign *wh* to it, so that if I want to question "Bill" in "John saw Bill," I assign *wh* to "Bill" and I get "John saw *wh* Bill," meaning that the position filled by the word "Bill" is going to be the position questioned.

The second operation, *wh* inversion, takes that *wh* element and puts it in front. Thus, we start with "John saw Bill" and get, by *wh* placement, "John saw *wh* Bill." We then place "*wh* Bill" in front, giving "*wh* Bill did John see." By other rules, "wh-Bill" (or, if we were being more accurate, "wh-someone") becomes "who." These two operations of *wh* placement and *wh* inversion will basically account for the formation of questions. If we want to form "Who saw Bill?" then, of course, *wh* inversion is vacuous, but we may

still say that it applies. The operation of *wh* placement and *wh* inversion will, in fact, with some minor, automatic changes, account for the formation of questions in English.

Precisely the same two operations will account for the formation of relative clauses. If we take the sentence "John saw Bill," we can form the relative clause "who John saw" or "whom John saw," in this case, by again taking the element "Bill," the second noun, assigning *wh*, and placing it in front; similarly, we can form "who saw Bill" by applying the same two operations (the second, vacuously) to "John." Both the question forms of sentences and the relative clause forms of sentences are formed by essentially the same two operations, namely, the operation of *wh* placement and *wh* inversion. Obviously everybody knows these rules—everybody forms questions and relatives using these operations with some elaborations that I omit.

However, notice that these two operations, namely, *wh* placement and *wh* inversion, differ from one another in the following way: *wh* placement is a free operation. I can apply it as many times as I like in a sentence. For example, if I have the sentence "John saw Bill," I can apply it twice to get "Who saw whom?"; or, I can form "Who gave what to whom?" and so on. I can apply *wh* placement as many times as I like, questioning as many aspects of the sentence as I like. On the other hand, *wh* inversion can be applied only once. That is, if I have the sentence "John saw Bill" and I apply *wh* placement twice giving "Who saw whom?" I can't apply the inversion twice to get, say, "Who whom saw?"

Similarly, if I say "John gave what to whom?" I have a possible question in English, but I cannot put both "what" and "whom" in front. I cannot say "What whom did John give to?"

The same is true of relative clauses. You can apply *wh* inversion once but you cannot apply it twice. You can have a *wh* element inside a relative clause, in which case you have a question like this one: "Mary saw the boy who was walking toward what?" Answer: "Railroad station." But I cannot put "what" at the point where the "who" was and get "what who was walking toward." A general constraint says that *wh* inversion can be applied only once.

Summarizing briefly, *wh* placement can be applied freely but *wh* inversion only once within a particular phrase. Actually, what I have shown so far is that *wh* inversion can be applied only once to form a question and only once to form a relative.

Can it be applied once to form a question and once to form a relative? Can I take a sentence with two *wh*'s and apply *wh* once to form a relative and a second time to form a question? The general constraint that restricts *wh*-inversion to a single application should exclude this. In fact, notice what happens if we take the three sentences, "Mary saw the boy walk toward the railroad station," "Mary saw the boy who was walking toward the railroad station," and "Mary saw the boy walking toward the railroad station." If we apply *wh* placement to "railroad station," this will give us the sentences "Mary saw the boy who was walking toward what?" "Mary saw the boy walking toward what?" and "Mary saw the boy walk toward what?"

In considering the sentence "Mary saw the boy who was walking toward what?" notice that in the embedded sentence "who was walking toward what?" I have already applied *wh* inversion once, vacuously, to form the relative clause. Therefore, the general principle should imply that I cannot apply *wh* inversion again, putting the word "what" at the beginning of the sentence. It should imply that I cannot form "What did Mary see the boy who was walking toward?" And this is, in fact, an impossible sentence. But now consider the sentence "Mary saw the boy walk toward what?" There has been no application of *wh* inversion in this sentence; therefore, I ought to be able to form the question by *wh* inversion, giving "What did Mary see the boy walk toward?" This is, in fact, perfectly acceptable.

Consider the third, ambiguous case, namely, "Mary saw the boy walking toward what?" And consider the associated question, namely, "What did Mary see the boy walking toward?" Observe that it is unambiguous. It can only have the interpretation of "what did Mary see the boy walk toward?" It cannot have the interpretation of "the boy who was walking toward the railroad station." So, clearly, it is true that *wh* inversion can be applied only once. If it is applied once to form a relative, it cannot be applied a second time to form a question. That is, it is true with respect to this very abstract operation which somehow we have represented in our minds, that we know how to apply it in such complex cases as this, and we know when it applies to give sentences and when it does not. The principle of this application is apparently something quite abstract. In fact, the explanation just suggested for these facts is not adequate, but this does not affect the point of the example.

These principles of *wh* placement and *wh* inversion, and so on, are what are called in the linguistic literature "grammatical transformations." The significant points about them are two. First, they relate deep structures to surface structure. Deep structures are extremely abstract objects which cannot be arrived at from data by any type of association or inductive procedure and are not represented in the data in any physical form. Second, these transformations, if you look at them as formal operations, are of an extremely special and peculiar kind, meeting very abstract conditions such as the condition of noniterability of inversion, just mentioned. When we acquire language, we acquire a system of operations of this type. We acquire the system of abstract structures that underlies them, the deep structures, and we acquire a set of abstract conditions on these operations, such as the condition of noniterability of inversion. The few examples given illustrate these facts.

It seems to be true that the underlying deep structures vary very slightly, at most, from language to language. That is quite reasonable, because it seems impossible to learn them, since they are not signaled in the sentence and are not recoverable from the signal in any nontrivial way by any inductive or analytical operation, so far as I can see. Since it is hard to imagine how anyone could learn them, it is pleasant to discover that they do not vary much from language to language. That fact enables us to postulate that they form part of the technic which a person uses for acquiring language; that is, they are part of the conceptual apparatus he uses to specify the form of the language to which he is exposed, and not something to be acquired. It is fortunate that this postulate is tenable, since it is difficult to imagine an alternative.

Second, it seems to be true that the abstract properties of transformation are also universal. This is what one would expect, again for the same reason, since it is difficult to imagine how operations of this type could be abstracted from data. There is certainly no process of generalization or association of any kind known to psychology or philosophy, or any procedure of analysis that is known in linguistics that can come close to determining structures of this kind. Again, it is to be expected that these operations and their general properties will be uniform across languages, and this seems to be the case.

From considerations of this kind, there are several basic conclusions, I think, that seem to emerge. A person who knows a language has represented in his brain some very abstract system of underlying structures along with an abstract system of rules that determine, by free iteration, an infinite range of sound-meaning correspondence. Possession of this grammar is a fact which psychology and neurophysiology must ultimately account for.

Second, investigation of the properties of such grammars seems to suggest that these systems are, to a significant extent, not learned, but rather that their basic properties constitute preconditions for learning. One is led to conclude that a grammar is no more

learned than, say, ability to walk is learned. There are certain aspects of walking, certain aspects of gait, that may be culture-dependent and may be learned. It is also true there are undoubtedly some superficial aspects of language which are learned and which vary from language to language, but it seems that the deeper properties do not vary and are so abstract that it is hard to imagine how they could be learned.

This raises a second question for ultimate neurophysiological or psychological investigation, namely, what are the mechanisms responsible for the structures which seem to be preconditions for acquisition for language?

It seems to me that there is no significant evidence of continuity, in an evolutionary sense, between the grammars of human languages and animal communication systems. I have no doubt that other cognitive systems, other aspects of human behavior, other aspects of animal behavior, share many of these properties, but it is unlikely that animal communication systems are the ones that share these properties in a most striking sense.

CHAIRMAN MILLIKAN: Dr. Lenneberg, will you open the discussion?

DR. ERIC H. LENNEBERG: Dr. Chomsky's presentation was stimulating as always, and was very rich, so much so that I have a difficult time picking out particular points that ought to be emphasized here.

What I would like to do is pick out those points which seem to me to have greatest relevance, partly to the papers which have preceded his paper and also in anticipation of those as yet to come. He stressed one important point, namely, the difficulty in accounting for various aspects of language in terms of simple association. I think this a point which has been frequently disregarded: that a simple associative process could only with great difficulty account for what we actually see in language learning.

Perhaps the most striking phenomenon in language acquisition can best be observed in various types of defective children, particularly blind children. Several years ago I tried to observe the language difficulties that congenitally blind children have. Making arrangements with the Perkins Institute in Boston, to my great surprise I found that there were no difficulties whatsoever. The nursery children, aged three, had just as much language as their sighted colleagues. There was virtually no difference in semantics which one could discover by listening and playing with these children. Occasionally something would occur, such as a color word being frequently, and naturally, misapplied, yet the general meaning of color words was apparently there. The word would occur in the right spot and the right connection. It was just factually wrong. This is rather strange, if you consider how much we believe we are bound to our visual input, to realize that language develops at the same time, with the same facility, at the same speed even in the presence of such a major disruption of sensory input.

Similarly, it is quite clear now that blindness, in addition to deafness, constitutes only a relatively minor obstacle to language acquisition. The problem is to get signals into these patients but, once this is accomplished through establishment of some appropriate signaling system, say a tactual one, then the particular mental activity—if you will pardon the expression—seems to be all present. The machine can start. Certainly all the major aspects and principles of language are established under these circumstances.

Also, a simple theory of sound and object association is put to great strain in the vocabulary acquisition of a child. Observation of children shows that a child has particular difficulty in learning that there is one object called "Daddy" and that this word applies only to one particular, unique individual. It seems to be much more natural to organize the world around him into categories, categories where each instance shows some similarity to other instances, yet where the nature of the similarity cannot be expressed in physical terms.

This, I believe, is what Professor Chomsky stressed a moment ago. It is so obvious, it hardly needs to be emphasized that learning requires peculiar organization of the world around us. Furthermore, the acquisition of language would not be possible if the child did nothing but learn to relate words to things. If he had no other knowledge, no other activity going on, he would be totally incapable of understanding what was being said to him. We speak in sentences, not individual words, and quite clearly the syntactic element in sentences is the important aspect for the understanding of communications. "Mary loves Johnny" is different from "Johnny loves Mary." If the child did not, *pari passu*, learn syntactic features with the semantic ones, he would not be able to develop language.

A similar point could also be made about the acquisition of phonology. Individual sounds in language—invariant sounds, I am tempted to say—do not exist; there is no such thing as an invariant speech sound. The sounds are interpreted in connection with other sounds, and a complex system of rules is necessary to interpret the acoustic reality that strikes us. This becomes much less abstruse than it may sound if we consider attempts to build a machine which is operated simply by speaking into it; human voiced speech would be the input, and the output would be international phonetic symbols. Such a machine has so far not been built, and it has not been built because the machine would have to be equipped with a very complicated set of syntax and rules for interpreting the sounds that it takes as input.

Another point which I think was implicit in Professor Chomsky's presentation is the role of imitation in language acquisition. This has reference to the question, "What is the peculiar motor that produces language acquisition?" Is it something that is artificial, put inside the child from the outside? Does the child simply imitate because he is rewarded for imitation? Or is it, rather, a machine that gets going which was there to begin with? "Imitation" is a very tricky word. Quite clearly children never imitate the way birds do. Typically the first utterances in the child are totally different—physically, syntactically, and semantically—from anything that occurs around them. You might say they are approximations but highly regular approximations and highly typical.

I could go into further detail but I think the point is quite obvious that what children do is to start with something you might call primitive, which is different from the paradigm language. They develop this further, differentiate it further and further, until only in the last stage do you get approximation, something which might even theoretically be considered as playing back. Imitation does not occur until language is totally acquired. Only at that point can you get children to repeat short sentences.

I think the association question that Dr. Chomsky raised—and I am simplifying—also has relevance to the study of aphasia, where I do not believe we find dissociation. I do not think that aphasic symptoms are interpretable as the snapping of links established between sounds and things. The most common aphasic symptom, difficulty in word finding, does not, I believe, represent such a simple severance, because most of the patients can recognize the word quite easily. If they are asked, "What is this?" they say "I can't remember" or "I don't know" or "It is too bright" or whatever the patients do. If they are asked, "Is it a shoe or horse or chalk?" certainly in the vast majority of cases they are able to recognize the right word. So, the word is not lost. I think that only by stretching the notion of association as studied in animal research in the laboratory can it be applied to human language behavior.

The last point that Dr. Chomsky made strikes me as extremely important, and that is the distinction between deep structure and surface structure. I think that we are dealing with something quite familiar to us in many different realms, where we also deal with deep structure and surface structure, or where we must assume deep structure, and where that deep something, whatever it is going to turn out to be, actually has a character.

Many years ago Lashley pointed out that we are faced with a serious and interesting problem in this kind of phenomenon: most of us have learned to write with the right hand; although none of us who are confirmed right-handers may ever in our lifetime have written with the left hand, we can right now take a pad of paper, close our eyes, put a pencil in the left hand—the nonpreferred hand—and not only write but write upside down. This is remarkably successful usually.

This poses the following problem: on the periphery, which is here tantamount to surface, entirely different muscles are being activated. The order is reversed because you are writing upside down. The direction of the pencil is reversed, and yet quite clearly a pattern is reproduced which you recognize as similar to that produced by the right hand. I think here, analogously, you have to assume that something is stored in the nervous system which corresponds to this patterning. Call it abstract if you wish, because we cannot see it. We cannot cut it out. In animal experiments we have great difficulty interfering by means of a scalpel with this type of neuronal event. These were problems raised by Lashley and confirmed many times since.

CHAIRMAN MILLIKAN: Questions or comments?

DR. THORPE: I would like to ask you questions on one or two points which seem to me to be of great interest. You said, I think, that everyone knows these rules without being taught, without their being formalized or specified. Are you, in fact, saying that thinking is not simply unvocalized language but that, on the contrary, thinking precedes language? When you refer to the underlying deep structures, would you not say that at least some of these deep structures must be present in animals before the acquisition of any language because they concern the very nature of the perception of or understanding of the world?

There is a good deal of evidence from the work of my colleagues and myself[387] which indicates the highly stimulating effect of mutual practice in promoting normal development towards the specific song pattern in the chaffinch (*Fringilla coelebs*) even though all the birds taking part are equally inexperienced. This suggests very strongly to me that something corresponding to your "deep structures" exists in relation to the development of vocal communication in birds.

DR. CHOMSKY: I think, in fact I am quite convinced, that thinking can proceed perfectly well without language, but I was not presupposing that here. Furthermore, I think one could design an automaton which never thinks but which has the capacity of acquiring any specific human language in a rather short time from a small amount of data.

I would want to put into the automaton an initial specification of what kind of formal object language is, what kind of operations, what kind of mechanisms it has, and leave the automaton just enough leeway so a small amount of data could select one of the possible languages. Having acquired this language, the automaton could produce sentences and assign them semantic interpretation. It would never do anything remotely like thinking. I think one could describe all these things without ever talking about thinking.

Similarly, I suspect if one knew enough about thinking, one could say many interesting things about it without referring to language. I am quite convinced that thinking is not dependent on language.

I would agree with your statement if you say that thinking precedes language; I am quite sure that is true. I don't doubt that an infant or a dog thinks in some sense and, therefore, that thinking precedes language. I was not presupposing that; in fact, I think the two things are logically, and in large measure factually, independent.

About the question of deep structure, it

seems to me, if we look at human beings and ask ourselves the empirical questions as to how they can acquire command of language, that we are led to the postulate, which seems to me fairly well confirmed by evidence, that significant aspects of these deep structures must be present in advance of language acquisition, that there is no inductive operation on language data which leads to the deep structures, but that, rather, the theory of deep structures provides part of a framework for interpreting signals which the organism uses to decide which of the possible languages is the one it is being exposed to.

As far as human beings are concerned, if we simply look at the empirical problem of accounting for the fact that they acquire command of the language, then we are led to the conclusion that they have a certain intrinsic mental structure, and this structure probably specifies the abstract, the general properties of language, of deep structures, and of transformations. We can then raise another question, namely, whether this system of mechanisms appears in any other organism, or, for that matter, the question of whether this system of mechanisms plays a role in any other aspect of human intellectual activity, in human cognitive processes, perceptual processes, and so on. I think it would be very surprising if it did not show up in other aspects of human intelligence and, also, somewhere in animal intelligence.

It would be surprising if this complex structure were so specific that it is there just for language and has nothing to do with anything else. I think it would be surprising, but it could be true. I do not think we have any evidence one way or the other.

DR. THORPE: It seemed to me to be rather satisfying to think that these deep structures, or some of them, could be present in animals before language ever evolved; otherwise the evolution of language would be almost impossible. If some of the deep structures can be acquired by normal linguistic experience, then it seems to me that you have got a possibility of language being evolved perhaps a number of times in the course of evolution, without any very great difficulty.

DR. CHOMSKY: I think most of the discussion of evolution of language is complete hand-waving. If one wants to give an account of how some complex structure is evolved, you have to say something more than that a lot of possibilities were tried and this one worked out. If you stop to think about the number of possibilities that can be tried, with no constraints given, then it is quite impossible that anything viable would ever work out.

So, I think if one really wants to give a serious account of the evolutionary process, he must first ask what kind of constraints there are upon the development of complex systems, given certain fixed conditions. Until those constraints are known, I do not see any point in speculation about the evolution of language.

It may turn out, when we learn enough about a complex organism like the brain, that we will discover the only way it can manipulate symbols, when it reaches a certain level of complexity, is this; perhaps this is even a consequence of physical law. If it is a matter of physical law, there is no point speculating about evolution. I am not proposing it as physical law; my point is that at the moment we have as much justification for saying it is physical law that at a certain level of complexity this particular kind of grammatical structure must appear—we have as much reason for saying that as we do for saying that language evolved in some fashion.

One could think of analogous situations in the physical world, where one would draw precisely this kind of conclusion. I am not convinced of the necessity of looking to selectional processes for an explanation of the development of language. If one is looking for an evolutionary explanation of language, I frankly do not see how his problem would be simplified if he were able to discover that other animals have systems analogous to language. I think if he were to discover this he would be faced with a new mystery, namely,

how these systems emerged. Adding a new mystery won't help to solve this one. There is a prior question, namely, whether other animals do have systems of this type. Maybe they do, but it does not seem to me that the communication systems of animals, at least, are of this type. If other animals do have systems with the formal properties of human language, I imagine the proper place to look for them is not in the communication systems but, rather, in systems for organization of perception or something of that type.

DR. EVARTS: You spoke of language as being a sound-meaning relationship. You would include, I suppose, sign language in all this. There is nothing special about the sound, if one communicates.

DR. CHOMSKY: I mean "signal." I should have said "signal-meaning correspondence." It is an open question whether the sound part is crucial. It could be but certainly there is little evidence to suggest it is.

DR. SILVERMAN: How can we tap these universals in creating a command of language in deaf children?

DR. CHOMSKY: One would expect that unless the appropriate stimulus conditions are realized, the instinctive behavior would not appear. It may be that the appropriate stimulus condition is hearing enough linguistic noises in your environment. So it just might be that there is no way to tap the system, any more than there is a way of initiating the system of flight in birds without putting them in the situation in which they have to flap their wings.

DR. RICH: Maybe you are not the one I ought to ask this question of. If I understood you correctly, there is a basic set of untransformed frames which the child would have at his command, prelinguistically, or very early. It seems to me at least possible that some transformations are, in a sense, more difficult than others.

Has a study been made of the ages at which the various transformations become available, and could one conclude from this anything about the successive psychic difficulty of the transformations?

DR. CHOMSKY: That is a very sensible question, one a lot of people have been worried about for quite a few years. I won't try to summarize the evidence. It seems to me that one general fact about the investigations that have been carried out is that there are two stages that are identifiable. There is a very early stage where in the child's production of speech you do not find many of the mechanisms, and there is a slightly later stage in which you find so many of the mechanisms you cannot begin to describe them, and the transition between these two stages seems fairly rapid.

There has been much careful analysis of language acquisition through its first few months, in which there is a slow increase in one-word sentences, two-word sentences, and three-word sentences, and then the experiment stops. The reason is that at that point development of language increases beyond any possibility of exhaustive description. I am not too convinced about the value of these studies of early stages of language development. These might be like the study of maturation of instinctive capacity before it reaches the appropriate time.

DR. LENNEBERG: I would like to comment on two points and pick up yours first. I am not particularly convinced, after having tried to study the development of language in children, that it is a good question to begin with to ask the time at which suddenly a child begins to use transformations. It makes perfectly good sense to say transformation is a special way of processing material that comes in, transformation of processing on a chronological level, transformation of processing involved in using words. This can be acceptable, if you think of it in this way. I think even a small child can divide those strings of words that are grammatical from those strings of words that make no sense. Here there is actually involved application of the deep structure that Dr. Chomsky talked about. You

apply it and it fits the pattern, and grammaticality is the common denominator.

I had originally planned to say that one can show, whenever you have a common denominator of this kind, that you can put this alphabet into this transformation of language where you transform the deep structure to abstract something in the structure into the reality of the sentence. Does this make sense? Let me try to state it another way.

DR. CHOMSKY: I think I agree with that. It seems to me that the deep structures are projected onto the signal by some kind of system of rules which I call transformations. One never produces the deep structures at the earlier stage of language. One does not produce the deep structures which are from the theoretical point of view abstract, and from the neurological point of view probably also deep. But there is some way of mapping these deep structures into signals. The way may differ for the young child, who does not have control of motor mechanisms, and for the child at a later stage.

It is also true, no doubt, that specific aspects of the deep structure and specific projection operations are not available to the child at an early stage. There are some respects in which English is different from German and Chinese, and so on. The child has to learn which of the possible languages is the one he is supposed to be talking. Before he has learned that, he has, I presume, just some kind of undifferentiated schema which can become Chinese or English or German, when enough data are presented to it.

Nobody knows anything about these mechanisms. It is plausible to assume there is an undifferentiated schema which becomes specified in one way or another and becomes specified and differentiated with more and more complexity and more and more uniqueness through some period of so-called learning. "Learning" is an inappropriate term for that kind of development.

At the latter stage of this process of acquisition, the process of projecting deep structure onto signals will be tremendously more extensive and more complex than at the early stages. There may be much more uniformity in the extensive and complex structure between different individuals than at the very early stages.

I think it is reasonable to suppose that the basic processes of formation of deep structures and projection are being utilized in a very undifferentiated and simple way at the beginning and in a more and more complex way at every stage, until, finally, the normal adult human system is achieved.

DR. CHASE: As I followed the discussion of the deep structure of language, Dr. Chomsky, it seemed quite clear to me that such a structure must exist insofar as we cannot explain the organization of the surface structure of language in its own terms. But it also seemed quite clear that we are not able to specify what the ordering functions are that impose organization on the surface structure of language. Insofar as we cannot specify these ordering operations, and I take it that the word "abstract" is really being used to say this, then it seems to me that we are not in a position to take a stand on questions of structure and mechanisms, and certainly not on the question of genesis.

It is the last point that I question most seriously, because I think the very best way not to discover the essential substrate in experience for acquiring a capability is to assume that it does not have a substrate in experience. It seems that you are inviting us to consider this possibility with respect to the deep structure of language.

DR. CHOMSKY: I would agree that if we could not specify the deep structures and we could not specify the projection operations, then it would be correct to conclude that we should not speculate about mechanisms and genesis. From what I said, there is no reason why you should guess that we can specify them. In fact, however, I think we can. Of course, anything we can now say is empirical hypothesis, and no doubt will be proved wrong in one respect or another. But I think we can, with a fair degree of confidence, say

something rather precise about the exact nature of deep structure and the exact nature of the rules that relate to it. This is the central question of linguistic work. Other linguists would not agree, but this is what I think, at least. It seems to me that a good deal of progress has been made toward giving a precise specification of a universal system of underlying structures and a universal schema which permits some variation from language to language, but not too much, and toward specifying in precise detail the rules of projection, if you like, that map these structures ultimately onto signals.

I have not said anything, really, to justify this, but I think I can refer you to work which would illustrate these claims. Furthermore, I should mention that there is nothing particularly new about this program or about these conclusions, at least in their general nature. In fact, much of what I have been saying was almost a cliché in the seventeenth and eighteenth centuries, and surprisingly good work was done in what is called universal grammar, a long forgotten tradition, in specifying underlying structures and specifying the abstract operations—by "abstract" I mean "removed from the signal," not "unspecifiable"—that relate them to surface form. Interestingly, this traditional theory developed out of a framework of rationalist psychology that made assumptions about perception and also assumptions about acquisitions of language that are extremely plausible and closely related to what I think would result from an unbiased investigation of how concepts and systems of this type are acquired. Of course, everything hinges on whether I can substantiate the claim that we can make precise some account of the deep structures and of projection rules.

MRS. RICHARD L. MASLAND: I would like to make a clinical comment about children who are late in developing language and then develop it. Miller[275] has pointed out how important it is to remember the sequence of auditory events. This point has been brought out. For instance, telling the difference between "Bear the eats," "Eat the bear," and "The bear eats." The interesting question is how a child with difficulty in keeping track of the sequence of auditory events can deduce the elements of the deep structures. This one sees clinically in operation in the child, and one deduces the confusion which may be the basis for the delay. This in a child with normal hearing acuity.

DR. CHOMSKY: I do not know anything about this.

MRS. MASLAND: Later, when some of the children do acquire language to the point of some fairly normal communication, the semantic elements still become scrambled sometimes. One case in point is a child who said, "My sister bike threw over fence" for "My sister threw her bike over the fence."

DR. CHOMSKY: Not knowing anything about it, I should not say a word. One can imagine all kinds of possible production defects, filtering defects, let us say, that would lead deep structures to appear not in their normal form but in other forms. For example, consider the phenomenon, which appears apparently with normal children, of producing just major words and not the "grammatical" ones. One might imagine that all that is happening is that there is a filtering device which throws out everything except stressed items. There might be a filtering device or a projection device of some kind that operates on deep structures in some non-normal fashion in the children to give other kinds of signals. One would have to study the material to draw any conclusion.

MRS. MASLAND: We think one of the devices that really can be demonstrated is shortened auditory-memory span.

DR. CHOMSKY: That sounds very plausible.

CHAIRMAN MILLIKAN: If there are no other comments, Dr. Irwin Pollack will discuss "Language as Behavior."

Language as Behavior

IRWIN POLLACK

Mental Health Research Institute
Ann Arbor, Michigan

I SHALL GO Professor Silverman one step further and announce my territorial abdication based upon my own lack of experience in this field. Several months ago when I was asked to speak on "Language as Behavior," I declined on the grounds of incompetence. I received back a firm but polite note from Dr. Millikan saying that I perhaps was incompetent to judge the competence of the Steering Committee in judging my competence, and I was expected to discuss "Language as Behavior." (Laughter)

Since we are immersed in a sea of language behavior, since our every waking minute is intimately associated with language-oriented behavior, there certainly is no lack of data for us to consider under the topic of language behavior. If anything, we are so swamped with our own language behavior that we are forced to develop concepts to describe this behavior.

Apparently the level of description of language behavior is crucial to its understanding. The decision made by the linguists, so beautifully exemplified by Dr. Chomsky, is at the level of the sentence. At this level of description the linguist sees commonalities across languages. He is impressed by the fact that children—for that matter, adults—utilize many of the complex rules of syntax without being able to verbalize or abstract these rules.

The level of description with which the experimental psychologists or, I should say, many experimental psychologists are most comfortable are those units which provide quantitative units of measurement. These units are usually the utterance or the word.

At his level of description the psychologist sees a long period of trial and error in the acquisition of language. He is impressed by the fact that his units of language behavior apparently obey many of the rules of any other form of behavior and are subject to the same contingencies for reinforcement and control.

In this controversy, the linguist and experimental psychologist are both satisfied with their own view of language. I personally feel sympathetic to both points of view and allow myself to accommodate both these divergent points of view, depending upon which level of description is appropriate.

On the other hand, if Chomsky is correct, the behavioral aspects of language are almost incidental, except in so far as they help reveal the underlying structural aspects of the organizational structure of language. To Chomsky what is important is the linguistic competence, not linguistic behavior. The fact that most of us speak ungrammatical sentences is irrelevant to him. What is important is that we can, indeed, when called upon, recognize the difference between a grammatical and an ungrammatical sentence. Moreover, Dr. Thorpe clearly pointed out that at the level of language behavior, animal communications possess many of the purposive features of human language behavior.

Thus, the features of language behavior which might throw light on the organization of the human brain are considered by these experts either as nonunique or as incidental. Therefore, I would like to reorient the topic of "Language as Behavior" and consider those more ephemeral aspects of behavior in which many of you as clinical psychologists, speech pathologists, developmental biologists, and linguists are much more knowledgeable than I, namely, the planning and the directive aspects of language behavior.

Now, it is very difficult to give a definition of the planning and directive aspects of behavior. It is much easier to point to it by a series of examples. I am reminded of the operational procedure of the psychiatrist in defining an optimist or pessimist. He places his subject in a room. If the subject is placed in a room full of toys and goodies, and he comes out crying a short time later saying that he cannot share all these wonderful toys and goodies with his friends and all the unfortunate children in the world, then he is a pessimist. However, if the subject is placed in a room full of horse manure and he comes out a while later happily exclaiming that, with all this manure, there must be a pony in there somewhere, he is an optimist. Your job is to find the pony. (Laughter)

As an experimental psychologist, I had originally come prepared to discuss various aspects of language behavior with you. I had come prepared to discuss a recent study from the University of Michigan which, with the aid of a digital computer, has analyzed the entire vocal output of a child in the first six months of life. This child was raised in a controlled acoustical environment and I believe the report provides a very interesting body of data. Such a report might have been of interest to the developmental biologist.

I had come prepared to discuss a recent study which, through the manipulation of acoustical feedback within an operant conditioning paradigm, demonstrates that fluent-speaking talkers can be reduced to stammering, stuttering speakers, whereas many of the worst stutterers and stammerers can have their behavior modified both within and outside the laboratory to be nearly fluent speakers. These technics of language behavior might have been of interest to the speech pathologist.

I had come prepared to discuss the beautiful work of one of our participants, Norm Geschwind, and his collaborator, David Howes, on another aspect of language behavior. They have been successful in developing quantitative measures of the language behavior of normal and aphasic speakers by the beautifully simple expedient of counting words from the utterances of their speakers and patients. Their methods not only differentiate between normal and aphasic speakers but also between different classes of aphasic speakers. The description of these results might have been of interest to the clinical neurologist.

I had come prepared to discuss the modification of verbal behavior through the use of other verbal behaviors. The skilled counselor who ignores the statement of his patient when he makes self-deprecating remarks and perks up his ears and leans forward when the patient makes approving remarks about himself can mold his patient's behavior. The molding and control of behavior might have been of interest to the clinical psychiatrist.

I had even come prepared to discuss how the experimental psychologist has attempted to scale how much nonsense there is in different nonsense syllables. Long after Ebbinghaus successfully employed the nonsense syllable to obtain quantitative measures of verbal learning, we have a large body—and I am ashamed at this point—of experimental psychologists investigating why some nonsense syllables are easier to learn than others. This material I am sure would have been of interest to few of you. (Laughter)

I had come prepared to discuss the language behavior in terms of the complex grammatical structures employed by speakers, but this was so much better done by our speaker and, besides, he is not interested in language behavior but in language competence. I had even come prepared to discuss Karl Lashley's love affair with the study of language behavior for the cues it might provide for the way the brain handles complex hierarchical functions. I even had a quotation from Lashley which succinctly described his views. Such discussion might have been of interest to the neurologists.

I can say I came prepared to discuss these and other topics because, indeed, I mimeographed my talk. I am not discussing these topics of language as behavior for the reasons originally outlined, but, even more important, because I would like to orient the discussion toward these aspects of the planning and directive functions of language.

Specifically, I would hope you could tell me what it is about the language environment of the so-called culturally deprived child that makes him culturally deprived. Dr. Hardy has alluded to this problem. Perhaps he can be persuaded to expand upon it.

I would hope you could tell me why certain aphasics emit apparently correct grammatical structures but seem to utter gibberish. I don't think Dr. Geschwind has to be urged too hard to discuss this. I hope he will discuss this for us.

I would hope you could tell me why certain patients live an utterly vegetative life because ordinary events are transformed by distorted language behaviors into highly traumatic situations.

I would hope you could tell me why it is said that German philosophy seems so much clearer in German than it is when translated into English. (Laughter)

I would hope you could tell me why scientists, with slightly different backgrounds, find it so hard to communicate with each other.

I would hope you could tell me how skilled motor behaviors, such as the swinging of a golf club or the driving of a car, are initially guided under strong verbal control but never become smoothly coordinated and integrated actions until the involvement of the verbal control is minimized. Parenthetically, the next time you bet on a golf game with high stakes, ask your opponent, just before he makes a crucial putt, which muscles he uses in making the putt. It will serve to break up his smooth action.

I would hope you could tell me how man effectively employs his verbal behavior to record his goals and aspirations and transmit a worthwhile culture to his grandchildren.

In short, I would hope you could tell me something about the planning and directive functions of language, its manifestations, its physiology, and its pathology.

The subject matter of this Conference is the relation between language and the functions of the brain. A very astute student of language, George Miller, has produced a provocative essay on this particular subject. He argues that, initially at least, the crucial aspect in man's evolution might not have been his large brain but, rather, his erect structure and his apposable structures. These structures permitted the use of the hands for the fashioning and manipulation of tools. But the time spent in fashioning tools is wasted unless there is a plan for their use. Presumably natural selection favored those individuals who could not only fashion tools but who could devise complex hierarchial sequences of behavior for their planned use. Language presumably served as the means for augmenting the plan. In this manner the evolution of a tool-using culture was not the result of man's large brain but, perhaps, the reverse.

The physical anthropologist, I am sure, does not look favorably upon this theory of culture modifying structure. Nevertheless, the theory provocatively causes us to re-examine most elementary assumptions of our own evolution and causes us to re-examine the role of planning and directive functions of language.

I have referred repeatedly to the planning and directive functions of language without defining these functions. Just as the psychiatrist defined his optimist and pessimist, I can only point in the direction which we might look by citing examples for its use, yet this is the area to which I would like to direct your attention. Could you please help me by answering some of my questions?

(The following paper, prepared by Dr.

Pollack, was made available to all Conference participants in mimeographed form. It was not orally presented and, therefore, was not the subject of general discussion.)

Man's involvement in language behavior is so utterly complete that it is difficult to dissect any waking behavior which is not, or was not at some stage, intimately related to language behavior. Even those motor acts which can be performed in a semi-automatic fashion—such as the driving of a car or the swinging of a golf club—were initially acquired only after much accompanying "talking-to-oneself" behavior. Man's involvement in language behavior is so pervasive that some theorists have suggested that the human brain not only made language behavior possible, but its evolution was fashioned by language.

In a fascinating essay Miller[274] suggests that the initial advantage of primitive man, *Homo erectus*, over his fellow apes was that his long, mobile arms and hands were freed for grasping tools. Presumably natural selection favored those individuals who not only could fashion tools but could also organize complex hierarchical sequences of behavior to fashion a plan for the use of their tools. Language served as the means for augmenting the plan, and consequently language and tool-making evolved together. In this light, language is not simply a result of man's large brain. Rather, the evolution of the human brain is a consequence of early man's success in making tools and in their language-directed use.

Miller's controversial hypothesis of culture modifying evolution leads us to re-examine the conventional view that human language is a function recently tacked onto a large brain. From this point of view, language evolved much earlier than heretofore accepted.

Linguists have been impressed by the commonality of languages over the face of the world. They have also been impressed by the fact that children utilize many complex rules of syntax without ever verbalizing or abstracting the rules. This has led some linguists to postulate that the brain has specifically evolved to accommodate language.

Neurologists also have been impressed by the fact that, despite widespread equipotentiality of function in the human brain, certain language functions are extremely localized. Stated differently, language behavior to the neurologist and linguist may be fundamentally different from the rest of the behaviors of the individual.

The experimental psychologist, perhaps because of his empiricist behavioral bias, strongly resists the argument that language universals are to be found over the entire human race and strongly resists the conclusion that language functioning has a strong innate component. He observes a long period of trial and error and conditioning in shaping the verbal responses of the child. He feels that language behavior obeys the rules of any other form of behavior and is subject to the same contingencies for reinforcement and control.

In this controversy perhaps each is right within his own field of interest. The linguist focuses upon the structural features of the language, and he finds early evidence of this development within the organism and across the human species. The psychologist focuses upon linguistic units such as words and finds that their acquisition obeys many of the rules associated with the acquisition of any arbitrary set of responses and is specific to the resident language community. There is also a fundamental difference in approach. The linguist is interested in competence for language performance, irrespective of the fact that most communicants do not strictly adhere to the rules at all times. The psychologist is interested in demonstrated behavior in terms of units which are manageable and quantifiable. This usually leads the psychologist to define units of verbal behavior in terms of the word or utterance, characteristics of language behavior which are of little interest to the linguist.

The approach of the experimental psychologist to the study of language as behavior will be illustrated by a few representative examples. The first examples examine the vocal output without considering subtle distinctions in the output.

Lane and Sheppard[215] have analyzed all the vocal behavior of one child (Sheppard's) from birth to six months. To collect this behavior, this child was reared in a controlled sound environment. His every utterance triggered a tape recorder. The collected output of the tape recorder was played to a computer which determined the fundamental frequency, amplitude, and duration of each utterance; and the variability of each of the measures. Of fundamental interest is their finding that, with the exception of an initial period of a few weeks directly after birth when breathing movements were being coordinated, neither the fundamental frequency nor the average duration per utterance changed appreciably in the first six months. In terms of these fundamental acoustic parameters, there was little evidence of a developmental sequence within the first six months.

Through an experimental analysis of stuttering behavior, Goldiamond[142] has been able to control such behavior by subtle manipulation of environmental contingencies. He has demonstrated increased nonfluent utterances in normally fluent speakers and decreased nonfluent utterances—and even their elimination—in severely stuttering individuals.

Before examining studies in which words are the unit of measurement, we should note the exalted place of the nonsense syllable in American experimental psychology. The scene is so weird that it borders on the ludicrous. In order to obtain standard units of verbal learning materials, Ebbinghaus devised the nonsense syllable way back in 1880. They admirably served his end and he did important work with these materials. But he would squirm in his grave if he could see the heritage he left behind. The outstanding feature of the nonsense syllable is that it is supposed to be relatively homogeneous and relatively neutral with respect to the subject's past experience. However, some nonsense syllables make less nonsense than others; for example, BOT makes less nonsense than QXZ. So, in our desire for precise measurement and scaling, psychologists have been busy little bees scaling nonsense syllables for all kinds of things—their meaningfulness, their pronounceability, their associativeness, etc. In each case, syllables which score high on one measure of nonsense score high on other measures. But there are enough discrepancies to keep us at the milk of this tit for at least another generation. Glanzer[140] has characterized this activity as a game where the experimenter tries to squeeze sense out of his materials while the subject attempts to put the sense back in. Hopefully there are encouraging signs that experimental psychology will go on to more interesting investigations of verbal behavior.

We now turn to a series of studies which examine the verbal output at a level above the crude utterance, but still fall far short of the complexities of language. Howes and Geschwind[175] have summarized their extensive investigations into the quantitative parameters associated with normal and aphasic speech. Basically their procedure is to record the verbal output of normal and aphasic speakers and then count the frequency of occurrence of the different words in their speakers' output. While aphasic speech obeys the same quantitative laws as normal speech, the quantitative parameters associated with the word frequency distributions differ between normal and aphasic speech. More importantly, different groups of aphasics may be characterized in terms of the derived quantitative parameters.

A large number of studies have been carried out on the modification of verbal behaviors by experimental control. In such studies the experimenter says "good" or "mm hmm" when a subject emits plural nouns. The purpose of the experiment is to determine whether or not the frequency of plural nouns is increased as the result of the experimental treatment. While verbal behavior may be easily modified (see Krasner[210] for a review of the experimental studies by these procedures), there is a dispute whether such modifications in verbal behavior can be established without an awareness by the talker of the reinforcement contingencies of the experiment.

Of late experimental psychology has become interested in the structural and hierarchical aspects of language behavior. In a remarkable enterprise which owes its academic roots to the Harvard Center for Cognitive Studies, it is now difficult to separate out the activity of the experimental linguist from that of the psychologist. In this enterprise the psychologist borrows heavily from the linguist in the design of his experimental materials. The linguist, in turn, draws upon the results obtained by the experimental psychologist to determine "natural" rules employed by communicants. However, since the linguist is interested primarily in language competence rather than language behaviors, the linguist is in the happy position of picking and choosing from among the results which fit his theoretical position.

Where this joint enterprise of linguistics and psychology will lead, no one can clearly foretell. I suspect it will continue to harvest rich dividends as long as George Miller continues to push the enterprise. But even if this enterprise fails—and no one expects this to —it will have performed a valuable service in rekindling the interest of students of behavior in complex structural and temporal behavioral sequences which meant so much to our common mentor, Karl Lashley. As did George Miller, I find the following quotation of Lashley's to be most relevant to the aims of this conference:

I have devoted so much time to discussion of the problem of syntax, not only because language is one of the most important products of human cerebral action, but also because the problems raised by the organization of language seem to me to be characteristic of almost all other cerebral activity. There is a series of hierarchies of organization; the order of vocal movements in pronouncing the word, the order of words in the sentence, the order of sentences in the paragraph, the rational order of paragraphs in a discourse. Not only speech, but all skilled acts seem to involve the same problems of serial ordering, even down to the temporal coordination of muscular contractions in such a movement as reaching and grasping. Analysis of the nervous mechanisms underlying order in the more primitive acts may contribute ultimately to the solution even of the physiology of logic.

CHAIRMAN MILLIKAN: Dr. Rosenblith, will you open the discussion?

DR. ROSENBLITH: First, I am puzzled by the size of this meeting. I know that meetings that want to settle issues or start large programs ought to be not larger than seven, plus or minus two times the appropriate number of dimensions represented. Otherwise, if they are of the order of 200, then the situation becomes very simple: the discussant or participant needs only to stand up for identification, the people in the audience who empathize with his viewpoint feel they have been represented, and all the rest is really done.

The second reason for my being puzzled is that Irv Pollack gave me a text; in contrast to all the people who complained, I cannot claim I have not had it. But he did not speak it! (Laughter) So, as far as I am concerned, this is the first time I have heard a society or profession that is not only well established but sometimes accused of being overprofessional, not only claim their territory but abandon it to the winds—the winds of the linguist.

So what should I do? How should I behave linguistically as a discussant? Can I do it by contrast? I do not think I can. By contrast, the well-known ploy, you show you have understood less than the rest of the audience, who thereby get the feeling of real fulfillment. Can I do it by enhancing the logical structure? I would have to repeat the structures my friend Irv gave. I might not even repeat them in as nice a manner as he gave them.

The next ploy is that you criticize the methodology. Well, he had a large wastepaper basket for the methodology. As he was talking, he discarded one technic after another. He did not even stick with quantification.

The only thing I can really do is the famous approach that says, "Let me add a few other facts of chronology." That turns out to be autobiography; since the man who speaks must be the expert, that gives a feeling of expertise.

Seriously, I think nobody will doubt that the only one who has spoken so far, and he has talked both from a position of theoretical strength and undoubted relevance, has been Professor Chomsky. It is clear that the rest of the people who have talked here—and I hope nobody will take this as a personal remark—kind of had to defend themselves as to what they had been doing before the linguists had been looking. And, in some sense, what Professor Chomsky has told us is, perhaps, a metaphorical rewriting of the Galbraith book on the affluent society. "Why," he has asked, "are you so data-rich and so theory-poor? Why have you kept on piling up the data and not worried about the public sector, which is the front where theory meets with other fields?"

I think that the only group, perhaps, who could have given him an answer are not represented here, and I shall not talk for them, but at least I shall evoke their image. They are the telephone engineers. They, more than anybody else, have shown how you can make an enormously successful, quantitative technology of measurement, as long as you can also run a telephone system profitably. But they have never had the burden of having to understand anything about the nature of language. So, when it really comes down to it—and, I think you all understand that my friend, Irv Pollack, has been extraordinarily modest—we find ourselves in the peculiar situation that the field of language, as such, has been dominated by a set of technologies of measurement.

Basically people have said, "Look, there are large problems here. We don't really understand them, but I can measure such-and-such." And it is better to measure something

honestly than not to measure anything. The more quantitatively honestly you can measure it, Calvin has taught our physicist friends, the more you know something positive. And we have, therefore, had related—and again I would like to stress that this is in no sense a personal critique of the people who have spoken here so far—a lot of facts that come from very good technic.

The kind of things that the rational man can say about language—the kinds of deep structures, the abstract operations, he can concatenate in some sense today—are still untestable. And they are untestable precisely because we do not have as yet a technology of what I might call his cognitive measurement. We can identify elements of technology of cognitive measurement but, most of the time, it does not deal with the cognitive part of it. Most of the time it likes to deal with it like kind of a festival in Rio: it deals with the costume instead of dealing with the underlying problem that it expresses. I think that, to a very large extent, we cannot really expect that the very beautiful, intellectual framework that linguists have built within the last few years, can be adequately tested, or that they can even get significant feedback to their thinking as long as there does not develop a cognitive technology that permits them to formulate experiments at a level that they will recognize as relevant and that the rest of us will recognize as relevant, too.

It is, for instance, not an accident that when you talk about the very relevant factor of behavior in time, you get very quickly into the fact that most of the things we know how to measure in time are either discrete events or involve tracking tasks. But we have no way of testing something that has, perhaps, superficially weak connections but deeply strong connections whether it be at the level of neurophysiology, of anatomy, of communication engineering, or of experimental psychology. In other words, how do you test for the temporal aspects of certain logical operations? You can determine their total length, and you can say, "Oh, this maybe could be parceled out" and so on.

I am saying this without in any sense disagreeing with what Dr. Evarts said about the puzzle of the 70 msec. we are talking about. Certainly here is an interval during which cognitive operations could take place, but do they? How can we test for them? I am struck with the fact of the gap that exists at the present time between the highly developed, quantifiable kind of technologies of measurements, and the basic facts of language, the development of language, the position of language, and the deterioration of language. All these things suffer from the fact that we have really no convertible currency that will lead us along from one level of measurement to another. There is nothing we have that is commensurable at these various levels.

We have, therefore, a set of not unrelated technologies, not unrelated quantifiables, but we have a set of things that meaningfully can only say to us, "Well, this is something which keeps us honest." It still is related to the speech event. It is related to the motor event. It is related to the information processing. Yet we have no way of making any contact with the now erased but, I suspect, irretrievable and irreversible imprinted deep structures in your brains.

I have also been impressed with the fact that, when the brain gets mentioned and when the word "evolution" gets mentioned, my friend Chomsky says "hand-waving." He does not quite believe in evolutionary tales for linguists. But, by and large, we do not really have any historical approach which might very meaningfully clarify how, even in recent evolution, languages have evolved. He has complained that it is perhaps not reasonable to say something about how it could be done as long as we do not know any physical constraints. I think, from the theoretical position of linguistics, that we also have to find some kind of constraints upon the concatenations of operations that might have to go on so that other fields could build a bridge towards this.

By no means am I impressed with the fact that this confrontation between students of language and students of the brain—and experimental psychologists are certainly among them—is going to lead automatically to a rapprochement.

I am impressed with the historical fact that, when Skinner developed his today, perhaps, overly-maligned technology of measurement, he looked at the brain—it is true it was before the Macy Conferences but still people talked about it—and he held it up and said it was kind of like the answer of the King of the Incas who took the Bible to his ear, threw it on the ground, and said, "It doesn't speak to me." Skinner decided he might just as well deal with an empty organism, later on called the black box.

So, in a sense, I think it is not necessary from here on forward that there come rapprochement between linguists and other students of the brain. Linguists are, by and large, bright enough, at least as long as they do not have very many students, to be able to invent their own brains and then live with them happily ever after.

My feeling is that, if a meeting such as this and similar meetings that undoubtedly are being held elsewhere have any potential impact for the future, it is because they lead to the fact that one cannot talk any more about the human brain without really trying to understand what linguists mean when they talk about language behavior. And if the word "behavior" is going to be used a little more broadly and, perhaps, less dirtily, a very deliberate effort has to be made by those of us who are here and by the constituencies from which we have been drawn as a nonrandom sample to find whether one can think of experiments that have a cognitive core and that make use of the very sophisticated technologies that have been developed by other brain students.

I think that the burden of proof is obviously not a one-sided one. I have the feeling that perhaps we are at a favorable phase, because students of the brain and students of language are both in a period in which they feel supported by a lot of young people, by a lot of curiosity, and by a lot of feeling that there is a great deal of change. I think if one of us were on the way down while the others were on the way up, this would have been a very unfortunate marriage. But the fact that there are grants supporting all of us—and the most important grants are the neurons that the young lend us—does not make for automatic success.

So not only am I puzzled by the circumstances that characterize Irv Pollack's speech, but I am kind of puzzled squared. I do not know that anybody here has the right answers, but I hope that this will be at least a point of departure where people will try to work out, in common, technics of measurement, and where the interaction between theoreticians and experimentalists is going to be a fairly fruitful one.

You see, physics is in a very strange position today because, by and large, there is nobody who invents experiments which they have to explain, except physicists. In principle, chemistry is really nothing but physics except that it is too boring for physicists to do. I think, in some sense, linguists are in a very similar position. Whatever remains of philosophy is in such full retreat that nobody is going to attack them from the rear. So, as far as they are concerned, their freedom and the lack of constraints on making of theories and making of models are restricted only by their own intelligence. I hope that they won't exploit that position by turning away from the laboratories instead of turning towards them.

CHAIRMAN MILLIKAN: Questions?

DR. HENRY W. BROSIN: I am encouraged by Dr. Rosenblith's challenge and the wide spectrum of discussion last night and today to report on recent work by four men at Pittsburgh. This work is a follow-up on that begun in December, 1955, in Palo Alto at the Center for Advanced Study in the Behavioral Sciences by the linguist-anthropologists Charles Hockett of Cornell, Norman A. McQuown of Chicago, Frieda Fromm-Reichmann, a psychiatrist, and myself. We were later joined by Gregory Bateson and Ray Birdwhistell in the task of detailed analysis at one-twenty-fourth (1/24) second intervals of the lexical, linguistic, and kinesic (body motion) components of human behavior in the clinical situation, and in ordinary social interaction as recorded by soundfilm and tape. There were films made by Bateson of three-, four-, five-, and six-person families, but most of the work was done on a three-person film of a mother, father, and child. This work resulted in a monograph which we hope will reach publication next year.[271]

We were motivated by the belief that psychiatrists, and probably most behavioral scientists in the human field, need better recording for the study of the therapeutic process and the measurement of change and related processes. We began with the conviction that human communication was more than dealing with words alone, or the linguistic-paralanguage components, which are the formal concern of linguists. Somehow we had to work in body motion studies, including posture, facies, and gestures. Eventually we would also have to deal with visceral reactions (autonomic nervous system), and I will enumerate quickly a series which may have value in the study of a stream of communication: hair position and secretions, skin color, blanching, pilomotor erection of the hair, sweating, temporal and carotid artery pulsations, pupillary size, and respiratory rate and depth.

One of the reasons that the behavioral scientists were willing to study a clinical interaction is that here one is acutely aware of contradictory signals within one system alone, as exemplified by Bateson's double-bind hypothesis in which a family of contradictory propositions may be uttered within one framework, or also by the phenomena of contradictory signals at the different levels (lexical, linguistic, kinesic, and visceral). These may cause a great deal of confusion not only in child-rearing and therapeutic situations but also in ordinary daily life.

There are reasons to believe that this broader way of study communication was initiated by Charles Darwin in 1872 when he published an extraordinary book, *The Expression of Emotions in Man and Animal*.[80] He advised, as program research strategies, or by examples, that scientists study the behavior of psychotics, child development, art, myths, and animal group dynamics, for which he is known as the father of ethology. It seems to me that with these leads, we should have fulfilled earlier some of Dr. Rosenblith's requirements during the intervening 93 years.

One clinical example of the need to follow Darwin's example is the study of what is called "flattened affect." Clinicians can agree on its presence, but it is not easily characterized in a "blind" study using tape alone, even by experienced linguists using current analytic methods. It seems probable that the effect called "flattened affect" is not merely an auditory phenomenon but may be inherent in a larger matrix which is as yet undefined.

Another clinical area requiring close study at various levels is the signalling by "neurotic" patients which involves sending contradictions, qualifications, scepticisms, and doubts at the linguistic-kinesic levels which alter the entire transaction in an otherwise apparently straightforward series of logical propositions at the lexical level. One example of such multiple signalling is that furnished by Charney,[61] who studied a half-hour film with tape for postural consonance between a patient and a therapist, either in the mirror or the parallel positions, which is also described by Scheflen.[343] They both find significant interaction and correspondence with the lexical content in independent studies.

We believe, as Dr. Chomsky does, that there is a complex hierarchical structure of patterned behavior and include here the kinesic systems for body motion, posture, gestures, and facies, as well as the lexical systems. I will cite one example furnished me by Dr. Birdwhistell. In the middle class American culture no healthy adult American male ordinarily changes the axis of his eyeball during an eye blink. Should he do so, he would be in danger of engaging in behavior which would be called "queer" in our culture. However, this is not an uncommon practice among females from the age of three to 20 or even later, particularly when they are in attitudes of being charming and seductive.

To support the profundity of Professor Chomsky's description of the "deep structure" and the mystery of learning, I would add that I doubt if any of you ever heard or saw a middle class American mother say to her little son, "Johnny, if I ever catch you moving the axis of your eyeball during an eye blink, I will punish you." You can see that we do not understand the nature or method of instruction, yet it is followed precisely. There are many other examples, particularly when seen cross-culturally, of the tremendous amount of learning which occurs in all modalities during the first 20 months, or the first four to six years in the classical Freudian schema. I am convinced that this learning occurs in a prepared nervous system which is programmed to take advantage of these potentials. Charles Hockett furnishes the example that Chinese children at 20 months have mastery of the basic Chinese intonation patterns, which differ widely from ours and which are very difficult for us to acquire.

There is no lack of hypothesis for these complex phenomena, a charge which may have been implicit in Dr. Rosenblith's comments. I have found Sapir[255] a most valuable guide in the study of language as a system among various communication systems in a culture, and I am pleased to learn that he remains well regarded in current linguistics.

Another investigator, Felix Loeb of Pittsburgh, using somewhat different methods, has also studied relatively large pieces of patterned behavior, called "making a fist," "the foot kick," or an arm movement (indicating) called the S_z, which have high correlation with the ongoing lexical content and congruence with the total body motions.

Sarles, a linguist-anthropologist at Pittsburgh, is dissatisfied with the models derived from other structural considerations such as pitch, stress, and time relationships. He would like to find other means to clarify these aspects of the dynamics of speech, methods having a more accurate designation and descriptions of aspects of intelligible "units." He is aware that oscillographic technics in this area have had a fairly long and quite unproductive history, as summarized by Pierce and David: "The trouble is that these records contain too much information even for a sophisticated sense, such as sight, to comprehend."[317] However, on careful re-examination of such records using primitive technics, Sarles finds characteristic changes in amplitude, frequency, and patterning which make it seem worthwhile to continue with oscillographic studies in spite of their unrewarding nature to date.

Another investigator of human communication, Condon of Pittsburgh, has accumulated a large amount of data during the past five years on the nature of the "units" involved using film at 1/24 second (24 F.P.S.) and 1/48 second, and plans to compare boundaries at 1/100 of a second. Here are some of his findings.

(1) He finds linguistic kinesic units in which there is relatively exact correlation between boundary points of speech segments and those of body motion, illustrating "self-synchrony" in the integrity of the behavior of the single organism.

(2) These units are distinguished from those of "interactional synchrony," which also reveal a precise synchrony between the speaker and his interactant. Patterns of movements on the part of the listener are observed to correspond to those of the linguistic-kinesic units of the speaker. There may be an auditory drive factor analogous to the photic drive. There are very few, if any, adventitious body motions. All are congruent except in some patients, such as

aphasics and schizophrenics, where by definition a different set of signal systems is invoked. That is the reason we call it an aberration or disorder. This recalls a definition of psychiatry current in 1900 but no longer in use, namely, the study of disordered emotions, thinking, and acting.

(3) "An assessment of the organization of the structure of behavioral units is underway. The behavioral process is seen to be simultaneously discrete and continuous without contradiction. The nature of this relationship can be illustrated empirically. The conceptual rubric of postulating a dichotomy of the discrete and the continuous is not a relevant, *a priori*, assumption for the study of process."

(4) Concomitant with self-synchrony and interactional self-synchrony, a third order of synchrony, also correlating with the preceding two, has been tentatively postulated. The EEG tracings (pen movements) of subjects and patients were found by Condon to be correlated with changes in overt behavior. Although much more verification is required, the neuroelectrical read-out during behavior seems to present a patterned analog of the patterns of behavior. The EEG markings are synchronous with the linguistic-kinesic segments. It may well be that other forms of read-out also exhibit this synchronous phenomenon. Furthermore, these EEG tracings of two interactants tend to illustrate the same synchrony as revealed in their overt behavior.

(5) "Many clarifying observations concerning units and unit organizations have been made using 48 F.P.S. film."

There has been considerable preoccupation for several years with the nature of the intelligible unit. It is a vexing problem, as you know, and no ready answer is in sight. These relatively early explorations need much more work to make them interesting to clinicians and theoreticians, but I thought you might be interested.

CHAIRMAN MILLIKAN: Other comments, questions, or discussion? Dr. Chomsky, do you have anything?

DR. CHOMSKY: I would just like to say, in

connection with Dr. Rosenblith's remarks, that I do not think anybody actually working on language can doubt the justice of his reminder that sooner or later—in some areas sooner, in other areas later—it is going to be necessary to discover conditions on theory construction, coming presumably from experimental psychology or from neurology, which will resolve the alternatives that can be arrived at by the kind of speculative theory construction linguists can do on the basis of the data available to them. That is, there will come a point, no doubt, and I think in some areas of linguistics it may already have been reached, where one can set up alternative systems to explain quite a wide range of phenomena. One can think that this or that system is more elegant and much more deep than some other, but is it right?

I hate to predict because somebody may come up with a bright idea which may upset it, but guessing from what we now know, it seems to me that in phonology that point may have been reached. We can set up quite elegant theories of phonological structure that can explain quite a remarkable range of phenomena. Most of the work I am referring to is not well known but I think it will be published fairly soon. I think rather striking explanations can be proposed for peculiar phenomena of phonetics. But they are proposed on the basis of theories which, although I think they are intellectually quite satisfying, have no evidence for them other than the fact that they explain quite a lot of phonetic data. Here, certainly, one hopes it will be possible to go beyond that, and you cannot go on beyond that on the basis of linguistics alone.

If the kind of constraints you are talking about, from psychology or from neurology, can be realized, that will be obviously all to the good. I do not know about the situation in neurology; I know a little about psychology. My feeling is that unless the character of psychological research changes fairly radically, not much help is going to come from psychology because of an insistence on attention to peripheral behavior and a refusal to try to do what every other science does, namely, to try to find some underlying theories that will account for behavior. Maybe this is too harsh a judgment, but it seems to me largely justified.

It seems to me some kind of shift of emphasis is needed in psychology, a shift which has taken place in certain areas of it but must take place over a much wider range, if these two fields—psychology and linguistics—are going to interrelate in some significant fashion.

CHAIRMAN MILLIKAN: Comments or questions?

DR. HIRSH: It seems to me that we have, even in the first day, heard quite a span of phenomena, from activity of single cells to the language behaviors Dr. Pollack asked about this evening. I exclude Chomsky because he doesn't talk about phenomena but, rather, about the structure on which certain classes of phenomena may be based.

Within any level of discourse, whether it be of cells or behavior of people or behavior of animals, there certainly are theories. People interested in cells worry about sodium and membrane theory, and such. People interested in the language behavior of people sometimes take their theory from more general psychological ones, on the assumption that a speaking person is still a behaving person and that speech is one aspect of behavior.

So, I cannot quite agree with my friend Rosenblith that we are lacking in theory. We may be lacking in a unification of these several levels of discourse in talking about language behavior. But I cannot believe that a sufficient qualification for such a theory builder is that he not be interested in quantitative data.

DR. ROSENBLITH: For somebody who has written about the quantification of the electrical activity of the nervous system, this is like beating him with his own bloody stump. This is not quite the point to which I tried to draw attention here. I was, first of all, careful to use the plural for "data" and the singular for "theory" and, in this respect, address myself not only to a unifying theory but to a theory that basically has the possibility of what you might call conceptual depth, namely, of commensurability across various types of phenomena.

I feel we have to be the total filter, the collective conscience, and ask ourselves, what is it out of the phenomena we observe, out of the particular theoretical involvement that we have, what is it that will contribute toward, not necessarily immediately a unified understanding, but an understanding of the focus of this conference, as I understand it. I am, just as you, one of the participants, and I am impressed with the fact that, whenever these discussions come up, there is relatively little that people who come from the various disciplinary fields have to contribute.

I think the important thing which has changed within the last 12 years is that 12 years ago, when Jakobson and Halle[185] were essentially trying to announce the theory of distinctive features, it looked like this was what we must work toward; and that once we ended up with a nervous system that has essentially the property of being able to categorize in fairly gross distinctive features, then we would have an understanding of speech. But the linguists have not stood still.

I have a feeling that the amount of relevant work that has been done in the established fields with respect to the understanding of language has, perhaps, not moved sufficiently fast because people have not really understood what has happened in linguistics.

There clearly has taken place in that particular decade—and I think Irv Pollack was really a bit too modest—a great deal of elucidation of pieces of behavior that have to do with the afferents of speech, have to do with the whole concept of intelligibility. I think that we have essentially gotten to understand how the concept of intelligibility fits into the whole picture. Irv was too modest to bring up this whole topic, but, once we have finished with this topic, I think we are still left faced with the facts of what language

is, and in respect to intelligibility, in this very technical sense in which it has been worked on, whether it be a signal-to-noise ratio thing, or whether it be the size of the ensemble, whether it be any of the other things, what little part of the total linguistic discourse it really occupies. I address myself to that and not to the other problem.

CHAIRMAN MILLIKAN: Other comments or discussion, or questions for Dr. Pollack? Dr. Pollack, do you have any concluding remarks?

DR. POLLACK: I did not bring up the work on speech intelligibility; actually I think we could have spun for you a very nice, pretty picture with respect to the activities in the area of the understanding of the intelligibility of isolated words out of context, some beautiful, quantitative results which unify whole blocks of data that have been arrived at. To me, however, that did not seem to fulfill the essence of the purpose of our discussion.

One of the things that has impressed me of late, after having spent about ten years examining the intelligibility of isolated words, is just to ask the question, "What is the unit of speech that we perceptually deal with?" An interesting trick is simply to record a speaker during conversation, speaking at a fairly rapid rate, and then excise out individual words. The surprising thing you get is a series of grunts and groans which, in the absence of a running context, are completely unintelligible. You ask yourself, "Is this the raw material from which speech is built up?"

I am reminded of a statement once made by Fred Frick at a symposium on the use of computers for speech recognition. (I think Dr. Lenneberg was referring basically to the same area here.) He told the engineers, "You will not successfully recognize speech until you understand the speaker's intentions," to which an engineer in the audience exclaimed, "We're having enough trouble trying to analyze the signal. How the hell can we analyze intentions?"

I think by "intentions" Frick was referring

to the fact that you need a minimal amount of running context to handle any speech analysis. It is this aspect of the running stream of speech that permits us to make sense out of materials which, when isolated, are completely nonsensical.

I was hoping that some of the more astute generalists in the audience might have commented with respect to some of the problems of the directive function of speech. We know very little about it but that usually does not prevent us from talking about it. I have no other comments.

CHAIRMAN MILLIKAN: Any additional comments or discussion? If there is no further comment, Dr. Geschwind will discuss "Brain Mechanisms Suggested by Studies of Hemispheric Connections."

Brain Mechanisms Suggested by Studies of Hemispheric Connections

NORMAN GESCHWIND

Veterans Administration Hospital
Boston, Massachusetts

HUMAN BEINGS produce an enormous amount of complex learned behavior in which they become highly practiced. As a result, the investigator may see only a deceptively smooth operation which may obscure the linkage of separate components. Many behaviors which appear to reflect a unitary mechanism may actually be the result of having learned to mesh smoothly the actions of separate regions. Furthermore, it may be difficult or impossible to realize that behaviors which superficially appear similar may be the result of quite different underlying mechanisms. Thus we have evidence that visual-motor tasks may be carried out in quite different ways in the brain. Such a function as comprehending written language may be acquired using different portions of the nervous system, depending on the circumstances at the time of learning, yet the final performances in adult life may be indistinguishable. In addition, so much of adult behavior, particularly in such functions as language, is made up of highly complex activities, that the simple foundations on which the superstructure is built may be concealed from view.

Often the only means available to us to study the components of apparently unitary behavior, to separate the mechanisms of similar-appearing behaviors, and to see the hidden foundations of highly complex activities is to study the brutal experiments of nature on the nervous system of man. This type of study has a special importance and like other branches of science its own special technical problems.

Wernicke[408] was one of the first to see clearly the importance of the connections between different parts of the brain in the building up of complex activities. He rejected both of the approaches to the nervous system which even today are often presented as the only possible ones. On the one hand, he opposed the doctrine of the equipotentiality of the brain; on the other, he rejected the phrenological view which regarded the brain as a mosaic of innumerable distinct centers. He asserted that complex activities were learned by means of the connections between a small number of functional regions which dealt with the primary motor and sensory activities. Although this third view dominated research on the neurological basis of behavior for a period of nearly 50 years, it has been omitted almost entirely from discussions of the higher functions in recent times.

My own interest in the importance of connections was stimulated by the early publications of Myers and Sperry on callosal functions. In early 1961, having heard Sperry speak, I began to look for parallels in man to the dramatic findings which had been described in animals. Only after we had seen our first case of a callosal syndrome a few weeks later did I discover that Liepmann and Maas[233] had many years earlier made the first brilliant description of such syndromes. When we carried our studies further, it soon became clear that the study of cortico-cortical connections not only clarified callosal syndromes but also many other syndromes of disturbances of the higher functions.

The first callosal patient that we saw[133] was discovered by accident. My colleague, Mrs. Edith Kaplan, examined a patient who six weeks earlier had undergone partial removal of a left frontal glioblastoma. For reasons not relevant here, she had tested writing separately in the right and left hand. Unexpectedly she found that the writing with the right hand was linguistically correct, that with the left aphasic.

On examination at this time the patient was alert, awake, cooperative, with normal speech, but he had a hemiplegia which was worse in the right leg. He had a marked grasp reflex in his right hand, some sensory loss in the right hand, and mild weakness in

his right hand. The left side of the body was perfectly normal in all these functions. When he wrote with his right hand, the grasp reflex affected some of the motor characteristics of writing, but as language his written production was perfectly correct. He also typed and did calculations correctly with the right hand.

By contrast, the writing with the left hand was strikingly different. The orthography was better than with the right but there were many linguistic errors. At the beginning some of the written production was undecipherable; later on he wrote clearly but aphasically. He typed incorrectly and performed calculations incorrectly with the left hand. It seemed obvious that the most likely explanation of this remarkable production of normal language with the right hand but

TABLE 9.

Right and left refer to cerebral hemispheres

	STIM. *RIGHT* RESP. *RIGHT*	STIM. *LEFT* RESP. *LEFT*	STIM. *RIGHT* RESP. *LEFT*	STIM. *LEFT* RESP. *RIGHT*
Objects Felt in Hand				
Supply object name verbally		+	− −	
Write object name		+	− −	
Draw object	+	+	−	−
Point to correct object	+	+	−	−
Tactually select object	+	+	− −	−
Describe texture of object		+	− −	
Tell function of object		+	− −	
Demonstrate use of object	+	+		
Oral Command				
Point to correct picture item		+		−
Perform verbal commands		+		− −
Writing on Oral Commands				
Alphabet		+		− −
Letters and numbers to dict.		+		− −
Words and sentences to dict.		+		− −
Punctuation symbols to dict.		+		−

+ = 15 per cent or less errors.
− = 16 to 49 per cent errors.
− − = 50 per cent or more errors.

Performance of patient of Geschwind and Kaplan.[133] A response is indicated in all four columns only for nonverbal tasks. As can be seen, a percentage of errors less than 15 per cent is achieved only when the response is demanded from the same hemisphere which receives the stimulus. Certain spaces are left blank since verbal stimuli and responses are treated as left hemisphere stimuli and responses, respectively.

aphasic language with the left was that the right hemisphere had been disconnected from the speech regions by a callosal lesion.

The other clinical findings in this patient are of interest. We were soon able to show that there were no elementary neurological findings on the left side and that the abnormalities we had at first thought to be present on this side were the results of incorrect examination. For example, when we first tested the patient for sensation on the right hand, he showed some mild impairment; when we tested him on the left side, he appeared to perform very poorly. When, however, we changed our technic and tested nonverbally for sensation on the left, it turned out that he actually performed much better on this side than on the right although we had to use quite complicated testing methods. For two-point discrimination we had him show one or two fingers with his left hand; for position sense we had him point up or down; for tactile localization on the left side we had him point with his left hand to the place touched. These nonverbal performances were perfect although in all these cases verbal responses were grossly abnormal.

In Table 9 are summarized the patient's performances, according to the hemisphere to which the stimulus was given and the hemisphere from which a response was expected. As you will see, the patient performed well only when stimulus and response both required the use of the same hemisphere. He did poorly on all tasks where the stimulus was given to one hemisphere and response was expected from the other. In particular, he performed badly when a verbal stimulus was presented and a response was demanded from the right hemisphere since verbal stimuli are evaluated only in the left hemisphere. Thus he made many errors in carrying out verbal commands with the left arm, but he performed well on verbal commands which demanded performance by the right arm. If an object was placed (concealed from vision) in the right hand, he named it correctly; if it was placed in the left hand, he named it

incorrectly, the response of naming being a verbal activity and therefore in the left hemisphere. We could prove, however, by the following maneuvers that recognition of the objects placed in the left hand was correct: (1) although he failed to name these objects, he handled them correctly; (2) he could, using the left hand, select the object afterwards from a group either tactilely or visually; (3)' he could draw with the left hand the objects he had held in that hand. He could not, however, with the right hand select from a group or draw an object held in the left hand and concealed from vision.

One exception was found to the rule that stimuli presented to one hemisphere could not elicit a response from the other. The patient could read aloud and comprehend words presented in either visual field.

We concluded that the patient had sustained damage to the corpus callosum resulting in disconnection of the hemispheres. We felt that this damage had, however, spared the splenium since the patient could read correctly in *both* visual fields. We faced the problem of accounting for the cause of the callosal lesion. We knew that preoperatively the patient had not had a paralysis of the right leg. Postoperatively he had shown paralysis of the right leg, together with a grasp reflex in the right hand and the signs of callosal disconnection which spared the splenium. In addition, over the period of observation he showed distinct improvement in the leg weakness, the grasp diminished, and the signs of disconnection decreased in intensity but did not disappear. All the above features appeared to fit most closely to the syndrome of infarction in the distribution of the anterior cerebral artery, probably on the basis of ligation of the left anterior cerebral artery at the time of surgery. At post mortem these predictions were confirmed. There was no tumor in the corpus callosum nor was there any tumor in the right hemisphere.

We learned several lessons from the study of this case. It had led us to realize that the usual methods of examination could be quite misleading. Thus we could have easily concluded, incorrectly, that the patient had sensory loss in the left hand because of his misnaming of objects held in that hand. Nonverbal testing in which we confined the stimulus and response within the right hemisphere rapidly showed that in fact sensation was quite intact in the left hand. The mistake of confusing this disturbance with astereognosis was probably made by Goldstein[144] in his description of the second case of callosal disconnection in man. He said that his patient had sensory loss on the left, but he did not use nonverbal testing in which stimulus and response were confined to the right hemisphere.

The fact that so obvious a misinterpretation could so readily be overlooked had another important lesson for us. It is quite common to hear the suggestion put forth that standard methods of testing disturbances of the higher functions should be adopted. But such a standardization could only serve to make it difficult to uncover new modes of testing which might cast further light on the mechanisms underlying clinical disturbances.

There was yet another lesson to be learned from this patient. Unlike most patients with elementary sensory loss he did not tell us that he did not know what was in his left hand but instead gave positive but incorrect responses. We have discovered since then that as a general principle those patients who have their lesions not in the primary sensory pathways (up to and including the primary sensory cortex) but in the sensory association cortex or in the association tracts will not tell you they do not know; they are quite likely to give you positive responses which are usually quite wide of the mark. These confabulatory responses can easily mislead the examiner.

One can be similarly misled by the patient's responses to demands for his introspections as to his reasons for failure. The patient with lesions in association cortex or tracts may be quite prepared to give you his "introspections" but these will be of no help and indeed may be actively misleading. Thus the patient with pure alexia without agraphia may tell you that he cannot read because he does not see the letters clearly, yet this same patient can copy correctly the very words he claims not to see distinctly! It is easy to see that if the cause of a disturbance is the disconnection of a particular region from the speech area, then "introspection" will be of little use since the speech area cannot give you an account of what is going on in a region to which it is not connected.

There are many instances in the literature of the higher functions in which neurologists have been deceived by the patient's so-called introspections. They have believed the patient when he told them that things were distorted or abnormal in some way. I do not mean to suggest that the patient is never telling us something useful, but it does mean that you cannot simply accept these so-called introspections without much further investigation. Why confabulatory responses are so readily produced in the presence of disconnections of association cortex or pathways is a fascinating problem which I cannot discuss further at this time.

The results of the study of this patient enable us to see the fallacy in what appears to be a very simple argument against localization of function. It is often stated that you do not learn to write with the right hand since you can write with your left hand or even with either foot without previous training. This would seem to suggest that the whole brain learns to write. Our patient, however, shows that this could not be the case. He could still write with his right hand but failed with the left. Thus it is obvious that when we write with the left hand we are using the right hemisphere only passively and are still actually using the left hemisphere in carrying out this task. We do in fact learn to write in one hemisphere and indeed probably only in the representation of one limb. There are other evidences which I will not cite here that the left hand is run passively. Liepmann[232] pointed out that while we usually think of the left hand as being clumsy, we do not realize how really clumsy it is since most of the skill it appears to possess is not its own. It is my guess that even the rules for the passive operation of the left hand across the corpus callosum are not built in but that one must learn by experience how to map movements of the right hand onto those of the left.

Let me turn briefly now to another more delimited callosal syndrome, of which, by strange coincidence, we saw an example only a few weeks after we had seen the patient described above. The anatomical lesions of this syndrome, alexia without agraphia, were described first by Dejerine[81] although this condition had been recognized clinically several years before. These patients cannot read but can produce normal spontaneous writing. They can copy correctly the words they cannot read. Dejerine's case showed destruction of the left visual cortex plus destruction of the splenium of the corpus callosum. He interpreted these findings as follows: the patient can see only in his right visual cortex, but as a result of the lesion in the splenium he cannot send the visual information across the corpus callosum to the speech area. In addition to Dejerine's case several other cases with the same clinical picture have come to post mortem and shown the same pathological findings. Fusillo and I[129,132] have studied a patient in detail and have recently had the opportunity to confirm the same findings at postmortem.

One important feature of well-studied patients with this syndrome is the remarkable pattern of preservation of certain tasks in the face of loss of others. Thus these patients tend to show in addition to loss of reading of words, loss of ability to read music[81] and loss of ability to name and comprehend color names[132] while preserving the ability to name objects and to name Arabic but not Roman numerals.[374] I have discussed these facts elsewhere[130,131] so that I will not enter into them here except for one comment. It is important to realize that two tasks which appear quite similar, such as reading a word and reading a number, may in fact be carried out in quite different ways by the nervous system.

Let me conclude by pointing out that I have attempted to show you very briefly two of the callosal syndromes which occur in man. Neither of the syndromes I have discussed here tells us anything about speech directly since in neither of them are the speech areas affected. However, in order to study effectively the neurological basis of language, we must learn to distinguish the effects of damage to the speech regions from those due to lesions which disconnect other portions of the brain from the speech areas.

CHAIRMAN MILLIKAN: Before we turn to a discussion of Dr. Geschwind's material, Dr. Sperry will present some additional data. His topic is "Language following Surgical Disconnection of the Hemispheres." Dr. Sperry.

Language following Surgical Disconnection of the Hemispheres

R. W. SPERRY
M. S. GAZZANIGA

California Institute of Technology
Pasadena, California

A FEW YEARS AGO we reported some observations on a commissurotomized human patient, a patient, that is, with surgical separation of the hemispheres.[36,37,134] These observations jibed nicely with the functional picture of the neocortical commissures that emerged from the animal studies,[366] and also conformed to the general interpretation of the now well-known Geschwind-Kaplan case just reviewed.

Since that time, during the past two years, that is, we have been foolish enough to start the study of another commissurotomized patient[35] and after that another, with results that have proved to be rather upsetting for the picture we had described for the initial case. The results as they now stand would seem to require a considerable shift in our general outlook on the disconnection syndrome for man. Whereas formerly we had stood, I suppose, maybe half-way between the Liepmann[233] extreme, on the one hand, and that of Akelaitis[4] on the other, we now find ourselves obliged, from this later evidence, to shift our position on a number of the important features of the syndrome well over in the Akelaitis direction, although we still find direct contradictions on a number of points making the present picture rather a hodgepodge of the earlier views.

Apparently these later patients have not read the recent literature or they are just being deliberate nonconformists, because we find them doing things like the following:[125,127] writing legible meaningful material with the subordinate left hand; drawing correctly with one hand the shapes of objects held out of sight in the other hand, even to the point here of recognizing and writing correctly with the left hand block letters placed in the right hand.

We find these people are able to guide purposeful, directed manual movements from visual cues in the opposite half of the visual field. Tactile localization of points on the thumb, the wrist, the palm, and little finger of the left hand can be discriminated verbally by a firmly right-handed subject. If these implications are not immediately clear, I am going to spell all this out in more detail as we go along.

With the employment of proper testing methods, one can show that these people are not "word-blind" in the left visual field nor are they "word-deaf" in the disconnected minor hemisphere. Many months and hours of testing later, we have come to believe that these and similar phenomena are probably not ascribable to incomplete surgery and that they represent, instead, genuine features of the cerebral disconnection syndrome for man.

It is very obvious that what we should have done, as you can see, was to have quit after that first case when the whole picture looked much simpler. I think the easiest way to present our current views is to just let the evidence speak for itself; following this "say it with data" approach, I will try to run very briefly through a few examples of the kind of responses that we see in these people, related to language functions, with some brief comments on the conclusions to be drawn, as we see them today. I emphasize the word "today" here because our testing program is still in full swing, and the overall picture continues to change from month to month. Just as our working picture at the moment is rather different from that of a year or two ago, so that of a year hence may be different still. I suspect just a word of caution may be in order here in regard to any attempt to apply this current view to interpretations of clinical material or to global value judgments regarding historical developments in the field. I am not sure that we really have the definitive picture even at this moment that would enable one to pass the proper long-term judgment.

All these patients—there are now six of them all told—are presumed to have a complete midline section of the cerebral commissures, including the corpus callosum, the anterior and hippocampal commissures, and in two cases, at least, the massa intermedia; hence a fairly complete disconnection of the right and left hemisphere. What I have to say in the following is based mainly on three of these patients, and mostly on two of them, in particular, whom we have singled out for language testing because of the relative lack of secondary complications like associated brain damage which we have come to believe is probably *the* big stumbling block to accurate interpretation of cortical conduction syndromes.

Since these latter two cases have relatively clean surgical disconnections without much secondary cortical damage, we have felt it worthwhile to do as thorough an analysis as possible, even though we do not have statistical numbers to deal with here. Furthermore, in view of the controversial nature of this whole area—and we have seen a few glimpses of it, I think, in this Conference—and in view of the almost intellectually paralyzing complexities and contradictoriness

of the literature in this whole field, we are very deliberately taking nothing for granted and are starting from scratch and working up the picture as we see it, in this population of two patients.

I am serving as spokesman here, for what has been very much a team project. All these patients are patients of Dr. Phillip Vogel of the California College of Medicine, who did the surgery at the White Memorial Hospital in Los Angeles to help control advanced epileptic seizures. Dr. Joseph Bogen has also collaborated extensively ever since he suggested the initial treatment. He does the medical aftercare and also most of the more standard neurological testing. Therapeutically the outcome at this date has been mixed. Three cases appear to have been definitely benefited; in the other three the results are dubious —or it is too soon to say. Dr. Michael Gazzaniga, who is present, has led the way in most of the functional testing I am going to describe, with myself collaborating in the background, and the two of us have collaborated about equally in the general approach and in writing up our joint material including that mentioned in the present discussion.

In defense of our West Coast Surgery (going back here to some remarks made yesterday) let me just insert at this point that case 3, like case 2, has made a good and rapid recovery. These two had not suffered any major brain damage prior to surgery, and this makes a difference. On the morning after surgery, case 3, a 13 year old boy, was able to recite "Peter Piper picked a peck of pickled peppers." He is a bright young fellow in many ways and also has a sharp sense of humor. That same first morning after surgery he was making quips to the doctors about having "a splitting headache." He and his family, of course, knew pretty much the pros and cons of what he was getting into.

Most of our tests relating to language have been conducted in the general testing apparatus illustrated in Figure 27. The subject is seated at a table on which is mounted a slanting shield that prevents the subject from seeing the top of the table. It prevents him from seeing the test items on the table, or his hands, or the examiner in the background. It also serves to hold a couple of ground glass viewing screens for the back projection of 2 x 2 slides set up in one or two automatic projectors in the rear. The shield also serves to hold cards and various other test items that one may want to set out in free view in front of the subject. Another examiner generally sits alongside the subject, recording his answers and his general reactions. Try now to keep this picture in mind, as I shall be referring back constantly in what follows to this general testing situation.

The subject is asked to fix his gaze on a central point on or between the screens. When the eyes are seen to be properly centered, one then flashes the visual stimuli, at a tenth of a second or less, too fast for eye movements. Two pictures may then be projected simultaneously, one to the left half field and one to the right half field, for example, a picture of a pencil on the left and of a knife on the right. This means, of course, that the

pencil image goes to the minor hemisphere and the knife image is projected to the left dominant hemisphere.

If the subject is asked what he saw, he will almost invariably and literally, in hundreds of such trials, assert that he saw the knife only and make no reference to the pencil. Similarly, in this same test setup, if one asks the subject to write below the screen his answers, instead of speaking them aloud, he again writes only the names of those stimuli that are flashed to the right half field and makes no reference to the stimuli presented in the left half field.

Or if one flashes only a single picture at a time, pictures of objects, colors, arrows pointing in different directions, lines, dots, and so on, and projects these serially and at random into right or left half field, similar results are obtained. That is, the subject describes normally in speech and writing only that material that appears in the right half field.

When a picture is flashed to the left field, the subject tells you he saw nothing, or "just a flash." He knows by this time that this

Fig. 27. Apparatus used for language testing by Sperry and associates showing subject (S) seated before shield which hides test items, his hands, and examiner (E).

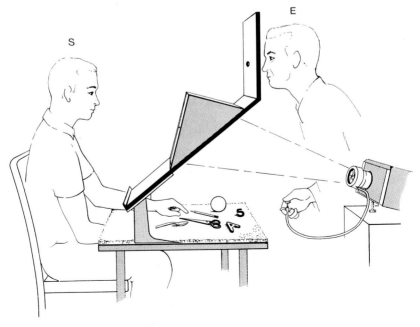

machine is rather erratic and that our series of test stimuli include blanks and plain lights to fool him.

One could draw quite a variety of different conclusions at this point from results of this kind. For the sake of brevity, let me forecast that the conclusion that seems to stand up in our testing experience is that these subjects are able to speak and write only about things seen in the right half visual field. In other words, with respect to the visual sphere of gnostic experience, verbal expression is possible only for that processed in the left hemisphere.

The same kind of result is obtained in this testing situation if, instead of using the two half visual fields, one tests the sensory surfaces of the right and left hands for stereognostic perception. The test objects themselves are now placed directly into the hand, the hand being held out of sight behind the shield. Again the patient does very well in naming and describing objects exposed to the right hand but is quite unable to describe items held in the left hand, the stereognostic centers for which are located in what we call, for convenience, the minor, that is, the right, hemisphere. These, and a large number of related tests, seem to support the conclusion that may be assumed to apply in what follows; namely that speech and writing in these patients, all of whom are right-handed, is firmly confined to the left hemisphere. Epilepsy apparently has not brought about any bilateralization of verbal expression in these cases.

The results are somewhat different within the same apparatus if, instead of having the subject tell you or write down what he sees in the projected slides, you have him reach out with one hand underneath the shield to search out blindly, by touch, an object that correctly matches the object pictured in the visual screen from among a series of ten or more test objects. Under these conditions, correct responses are obtained not only for the right half field but also for the left half field. The left field responses are correct, even though the subject denies verbally having seen anything and has to be urged and prodded to go ahead and put his hand out and give it a try. He then comes up with the right object.

In this test, however, it makes all the difference which hand is used to retrieve the matching object. The left hand can be used to gather items flashed to the left visual field and the right hand can be used to gather objects seen in the right field, but cross combinations do not work. If one tries to force the subject to use the right hand to find an object that he has seen pictured in the left half field, he is lost, and the converse is true here, provided that audible cues are eliminated. You have to be careful that the one vocal hemisphere does not start talking to the other to give the answer through auditory channels.

When the subject is thus made to use the wrong hand in this inter-modal task, the hand is moved proficiently enough, and from other tests we know that the objects it explores are perceived and recognized. However, the hemisphere that perceives in this situation does not know what it is looking for, and the hemisphere that knows what it is looking for does not get the correct feedback information. Consequently the two never match, and the performance fails.

From this and related tests we conclude that the minor hemisphere senses, perceives, learns, and remembers visual material, even though it is unable to talk or write about such experiences. The same conclusion applies for stereognostic discriminations performed with the left hand-minor hemisphere combination. And, as we will see shortly, it applies in the auditory as well as in the visual and tactual spheres. Let us say now that the subject has located correctly and is proudly holding up in his hand the correct item, say, a little flashlight bulb. He is asked casually what it is that he has selected. His reply is apt to be, in accordance with what we have said about stereognosis in the left hand, almost anything, like nail clip or cigarette lighter or what-not. Thereupon, as soon as the dumb hemisphere hears the vocal hemisphere reply with what the dumb, minor hemisphere recognizes to be an error, the subject will then usually wince and make another try. The next try at naming the object, however, will be as bad as the first one, and this kind of confusion continues. Such "confabulation" tends to be more prevalent it seems in the stereognostic sphere than in the visual. Another question arises here, as to whether some very simple, familiar, or emotionally toned words might not come out of that minor hemisphere. Simple "Yes," "No," swear words, lyrics and expletives, for example, might be possible. We have not pushed this question as yet and do not know the answer.

In this same testing situation if the subject if asked to write the names of objects flashed to left and right visual fields, using now the left hand instead of the normal writing hand, one finds that the subjects are able to write with the left hand at a rather clumsy and low level of penmanship, of course, but only for stimuli presented in the right half visual field. The same applies to left-handed writing of the names of objects placed in the left and right hands. It goes only for objects identified by the right hand.

From these findings and various tests not aimed specifically at language, it seems that the major hemisphere can govern the movement of the subordinate or homolateral hand. This is another example of what we reported earlier, the bilaterality in motor control. It follows, then, that the left-hand writing in these patients is not contradictory to the earlier conclusion that writing is organized in the major, left hemisphere only.

So now, with this general background, we can turn to some more specific questions concerning language comprehension, where verbal material, words, sentences, letters, numbers, and so on, are used as the stimuli. With free vision our two cases have no particular trouble in reading the page of a book, for example, or in reading signs provided

they can scan adequately to the left, which they seem to pick up easily.

If words, letters, phrases, and numbers are flashed separately to right and left half fields of vision, and the subject is asked to read these, there is no particular problem with respect to the right half field. In the left half field, however, the subject appears to be alexic and word blind. The same applies to the stereognostic perception of cut out, blocked letters, numbers, and so on, presented to the hands. That is, the subject can read off such stimuli correctly only when using the right hand-major hemisphere combination but not when using the left hand. But remember now that these people lack verbal expression for any kind of mental activity in the minor hemisphere. This result therefore does not prove that the minor hemisphere is not comprehending this verbal material.

The big challenge in most of our testing, of course, is to find out what goes in that silent, mute, speechless minor hemisphere, and, particularly for the purposes of the Conference, how much, if any, language comprehension may be present there.

As I have already indicated, it is possible to show, with the use of adequate testing methods, that the disconnected minor hemisphere in these two patients is, in fact, not word-blind nor is it word-deaf, nor word-dumb, in the tactile sphere, if you want to use such terminology. Actually, even when applied correctly in the accepted manner, this terminology seems highly questionable. There really is not any blindness nor any deafness involved in the standard use of the term. We could use some better words here.

Let us look closer now at the comprehension problem in the minor hemisphere. The subject is asked to reach out blindly with his hand to search out an object that has been vocally named aloud by the experimenter, say, a rectangle, after a rectangular block has been placed out of sight behind the shield along with a series of other geometric shapes or other objects. There is no problem for the right hand in this, of course, but we find that the left hand also can perform correctly. The subject reaches out; he explores carefully among the test items, rejecting and bypassing maybe up to nine of them if necessary, until the hand finally contacts, explores, and holds up the correct item. Since other evidence tells us that stereognosis in the left hand is processed in the minor hemisphere only, it may be inferred that the minor hemisphere must, therefore, in this performance have perceived and comprehended the verbal instructions of the experimenter.

With this technic words like the following appear to be understood in the minor hemisphere: pyramid, cylinder, tack, coin, pliers, flashlight bulb, screwdriver, fork, cup, and so on, plus more complex phrases like "measuring instrument" for ruler or "eating utensil" for spoon. It also responds correctly to not so simple definitions like "used to drive nails" for hammer, or "kept in the bank" for coin, and so on. The minor hemisphere has at least a moderate vocabulary.

Since the spoken stimuli here are surely recognized also in the major vocal hemisphere, one always wonders if there is any way in which the minor hemisphere may be getting assistance from the other side, like feedback from subliminal speech or something of the type. We became somewhat worried about this the last time case 2 was in for tests of this kind. She had been retrieving objects correctly with the left hand to vocal descriptions like "writing instrument" for pen, "unlocks doors" for key, and so on for some seven correct out of seven trials. But when she directly sought out a quarter by touch from among some 15 other objects upon hearing "inserted in slot machines," this seemed to both Dr. Gazzaniga and me to be well beyond the expected capacity of the minor hemisphere—as if there must be something radically wrong either with our testing methods or our whole working hypothesis.

Upon indicating our surprise that words like "inserted" and "slot machine" should be so easy, the subject came back quickly, "What? Las Vegas! Where all our money goes!" (It seemed obvious that enough experience with slot machines had occurred even after surgery that we need not seek new hypotheses on this count.)

In any event, we find that this comprehension of the spoken and written word by the minor hemisphere proceeds under conditions in which only the minor hemisphere has the answer, unlike the foregoing case with auditory input. For example, if we flashed to the left half visual field-minor hemisphere combination a short word in print like spoon, cup, match, pin, comb, and so on, we find the subject is then able to reach out and identify the corresponding object, using the left hand, whereas he or she is not able to repeat that performance when made to use the right hand or to do the same task in separate trials with the right hand. This latter shows, you see, that the major hemisphere could not have read this material; it does not know the answer.

Furthermore, if the subject is asked, immediately following a correct response with the left hand, what the object is that he has chosen and is holding, he is quite unable, with the dominant hemisphere, to tell you what it is. In other words, the dominant hemisphere in such instances has no idea what the minor hemisphere has been doing in the performance of these tasks. We see this so consistently—that is, the complete agnosia in one hemisphere for the mental activities that have just taken place in the other—that we regularly rely on this in our testing procedures to check on cheating. For example, in presenting visual material, if the subject can tell you about something that was presented in the left half field, as may happen on rare occasions, you immediately suspect eye movements and discount that particular trial.

In another type of test a list of ten or more printed names of objects is laid out in free view in front of the subject for reading. Then pictures of these same objects are flashed one at a time into the left half visual field, that is, to the minor hemisphere. The subjects are then able to point out the correct name on the list for an object that was seen only by the minor hemisphere. This is also true for tests in which an object is placed in the subject's left hand with vision excluded. In tests of this kind the moment the finger comes up and points to a chosen name, the vocal hemisphere immediately reads it off, as if it also had known the answer all the time. But if you ask the subject to give you the correct answer before he has pointed, and before even his eyes have had a chance to fixate on the correct name, you then find that the major hemisphere is lost. Since the major hemisphere does not know the answer here, we deduce that the minor hemisphere is reading and comprehending the printed list of names. From such performances, we conclude, then, that the subjects are able to read and comprehend the printed list of words with both hemispheres, the minor as well as the major.

The minor hemisphere can also spell on a very low level, simple words like hat, how, dog, and what, when large, cut-out letters three to four inches high are presented in scrambled order, out of sight, to the left hand. It is not the major hemisphere that is doing the spelling here, because it vocalizes a running commentary on the progress of the left hand, like "This is A" when it really is "T," and so on. This vocal commentary is entirely off on the progress of the left hand, except for accidental coincidences. This in itself is of some interest here, namely, that the minor hemisphere can concentrate and carry on tasks of its own, ignoring the erroneous and distracting chatter of its better half. Other tests show that calculation is restricted almost entirely to the major hemisphere—and so it goes.

In general, as you can see, we have been concerned here mainly with the grosser features of interhemispheric integration. We have not applied as yet the more refined types

of tests that might detect more subtle differences between the hemispheres, of the kind that Dr. Milner, Dr. Hécaen, and others have used.

In closing, I would like to emphasize just one further point. I understand there have been objections to speculations that we have made in years past regarding the coexistence of two rather separate mental entities operating simultaneously in parallel in the two disconnected hemispheres.[366,367,369] Eccles,[96] I understand, now favors the view—which goes back to a comment made by MacKay[269]—that consciousness in these cases remains single and is centered mainly in the major, the dominant hemisphere. The subordinate hemisphere is conceived to carry on in a kind of an automaton state.

Recall in this connection some of the points that I have mentioned here regarding the capacity of the minor hemisphere; it carries on inter-modal associations between visual, tactile, and auditory spheres and can even go from words, visually or audibly presented, to objects, and vice versa. It makes generalizations and certain mental associations that look like ideation. In the testing of mental associations, for example, it will go from "shoe" to "sock," from "cigarette" to "ashtray," from "hand" to "ring," from "dollar bills" to "metal coins," picking out these related items in each case from an array of others not related.

Furthermore, the minor hemisphere is superior to the major hemisphere in some performances like visual constructional tasks.[123] The minor hemisphere also shows emotional reactions in response to pinup shots.[122] For example, one flashes a series of pairs of pictures to right left visual fields and the subject reads off the names, but only, of course, for those that appear in the right half field. Into this series of paired presentations of triangles, umbrellas, horses, houses, cigars, and other neutral stimuli one then flashes a vivid pinup shot of a nude that projects into the minor hemisphere only. At the same time a tree or horse or some such appears on the right side. The subject says, of course, that she saw a horse—with no hesitation. But then you notice that a kind of sneaky grin has begun to spread over the subject's features, and even the tone of voice changes. This emotional effect then carries on through the next several trials. If you ask her what she is grinning at, she does not know, and says, "Oh, that light!" In this situation recall that the major hemisphere meantime is going along in parallel and is calling the correct names of these objects in the right half field.

To continue with the automaton interpretation, recall that the minor hemisphere learns and remembers, that it holds an immediate memory even when long delays are imposed in these retrieval tests that I have been talking about. A distracting conversation is deliberately interjected and the subject is allowed to get up and go down the hall and come back again. After this he sits down and again makes the correct response with the minor hemisphere.

The minor hemisphere carries out reaction times as fast as the major hemisphere where a visual discrimination of color is involved, and the other hemisphere is working in parallel just as fast as it can.[126] The minor hemisphere also triggers facial expressions, grimacing, and wincing when an error is made by the vocal hemisphere and where the correct answer is known only to the minor hemisphere. The minor hemisphere seems definitely bothered in the situation. One wonders if a mere automaton would be so annoyed by an error in this kind of testing situation. If all the foregoing represents the behavior of an automaton, one wonders if it will not be difficult indeed to show that the separated dominant hemisphere or even the undivided brain is more than an automaton.

DR. BENTON: Before you leave the podium, tell us about the patients. Where were their lesions? Are these epileptics?

DR. SPERRY: Yes, these are all advanced epileptics.

DR. BENTON: I wanted to know if there are foci in the left hemisphere.

DR. SPERRY: In that early first case there was major brain damage, prior to surgery, and seen at operation, in the minor hemisphere in addition to an apparent focus in the parieto-temporal area of the left hemisphere. We tried to warn our readers—I think Dr. Myers and apparently Dr. Geschwind probably did not see our warning sentence—to the effect that many of the symptoms described were presumably exaggerated by the presence of this brain damage. We probably should have italicized that. In case 2 the x-ray showed a small calcification beneath the right central cortex about a centimeter or so in diameter associated with a little hypesthesia in the left hand. The other patient I've been talking about, case 3, had no visible damage prior to surgery. The others have complications that make them less suitable for studying language.

DR. ETTLINGER: Are these patients more or less normal?

DR. SPERRY: Under ordinary conditions, yes.

DR. LENNEBERG: How did you make sure of the visual input?

DR. SPERRY: The image projected to the right side of a visual fixation point is projected to the left hemisphere and vice versa. This division, incidentally, runs very nicely down the midline with little or no central overlap or central sparing.

DR. LILLY: How did you maintain fixation?

DR. SPERRY: By eyeballing the eye. The subject is told to fixate and the examiner looking directly into the subject's eyes, watches his gaze, and clicks in the slide when the gaze is properly centered. Occasionally one sees eye movements, and, as mentioned, these can often be checked out.

DR. ROSENBLITH: Dr. Sperry, you said something about calculation being confined to the right hemisphere. Have you tried to do psychophysical scaling independently on both sides?

DR. SPERRY: All of this is pretty gross. Calculation tests for the minor hemisphere were run with one to four dots for visual input and one to four pegs for tactual input; the subject was asked to add or multiply using this input.

CHAIRMAN MILLIKAN: Dr. Grey Walter, will you continue please?

DR. GREY WALTER: Like Dr. Sperry, I would like to present some data from observations in human beings following surgical implantation of multiple chronic electrodes. I would like to skip the clinical aspects. These data relate to the general question of inter-hemispheric interaction and were derived from very tedious computations of responses to electrical and sensory stimuli by a colleague from Budapest, Imre Tomka, on a World Health Organization Fellowship. We have studied some thousands of electrode implants in the brains of organically normal patients and developed a kind of hypothesis. We have used electrical stimuli to the cortex, in all parts of the brain, covering a wide area in the frontal and anterior temporal lobes.

Figure 28 shows the general summary of results. The central diagram indicates the position of the electrodes. We have studied the electrical responses from all the electrodes, with a view to developing an idea of the connectivity of the human cerebral cortex. In simple terms, we are asking a topological question; we want to know how you get from here to there in the brain. Occasionally we get the answer of the peasant who when asked this, said, "If you want to get there, you shouldn't start from here."

In general, we do find considerable reciprocal connectivity in the cortex. For example, the record in the bottom left hand corner shows stimulation of electrode 30 in the left temporal tip, and responses at electrode 6, which is in the orbital frontal cortex on the

Fig. 28. General summary of results of study of the connectivity of the human cerebral cortex.

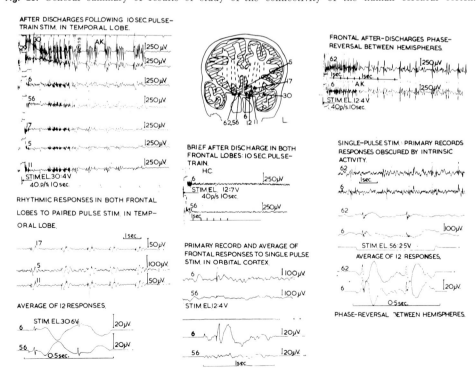

same side, and also at 56, which is in the homologous region in the other hemisphere. Similarly, in the bottom right hand corner stimulation of electrode 56, which is on the right side, produces responses at electrode 62 nearby and also across to 6 on the other side. We have made a very large number of such observations, with surprisingly consistent results. The first is that there is an enormously elaborate reciprocal connection between orbital cortex and anterior temporal lobe, and second, perhaps the most important, invariably in all these thousands and thousands of stimulations there is this peculiar inverse phase relation between the left and right hemisphere. With all the electrodes, the potentials are referred to the average of all the others, so this is not a question of one electrode being affected by inverted potentials.

What we think may be happening is that activity started out in the cortex by our electrical stimulation invades the adjacent cortex quite slowly. If one measures the latency of the responses in the opposite hemisphere, the response is not merely upside down but often starts slightly *before* the activity in the cortex near the stimulation point on the ipsilateral side, as though the activity had spread rapidly through a commissure, presumably the corpus callosum, and invaded the opposite hemisphere from the inside as it were through the white matter instead of spreading slowly through cortex as in the ipsilateral hemisphere.

Figure 29 is a diagram of these connections in one patient. This illustrates the pattern of connectivity in the temporal and orbital frontal cortex with lines running also from one hemisphere to the other, but not always to homologous regions and not always with reciprocal relations either.

Bearing in mind the consistency of these patterns and the peculiar time- and phase-relations between hemispheres, I would like to suggest that the hemispheres may act as a double storage-buffer in which information can be tossed from one side to the other and

Fig. 29. Diagrams of connections in temporal and orbital frontal cortex in one patient.

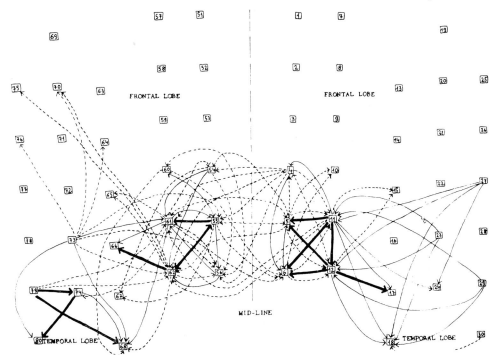

read out or registered in the process, possibly with destructive write-out. Thus, for any particular set of experiences one hemisphere would be accumulating the information for a while and would then transfer the relevant sections to the other hemisphere, clearing its register at the same time. This sort of procedure is used in some computers and can be an economical way of selecting and storing information in a system of limited capacity.

I wonder if some of Dr. Sperry's brilliant and provocative observations might be explained in terms such as this.

DR. EFRON: I do not know whether this is a question to Dr. Sperry or a statement describing my own confusion. It seems to me, unless I have misunderstood Dr. Sperry rather profoundly, that his point is very strongly confirmed by the fact that he is instructing his patient to use his left hand. Let's say the patient comes into the box on a given day; Dr. Sperry speaks to him; he has to communicate with the patient. He tells the patient to reach out with his left hand and do something. Since these patients have a callosal section their ability to follow this verbal command at the onset of the testing session must indicate that "the right brain must have understood the set of instructions." It would seem to me that the rather complex tasks Dr. Sperry has described merely confirm what could have been proved the moment the patient did the first task correctly. Have I misunderstood Dr. Sperry in this respect?

DR. SPERRY: There is the matter of ipsilateral control on which we may have different views and also various other factors in the testing situation that would make conclusions on this basis a bit shaky.

DR. LILLY: I have a question and a comment to Dr. Sperry. In any of your cases was there any evidence whatsoever that the non-dominant hemisphere had had access to language and speech? Now I am talking about all of proto-speech, all of noise-making, and the elements of speech that we have discussed

here, as well as concept formation, cognition, and so forth.

DR. SPERRY: We cannot be certain at this time that the minor hemisphere cannot utter some simple, familiar, or emotional material.

DR. LILLY: I just wanted to get that straight. Then I just want to report that recently we have found the dolphin can use two separate phonation mechanisms, one on the right, which is innervated completely from the left hemisphere, and one on the left, which is completely innervated from the right hemisphere, quite independently, and at least make noises of very high complexity equally with each side.

They can also, as we have recently discovered, link the sounds from the two sides so that one gets an apparent source which shifts from the right to the left and back again. This is most dramatically shown by stereophonic listening to a dolphin in air with two pick-ups, one on the right phonation side and one on the left. If one now listens with stereophones, one can hear sounds alone on the right, alone on the left, or an apparent source moving through one's head from right to left and back again.

I think that this suggests an experiment— and I hope some day Dr. Sperry will come and do it—of splitting the brain of the dolphin and seeing if one can disconnect, as it were, the stereovocalization and see if the two independent vocalizations still exist.

DR. EVARTS: I just wanted to pick up a point that Dr. Sperry mentioned, the point that the dominant hemisphere does, in fact, have some access to both sides of the body in terms of control of the hand. Didn't you say that, Roger? In terms of Dr. Efron's questions, one has to keep this in mind. I believe that Dr. Efron proposed that if a subject reaches out with his left hand in response to a verbal command, this means that the right hemisphere must have had access to the verbal information. One can propose, however, that for certain types of acts the left hemisphere can in fact control either hand.

DR. GAZZANIGA: Dr. Evarts is quite right

and from some related studies of ours it is clear that each disconnected hemisphere can control with almost equal ability both the ipsilateral and the contralateral hands if one excludes from consideration the individual control of the fingers ipsilateral to the hemisphere in command. In addition, it is of interest to note that results from some animal studies show that split-brain monkeys demonstrate marked ipsilateral eye-hand impairments when, in addition to the pure midline surgery, unilateral lesions are made in motor and premotor areas.[128] That is to say, ipsilateral visuomotor control is dependent on the integrity of the motor cortex contralateral to the responding hand. This type of evidence goes a long way to explain the difference between our first case—as well as the Liepmann-Geshwind type—versus our latter two cases. It also hints at the underlying mechanisms of ipsilateral control. That is, these studies argue against the view that ipsilateral control is managed by only motor systems originating in the ipsilateral hemisphere. Rather they suggest that much of the ipsilateral control could take place in the opposite visually deprived hemisphere, which is possible because of a cross-over of target information originally established and determined by the ipsilateral hemisphere.

CHAIRMAN MILLIKAN: Dr. Sperry, do you wish to comment on that suggestion?

DR. SPERRY: Thank you, not now. I only hope we've not encroached on Dr. Milner's time as a result of this.

DR. ETTLINGER: I would like to ask a brief question. Do I correctly understand from your presentation, Dr. Sperry, that your data suggest the following types of organization for the minor hemisphere, namely, that the minor hemisphere cannot evoke names or language (which is what you had also previously reported for your other patients, and I understand that you have confirmed this) but the minor hemisphere can be used in the recognition or reception of language? The nominal aphasic patient cannot find the name but, given the name, he can recognize it from

a selection. Also severe comprehension defects are more rare than severe disorders of expressive speech. I wonder whether you feel this information is correct or whether your observations imply that transfer can occur after callosal section in one direction between the hemispheres but not in the other.

DR. SPERRY: Yes, it would seem to be the executive and more motor or expressive aspects that are mainly lateralized. Other evidence shows this going in the reverse direction in visual constructional tasks in which the right hemisphere is more proficient.

DR. EFRON: To follow-up the same question: I think I am still confused. If you instruct the patient verbally, "Move your left hand upward if a coin is present; move your hand sideways if a dollar bill is present" what will such a patient do?

DR. SPERRY: There is no problem. He could do that from the one hemisphere, that is, comprehend the instructions, feel around, locate the coin, and respond accordingly. Presumably he does this all from the minor hemisphere. What was the rest of it?

DR. EFRON: That will do.

DR. MURRAY A. FALCONER: Dr. Evarts raised the question of bilaterality of representation in the hemispheres. In these cases that you were just talking about where the patient with split commissure can reach out with the left hand: that action must involve the right hemisphere and not just the left, because in patients after a right hemispherectomy, the only movements possible in the left arm are feeble movements of the shoulder and the elbow, while the finer movements of the hand go. Therefore if a patient, after the commissure is split, can reach out in purposeful directions, the action must be coming from the right hemisphere.

DR. SPERRY: We have shown in experimental work in monkeys and the same thing in the human that for efficient ipsilateral control, one hemisphere working the ipsilateral hand, you need the integrity of the contralateral motor cortex. In our first case we can probably explain poor ipsilateral control by the fact that he has quite severe extracallosal brain damage. In this regard, we notice there is no dysarthria in these patients. Where you do get dysarthria is with right hemispheric lesions. In order to control the speech mechanism, leave intact the right motor hemisphere.

DR. HIRSH: May I put a question about very fundamental neuroanatomy. We know about the confusing bilateral representation of the auditory inputs in the two cortices, but about the fine motor control of the speech mechanism, for example, the tongue and the laryngeal musculature: are the two sides of this speech mechanism represented separately in the same way that the two hands are represented separately on the two sides?

DR. GESCHWIND: There is some interesting evidence to show that there are separate pathways descending in both the left and right internal capsule for bilateral innervation of the speech musculature. The left is normally used but the right can substitute.

The evidence for this comes from the description by Bonhoeffer[38] of one of the early cases of callosal disconnection. On clinical criteria Bonhoeffer had predicted during the life of the patient the presence of a callosal lesion. In addition he had expected a Broca's area lesion because of the patient's aphasia. At postmortem the expected callosal lesion was found but Broca's area was intact. There was, however, an infarct involving the left internal capsule. Bonhoeffer interpreted this very astutely. He pointed out that lesions of the left internal capsule do not produce aphasia. The reason is that if this left-sided pathway is destroyed, you can still use the alternative pathway from Broca's area via the corpus callosum to the corresponding region in the right frontal lobe and eventually down the right internal capsule. In Bonhoeffer's patient the callosal lesion cut off this alternative route. This type of lesion is probably quite common but not in this neat form. Thus many subcortical lesions which are beneath Broca's area produce aphasia by the same mechanism. Although Broca's area is

intact, the lesion simultaneously destroys descending fibers and callosal fibers and has the same effect as the two lesions in Bonhoeffer's case.

The same type of mechanism probably holds for other bilateral movements such as walking for which there is evidence that it can be triggered from either hemisphere alone.

DR. HIRSH: I put the question wondering whether some of the gentlemen who have patients of the kind described this morning ever observed anything like or anything analogous to the one-sided clumsiness Dr. Falconer just referred to, either with a canted tongue or one-sided phonation. Is the innervation so separate that this kind of articulation can be observed?

CHAIRMAN MILLIKAN: Can you respond to that question?

DR. SPERRY: Not in the cases that have the opposite hemisphere intact. Very briefly after the surgery there is a short period of recovery.

DR. EVARTS: I just wanted to follow this up. Dr. Sperry has said that one does not see this effect in cases where the opposite hemisphere is intact. Dr. Falconer pointed out that for a movement to take place, it is essential that the opposite hemisphere be intact. However, granting that the integrity of the contralateral hemisphere is essential to the operation of the extremity, it remains a possibility that information concerning guidance of movement could arise in the ipsilateral hemisphere. In the work I have done on hand movements in the monkey, the monkeys were trained to use either hand. The units I showed you yesterday were active in relation to the contralateral hand. However, when one records from PTNs in association with ipsilateral hand movements, one sees that there are certain neurons, small in number perhaps but definitely there, which are locked onto and related to the ipsilateral hand movements only. Thus, given the integrity of the contralateral hemisphere, the ipsilateral hemisphere may send down information which for certain sorts of movements, perhaps the elementary, is sufficient. The fact that the ipsilateral is able to provide information for certain kinds of movement, given the integrity of the contralateral, may explain some of these observations.

DR. HÉCAEN: This is just a very brief question about the recognition of a familiar human face, as in a picture, by the minor and the major hemisphere.

DR. SPERRY: This is one of the more subtle tests we have not gotten to. We are going to hear about it later on.

DR. LENNEBERG: Just a brief comment on the question of dysarthria. It seems to me that dysarthria is not a prominent feature of high lesions. In the patients that Dr. Penfield described, dysarthria is certainly not even a transient symptom according to the clinical descriptions. In the hemispherectomy cases reported in the literature, again, dysarthria does not seem to be figuring—correct me, if I am wrong—in the clinical picture. On the other hand, dysarthria is very prominent and dramatic in diencephalic lesions, surgical interference, and stimulation and also in mesencephalic lesions and stimulation experiments. I think all this indicates that motor integration is a very low phenomenon, and the role the cortex plays in just the motor output is something we do not really understand completely. It does not seem to be a matter of immediate integration of individual muscles. It seems to be something much more general. Possibly speech may be slowed down somewhat in the case of high lesions, but I do not think you really see dysarthria, strictly speaking. It is very much different from the dysarthrias of lower lesions.

CHAIRMAN MILLIKAN: Dr. Geschwind, a final comment.

DR. GESCHWIND: I was fascinated by the studies presented by Dr. Sperry. He says that these cases are much closer to the Akelaitis pole than to the Liepmann pole. I would like to suggest that in fact he has not moved very far from the Liepmann pole. As Dr. Ettlinger pointed out, he has in fact practically refuted Akelaitis on all major points. What is important is the evidence that in some callosal cases the minor hemisphere can perform to some extent, particularly in comprehension tasks.

The problem of variations among patients is one that has always concerned students of the higher functions. Thus Liepmann and Maas's[233] original case of callosal disconnection showed poor object handling in the left hand, yet the second case[252] handled objects well in the left hand. I cannot go into all the possible reasons for this. I would, however, suspect that many of these variations are not due to differences in the lesions but rather to pre-existing differences in the brains. There is evidence from other sources that the capacities of the minor hemisphere vary from patient to patient, particularly in its ability to comprehend language.

It is encouraging that individual difference need not be regarded as purely an *ad hoc* hypothesis since there is some evidence from animal experiments that shows such variation. I was fortunate to hear Dr. Myers present some elegant experiments which are relevant. Among a group of monkeys with the same lesion (cutting of the splenium) some were less impaired than the majority were but then showed impairment when an anterior commissure section was added to the splenium section. Hence the extent to which anterior commissure can support interhemispheric transfer of visual learning varies from animal to animal. I hope we will, similarly, be able to devise better techniques to study such variation in man.

CHAIRMAN MILLIKAN: We will continue with "Brain Mechanisms Suggested by Studies of Temporal Lobes." Dr. Milner.

Brain Mechanisms Suggested by Studies of Temporal Lobes

BRENDA MILNER

Montreal Neurological Institute
McGill University
Montreal, Canada

THE AIM OF THIS REPORT will be to review for you as succinctly as possible the results of 15 years' study of temporal-lobe function in man. Since this symposium centers on problems of language, I shall give the bulk of my attention to the effects of lesions of the left temporal lobe (that is, of the temporal lobe in the dominant hemisphere for speech), rather than of the right. Yet, this emphasis on the left hemisphere poses problems, as we have accumulated considerable evidence of the important role of the right, or minor, hemisphere in many nonverbal skills; and only recently Dr. Sperry was suggesting that the right hemisphere had been unduly neglected. I shall resolve the dilemma by contrasting the effects of right and left temporal lobectomy, beginning with a brief account of the many tasks—visual, auditory, and even somesthetic—on which deficits appear after right temporal lobectomy but not after left. Then I shall go on to describe in more detail the specific contributions of the left temporal lobe to verbal processes, comparing the effects of left temporal-lobe lesions not only with those of right, but also with the effects of similarly elective lesions of the left frontal and left parietal cortex.

By way of introduction, I should point out that the patients studied were all undergoing unilateral brain operations for the relief of focal cerebral seizures dating from early life.

This work was supported by the Medical Research Council of Canada and by U. S. Public Health Grants NB 02831 and M5774 to the author.

Except for one case of brain tumor (discussed separately), all had atrophic lesions. They were a young group, with an average age of 26 years (ranging from 14 to 54 years) and were neither mentally retarded nor suffering from obvious personality disorders.

For data analysis the patients were subdivided into different groups according to the laterality and locus of cortical excision. We shall be concerned primarily with the right and left temporal, left frontal, and left parietal-lobe groups, the left hemisphere being dominant for speech in all cases.

Some representative unilateral temporal lobectomies, left and right, are shown in Figure 30. The total area ablated varied from patient to patient, but, contrary to what is often supposed, the excisions on the right were not significantly larger than those on the left. In both groups some removals extended back far enough to include the transverse gyri of Heschl in the depths of the Sylvian fissure; others were more limited in lateral extent. On the mesial surface the removals always included the amygdala but varied in the degree to which they encroached upon the hippocampus.

The brain maps in Figure 31 illustrate other representative removals in the dominant hemisphere. The left frontal lobectomy (case H.M.) spares Broca's area on the lateral surface but is otherwise quite radical; it extends to include parts of the cingulate and subcallosal gyri on the mesial surface of the hemisphere. In the left parietal lobe the excisions were more variable in locus and extent; two examples of these relatively small removals are shown here.

The left-hemisphere removals described above do not cause any lasting dysphasia, since care is taken not to invade the primary speech areas, which are mapped out at the time of operation. Figure 32 shows a composite diagram of the areas of the left cerebral cortex within which electrical stimulation has elicited dysphasic responses from conscious patients. It is evident that the temporal lobectomies of Figure 30 lie anterior to the temporal speech zone and, similarly, that the removals in Figure 31 spare the frontal and parietal speech zones.

Comparison of Effects of Left and Right Temporal-Lobe Lesions. The left temporal lobe appears to be remarkably specialized in its essential functions, and on a variety of nonverbal tasks the performance of patients after left temporal lobectomy has been found to be indistinguishable from that of normal control subjects. Right temporal-lobe lesions, on the other hand, are associated with low scores on a number of perceptual and memory tasks, the nature of which will be briefly described.

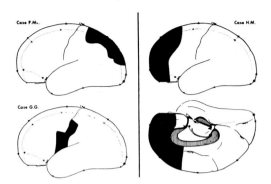

Fig. 31. Cases P. Mo., and G. G.: partial left parietal lobectomy, lateral view; case H. M.: left frontal lobectomy (lateral view above, mesial view below).

In vision, we find a consistent impairment in the perception of irregular patterned stimuli, particularly those to which a verbal label cannot readily be attached. The defect is a subtle one, only evident when the normal perceptual cues are reduced. This goal may be achieved by brief exposure, as in a tachistoscope,[201] or by eliminating some of the contour lines. Thus, patients with right temporal-

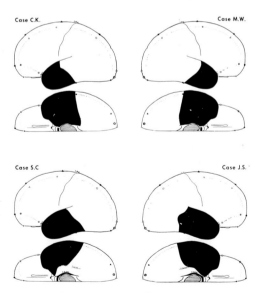

Fig. 30. Representative unilateral temporal lobectomies, lateral and inferior views; above, hippocampus removed; below, hippocampus spared.

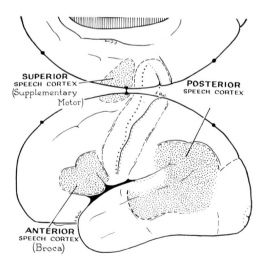

Fig. 32. Brain chart showing areas in the left cerebral cortex from which electrical stimulation has produced dysphasic responses at operation. (Adapted from Penfield and Roberts,[309] p. 201.) Reprinted by permission of Princeton University Press. Copyright 1959, by Princeton University Press.

lobe lesions are confused by sketchy cartoon-like drawings,[279] cannot easily organize patches of black and white into a distinct human face,[219] and are impaired in the discrimination of fragmented concentric circular patterns.[272]

On visual memory tasks the defect after right temporal lobectomy is more pronounced and can readily be demonstrated by the use of visual memoranda which cannot accurately be described in words. Thus, patients with right temporal lobectomies have difficulty in recognizing snapshots of human faces which they can easily discriminate and which they have had ample time to inspect less than two minutes prior to testing. They make abnormally many mistakes when asked to pick these faces out from a larger array and are apt to complain that the task is too difficult, because, for example, all the girls have long hair and necklaces, and therefore the individual faces cannot be remembered by such verbal simplifications.

Much evidence has now been compiled for a defect in remembering unfamiliar nonsense patterns after right temporal lobectomy. This impairment may best be illustrated by describing one task especially sensitive to right temporal-lobe damage, the Recurring Nonsense Figures test devised by Doreen Kimura. Figure 33 shows a difficult item from this test.

The test material consists of a series of 160 cards, on each of which an unfamiliar design is drawn;[201] this may be geometric, or, as in Figure 33, completely irregular. Eight designs recur within each 20 cards, intermixed randomly with designs that appear only once. The cards are shown one at a time to the subject, who has to say "Yes" if he thinks that the design has appeared before and "No" if he thinks that he is seeing it for the first time. The task is a rather difficult one initially, but normal subjects rapidly learn to identify the recurring figures and to disregard the others.

Figure 34 shows the postoperative mean error scores for the various patient groups and for normal control subjects, the error score being the sum of the false positive and false negative responses. Analysis of variance yielded highly significant intergroup differences ($F = 15.3$, $p < .001$), the right temporal-lobe group being impaired relative to

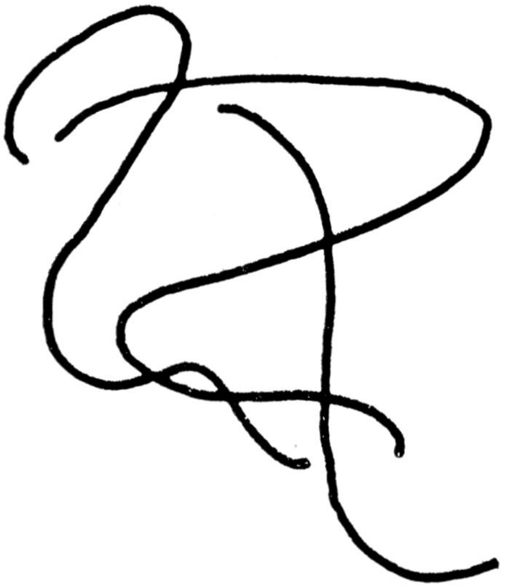

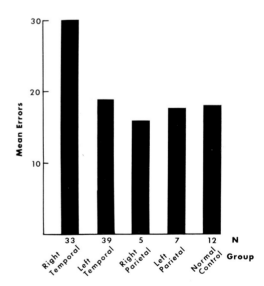

Fig. 34. Recurring Nonsense Figures test: mean error scores for different lesion groups, showing significant impairment after right temporal lobectomy.

Fig. 33. Example from Recurring Nonsense Figures test (Kimura [201]).

each of the other groups, who did not, however, differ from one another. On this, as on the other nonverbal tasks sampled, the left temporal-lobe group performed normally; so also did the small group of patients with right parietal-lobe lesions. Thus, there is evidence of a selective impairment in visual pattern recognition after right temporal lobectomy in man, a defect which may be considered analogous to the visual-discrimination loss produced by bilateral excision of the inferior temporal cortex in lower primates.[69,287]

Turning now to audition, we again find defects on nonverbal tasks after right, but not after left temporal lobectomy. Simple pitch discrimination is unaffected by the lesion, but there is an impairment in the discrimination of tonal patterns and of tone quality or timbre.[278] These results are illustrated in Figure 35, which shows the increase in mean error score after right temporal lobectomy on two of the Seashore Measures of Musical Talents.[341] On the Tonal Memory test a short sequence of notes is played twice in rapid succession, and the subject has to decide which note changed in pitch at the second playing. Here again the disability shown by patients with right temporal-lobe lesions seems to resemble the tonal pattern discrim-

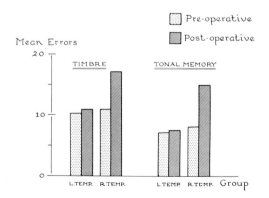

Fig. 35. Seashore Timbre and Tonal Memory tests: mean error scores before and after operation for left (L) and right (R) temporal-lobe groups, showing postoperative impairment after right temporal lobectomy but not after left (Milner[278]).

ination loss produced by bilateral temporal-lobe lesions in cat and monkey.[296]

The auditory-discrimination deficits produced by right temporal lobectomy appear to be permanent, since they are still detectable several years after operation. Moreover, they are not contingent upon removal of the transverse gyri of Heschl, the main auditory projection area. By now we have assembled a large enough group of cases to permit us to compare the effects of lesions sparing and of lesions destroying Heschl's gyri. Dr. Chase will be interested to know that the defects after right temporal lobectomy are significantly greater when the projection area is spared than when it is removed. There is no defect after left temporal lobectomy, in either subgroup.

In addition to the selective disturbance of pattern discrimination, visual and auditory, which we have been considering, there is evidence of an impairment in stylus-maze learning after right temporal lobectomy, but not after left. This is true both for visually-guided maze learning[282] and for maze learning with vision excluded and responses guided mainly by proprioception.[75] On these maze tasks the behavior of patients with right temporal-lobe lesions does not suggest spatial disorientation but, rather, difficulty in retaining the correct sequence of turns from one trial to the next. Unlike the defects of pattern recognition, the maze-learning impairment after right temporal lobectomy requires that the removal include radical destruction of the hippocampus. After left temporal lobectomy, maze learning is entirely normal, even if the hippocampus is excised and even if the patient is dysphasic at the time of testing.

What, then, are the defects associated with left temporal-lobe lesions? Quite consistently patients with such lesions show impairment on verbal memory tasks, regardless of how retention is being tested, whether by recognition, free recall, or rate of associative learning. In cases of longstanding epileptogenic lesions of the left temporal lobe, the memory defect is demonstrable preoperatively and increases markedly after removal of the temporal lobe. A residual postoperative loss is evident on follow-up examination, from one to ten years later, although there is no dysphasia at that time and little if any disability on other kinds of verbal task. It is true that under special conditions of testing, as with the dichotic listening technic of Broadbent,[54] in which different digits are presented simultaneously to the two ears by means of stereophonic earphones, patients with left temporal-lobe lesions show a mild impairment.[202] Any verbal perceptual difficulty is, however, relatively trivial; individual words clearly enunciated are easily understood and written sentences easily read. There is, on the other hand, a difficulty in learning verbal material in excess of the immediate memory span that is quite disproportionate to any verbal discrimination defect.

We showed this verbal memory difficulty first by the oral presentation of short prose passages, which the subject was required to retell immediately afterwards. These stories were too long for perfect one-trial repetition by normal subjects, and some patients with epileptogenic lesions of the left temporal lobe found this initial recall quite difficult. Their impairment became unequivocal, however, when they were tested for delayed recall, without forewarning, one hour later, the interval having been filled with other testing.[279] A similar defect in verbal associative learning was later demonstrated, and we then combined the delayed recall scores for these two tests (the mean number of items correctly recalled from the two prose passages plus the number of correct word associations) to yield one "delayed verbal recall" score. When patients with epileptogenic lesions in different cortical areas were compared with respect to this composite measure of verbal memory, only the group with left temporal-lobe lesions was found to be impaired. Similar results were obtained after operation, on long-term postoperative follow-up testing, and at that time there was also an impairment in the immediate recall of the two stories.[278]

These findings resemble those obtained by Meyer and Yates[273] with Mr. Falconer's temporal-lobe patients. Meyer and Yates had, however, emphasized the auditory character of the tests on which patients were impaired after left temporal lobectomy, whereas we had always assumed that the critical feature was the verbal nature of the test material, rather than the sensory channel. Our next task was, therefore, to show that the verbal learning defect was not specific to the auditory mode. This was done in two ways.

Preliminary evidence came from a visual-verbal task modelled on Kimura's Recurring Nonsense Figures test. By this continuous recognition method, patients with left temporal-lobe excisions were found to be impaired in learning to recognize words, nonsense syllables, and three-digit numbers, although the same patients obtained normal scores on the more difficult task of recognizing nonsense drawings. After right temporal lobectomy there was no deficit on the verbal recognition task, but the expected impairment with nonsense figures.[285]

Data more directly comparable to the auditory verbal-learning scores have since been obtained by the more straightforward method of having the patient read two eight-line stories, writing down after each one all he could remember of it. Only two lines were visible at a time, and the paper advanced by one line every five seconds, thus providing ample reading time. A paired-associates task modelled on the auditory one was also devised, ten pairs of words being exposed successively, one pair every two seconds. Retention was tested by following each learning trial with a test trial in which the first word of a pair was presented and the subject was allowed five seconds in which to write down the other member of the pair. Three learning trials were given and the responses were scored in the same way as for the auditory test. Delayed recall was obtained by requiring the subject to write the stories out again after 40 minutes of other testing, and also to complete the ten word-pairs. The subjects

TABLE 10.

Group	N	Auditory		Visual	
		Pre	Post	Pre	Post
Left temporal	21	11.2	6.6	13.2	9.6
Right temporal	23	14.8	15.7	17.1	17.2

Delayed verbal recall: preoperative and early postoperative mean scores.

were not permitted to repeat any of the visually presented material aloud, although they may well have carried out some silent rehearsal during the original reading.

Table 10 shows the preoperative and early postoperative delayed-recall scores for both aurally and visually presented verbal material, obtained from a group of 44 patients undergoing unilateral temporal lobectomy for epilepsy. The auditory scores replicate exactly our earlier findings, confirming the defect in the left temporal group. As we had predicted, the visual recall scores parallel the auditory ones very closely. The left temporal group obtained significantly lower scores than the right preoperatively (t = 3.42, p < .01), and after operation there was the expected sharp drop, corresponding to the stage of postoperative dysphasia. The scores of the right temporal group were normal throughout.

Residual Defect after Left Temporal Lobectomy: Comparison with Other Brain Lesions. The evidence for a residual impairment of verbal memory several years after left temporal lobectomy is compelling and contrasts with the normal verbal recall of patients with comparable excisions in other parts of the cerebral cortex. Table 11 shows the mean delayed recall scores and mean Wechsler-Bellevue I.Q. ratings for 56 patients tested in long-term follow-up and subdivided according to locus of cortical excision. On the verbal recall measures there are significant intergroup differences, not only for auditory material (as already known), but also for visual (F = 15.4, p < .001). The left temporal group has a deficit on both tasks; the right

temporal and the large minor-hemisphere groups do well on both. Moreover, patients with lesions in other parts of the left hemisphere (though admittedly in regions which lie outside the speech areas) also obtain normal scores. Thus, it can be seen that the left frontal group does particularly well on both forms of verbal recall; the small left parietal group does a little less well but makes significantly higher scores than the left temporal group (p < .02). Yet, on standard intelligence testing the level of the left temporal group is either equal or superior to that of the other groups tested.

It will be noted that Table 11 includes an individual case of left occipital lobectomy. This young girl, unlike the other patients studied, had a brain tumor, but her test performance was considered to be of sufficient interest to merit her inclusion here. This patient, case C.Be., had had seizures since the age of seven, characterized by marked receptive dysphasia for many minutes postictally, even though she could speak fluently at the time. At operation the surgeon, Dr. Charles Branch, discovered that she had a slow-growing tumor (an oligodendroglioma) which was thought to have been satisfactorily excised in the ensuing radical occipital lobectomy. After the operation the patient was at first unable to read and she has remained a poor reader. Nevertheless, when she returned

TABLE 11.

Excision	N	Verbal Recall		Mean I.Q.
		Auditory	Visual	(Wechsler)
Left temporal	22	9.6	10.0	110.3
Right temporal	13	16.5	17.4	110.1
Minor hemisphere (large)	10	17.4	16.2	101.3
Left frontal	6	18.1	18.4	109.8
Left parietal	4	15.0	15.4	111.5
Left occipital	1	20.0	16.0	96.0

Delayed verbal recall: follow-up mean scores.

for reexamination one year later, having had no seizures or other evidence of tumor recurrence in the interim, she obtained the high verbal recall scores shown in Table 11. It is noteworthy, however, that the visual recall score is slightly lower than the auditory one, as is also the case for the group of patients with large minor-hemisphere lesions; this is a reversal of the trend shown by the other groups.

The efficient visual-verbal recall of case C.Be., in the presence of marked reading disability, made it seem unlikely that the low scores of the patients with left temporal-lobe lesions were due to the fact that they were slow readers. It seemed desirable, however, to test more systematically the hypothesis that slow reading is compatible with normal achievement on our visual-verbal memory tests. The outcome of this study is illustrated in Figure 36, where speed of reading-comprehension is compared with efficiency of visual-verbal recall for three groups of pa-

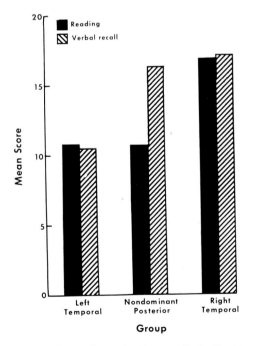

Fig. 36. Comparison of Chapman-Cook Reading Speed and Visual-Verbal Delayed Recall mean scores for different follow-up groups.

tients tested several years postoperatively. In addition to the right and left temporal-lobe groups, there is a small group of patients with extensive removals in the posterior cortex of the minor hemisphere.

The patients with posterior lesions had been selected for study because, unlike the temporal-lobe groups, all had contralateral homonymous visual field defects, involving more than one quadrant. It was thought that these large scotomata might handicap the patients on a speed-of-reading test, without, of course, affecting memory for what they had time to assimilate. Reading speed was, therefore, assessed independently of the visual-verbal memory tasks, using the Chapman-Cook Reading Speed test in which the subject has to discover and cross out the inappropriate word in each of a series of short paragraphs. The score is the number of words correctly crossed out within the time limit of $2\frac{1}{2}$ minutes. It can be seen from Figure 36 that the left temporal and the nondominant posterior groups show equal impairment on this task, as compared to the right temporal group, who perform normally. On the visual-verbal memory tasks, on the other hand, the left temporal group alone is impaired, the group with large posterior lesions achieving as high a mean score as the right temporal group, despite their lower reading speed. This finding is not altogether unexpected, in view of the very slow pacing used on the memory tests. It does, however, suggest that the slow reading of the left temporal patients is secondary to their verbal memory defect, making them refer back to the earlier parts of a paragraph more often than the average reader.

So far we have been treating the left temporal group as a homogeneous one, but there was, of course, considerable individual variation with respect to verbal memory and it seemed worthwhile to determine whether these individual differences were in any way related to the amount of tissue destroyed. In particular, we were interested in investigating the role of the left hippocampus in verbal learning and recall, since we had seen that after right temporal lobectomy the impairment in maze learning was found if, and only if, the bulk of the hippocampus had been removed. It is also known that bilateral lesions of the hippocampus and hippocampal gyrus cause remarkably severe and generalized memory disorders in man.[281,348] Accordingly, we analyzed our verbal memory data afresh from the standpoint of whether or not the hippocampus was destroyed. At the same time we took into account the extent of removal along the first temporal convolution by subdividing the temporal-lobe patients into those with Heschl's gyri spared and those with Heschl's gyri removed.

Table 12 shows the mean verbal recall scores in follow-up study after unilateral temporal lobectomy, for groups subdivided according to both side and size of removal. It is clear that the larger lesions on the left are associated with the more severe verbal memory impairment, whereas on the right all scores are within the normal range and there is no consistent relationship to lesion size. Although there is some hint that left hippocampectomy may increase the verbal learning deficit in left temporal-lobe lesions, the extent of lateral neocortical excision (as exemplified by complete ablation of the transverse gyri of Heschl) appears also to be a relevant factor.

Illustrative Cases. In Figure 37 some of the points which we have been considering are illustrated for four individual cases of left cerebral excision which seem to me instructive. In addition to the extent of cortical excision (shown in black), the brain charts show the points from which the surgeon elicited dysphasic responses at the time of operation, thus indicating how close the excision came to the speech areas. The delayed verbal recall scores for each patient are also given, together with their scores for the Broadbent dichotic digits test, another task sensitive to left hemisphere damage.

On the left of Figure 37 are shown two sharply contrasting instances of left temporal lobectomy. Case P.W. (above) had a radical excision limited to the neocortex and sparing the hippocampus by a wide margin. He represents one extreme of the left temporal group, since the lateral removal is unusually large and the mesial sparing quite unequivocal. This young man still has slight residual postoperative dysphasia and his score on the dichotic digits test is very low, as is his digit span measured in the conventional way. Nevertheless, his delayed verbal recall scores are in the upper range of the left temporal group and represent only mild impairment.

Case G. DeL., on the other hand, whose removal is shown in the left lower brain charts, presents a very different test pattern. This patient, a young engineer, had a considerably smaller lateral-temporal removal

TABLE 12.

Excision			Left Temporal			Right Temporal	
Hippo-campus	Heschl's gyri	N	Auditory	Visual	N	Auditory	Visual
Spared	Spared	9	10.7	12.2	3	16.0	16.8
	Removed	5	9.1	9.8	4	13.9	16.1
Removed	Spared	3	8.8	9.5	3	19.5	19.5
	Removed	5	8.5	7.3	3	17.7	17.7

Delayed verbal recall: follow-up mean scores as related to locus and extent of temporal lobectomy.

than P.W., but the hippocampus was radically excised. His score on the dichotic digits task is superior, indicating that he has no difficulty attending to auditory verbal input, even under the difficult conditions of rivalry between the two ears. His delayed verbal recall scores are, however, extremely low for both auditory and visual modes, and this despite the fact that these tests were carried out five years postoperatively. These findings encourage me to hope that when we have collected more cases like these two, with such clearly demarcated and contrasting lesions, we may yet shed some light on the functional relationship between the left hippocampus and the overlying temporal neocortex.

On the right of Figure 37 are two rather different excisions, both of which spare the temporal lobe and neither of which is associated with verbal memory impairment. The upper brain charts show the occipital lobectomy in case C.Be., the young girl whose

high verbal memory scores have already been mentioned. She had marked defects in reading and calculation and her dichotic digits score was low. Finally, the lower right-hand chart (case J.Al.) shows a removal of the pre- and postcentral face area. Unlike the other cases shown here, these test results are for the early postoperative period (about the seventeenth postoperative day), at which time this boy showed a complete disintegration of stereotyped verbal sequences, such as counting and saying the alphabet, and both spelling and writing were poor. Nevertheless, he obtained normal scores on both verbal-recall tasks, the lower score on the visual task being clearly related to his writing difficulty. Fortunately he was left-handed, otherwise the transient weakness of the right hand would probably have prevented him from performing the visual task. Preoperative intracarotid amytal tests had demonstrated speech to be represented in the left hem-

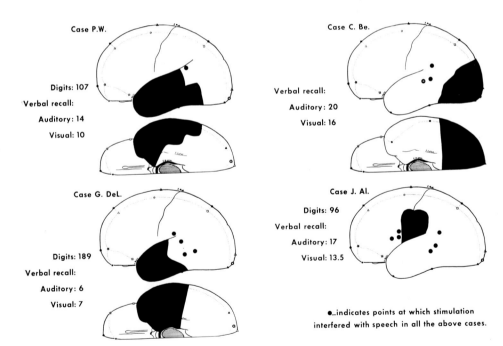

Fig. 37. Brain charts showing four different cases of cortical excision in the left hemisphere together with the corresponding Dichotic Digits and Delayed Verbal Recall scores. Case P. W., large temporal lobectomy, sparing hippocampus; case G. DeL., temporal lobectomy including hippocampus; case C. Be., occipital lobectomy; case J. Al., pre- and postcentral face area excision.

isphere and, as can be seen, stimulation of the exposed cortex interfered with speech in both Broca's area and the posterior temporal region, confirming that this was indeed the dominant hemisphere.

Differential Effects of Left Temporal and Left Frontal Lobectomy. The disturbance of verbal memory which is so characteristic a finding in lesions of the dominant temporal lobe is relatively rare in other cortical lesions, apart from those causing dysphasia, in which case the verbal memory defect forms part of a more complex language disturbance. The results for case J.Al., with a central area lesion, show, moreover, that some forms of dysphasia are compatible with normal verbal recall. What we do find, however, is that dominant-hemisphere lesions sparing the temporal lobe and sparing the speech areas do produce specific verbal defects, which differ from those seen after left temporal lobectomy. This point will be illustrated with reference to the left frontal lobe, anterior to Broca's area.

We saw earlier (Table 11) that the small group of patients tested in follow-up after left frontal lobectomy obtained superior scores on both the auditory and visual forms of the verbal memory tests. It does not follow, however, that the removal of the left frontal cortex causes no verbal deficit; indeed, one of the first things one notices about such patients is their lack of spontaneous speech. This observation is not new. Luria[249,250] has attached considerable importance to the impairment of spontaneous monologue, or narrative speech, in patients with tumors of the dominant frontal lobe, and, among earlier workers, Kleist[205] has commented on the poverty of spontaneous verbal expression in patients with lesions of the left anterior frontal region, although they are not dysphasic in the usual sense.

We set out to demonstrate the expressive defect quantitatively, in a very simple way, by means of the Thurstone Word Fluency test. In this test, the subject is first required to write down as many words beginning with the letter "S" as he can in five minutes; he is then allowed four minutes for the slightly harder task of writing down four-letter words beginning with "C." The score is the total number of words produced on the two tasks within the time limits. In a preliminary study[280] patients with left frontal lobectomy obtained abnormally low scores on this test, whereas patients with right frontal-lobe lesions obtained scores more appropriate to their I.Q. ratings. A small left temporal-lobe group, matching the left frontal group in intelligence, showed no word fluency loss.

Table 13 gives the word fluency scores for 40 patients in the present study, who were tested several years postoperatively. The patients are grouped according to locus of cortical excision, and the corresponding mean scores for delayed verbal recall, both auditory and visual, are also listed. The results completely replicate our earlier findings, although the groups are still quite small. Analysis of variance confirmed that the inter-group differences in word fluency were significant ($F = 6.75$, $p < .01$), the left frontal group obtaining significantly lower scores than either the left temporal ($t = 2.70$, $p < .02$) or the right temporal ($t = 3.67$, $p < .01$) groups. Only the left temporal group was impaired on the verbal memory tests. There is thus a differential effect of left frontal and left temporal lobectomy upon verbal fluency and verbal memory, both defects falling within the domain of language.

TABLE 13.

Excision	N	Word Fluency	Verbal Recall Auditory	Visual
Left temporal	18	49.3	10.1	10.5
Left frontal	6	28.7	18.1	18.4
Left parietal	4	44.3	15.0	15.4
Right temporal	12	58.4	15.4	17.0

Word fluency and delayed verbal recall: follow-up mean scores.

If we look once more at the map of the speech areas (Fig. 32), we see that even in the unshaded regions some specifically verbal functions are being mediated, although these parts of the left cerebral cortex can be excised without producing lasting dysphasia. If we consider that the defects shown by patients tested some years after operation (and when they are no longer having seizures) provide clues as to the essential function of the areas removed, then the anterior temporal region of the left hemisphere appears to be highly specialized for verbal learning.

CHAIRMAN MILLIKAN: Dr. Grey Walter, will you open the discussion, please?

DR. GREY WALTER: It is difficult for me to comment directly on this elegantly presented and statistically convincing material. There have been so many inadequate and anecdotal studies of temporal-lobe stimulation and excision that it is refreshing and reassuring to see figures which are so clear and convincing. Perhaps I can supplement them with some studies of people with implanted electrodes, in which we have proceeded, in most cases, to excision but in whom we have investigated temporal-lobe function by stimulation and recording technics and by measurement of local changes in metabolism. We have reached some conclusions which, in general, support Dr. Milner's thesis but also indicate some of the difficulties in interpreting observations of this type made in the operating room or the clinic.

The first is that in the whole brain we are dealing with a very richly connected system. For example, as I described earlier, the temporal lobe has very intimate reciprocal interconnections with the orbital cortex and other regions. It is a basic principle of interpretation and technic that, if you remove a particular component in a circular or feedback circuit, the circuit or function may be interrupted, but this does not prove that the region you have excised or damaged or stimulated is the essential component. It

is only one of the components. In studying normal function in man, this can be an almost insuperable barrier to direct interpretation. This applies both to interhemispheric and intercortical connections.

The other difficulty Dr. Milner mentioned; inevitably, in most cases of this type, one is dealing with a region of the brain already diseased, with a tumor or other lesion producing seizures or, in some of the cases we have been studying, intractable behavior disorders, as well as seizures. Also, the patients are usually under medication, often under heavy medication, in the hope of controlling both seizures and behavior and they come to operation because this medication has failed.

Figure 38 shows an x-ray of a patient with temporal-lobe epilepsy in whom sheaves of electrodes have been implanted in the frontal, temporal, and occipital lobes on both sides. There were 68 electrodes all together at 8mm. intervals along these sheaves. In this way we hoped to be able to identify the primary source of the electrical disturbances we had seen in routine scalp records which involved nearly all regions from time to time over several years of study. We have also had patients with thalamic implants for various types of dyskinesia. The advantage of this procedure is that one can observe the effects of stimulation in subjects who are quite normal and relaxed—with telemetry they can be free-ranging and engaged in everyday activities.

Starting at the lower level, stimulation of some thalamic centers (and we do not know exactly which because we have only x-ray geometry to locate the electrodes) can evoke sensations which seem to replicate the prodromal signs and symptoms of a temporal-lobe seizure. This suggests that some of the functions which we generally relate to temporal-lobe structures may involve other deeper midline or bilaterally represented circuits. Furthermore, sensory tactile stimulation of, say, one hand evokes a bilateral response in these thalamic regions, but on the contralateral side it is a typical "evoked response" while on the ipsilateral side the first response is a brief *suppression* of the *intrinsic* activity, followed by a complex response in phase with the contralateral components. This observation illustrates a serious limitation of the familiar and convenient "averaging" technics; an average of large numbers tends to conceal changes in amplitude of unsynchronized or random activity, but these may well be as significant to the brain as the more obvious synchronized responses, just as the silence of an audience is as significant as the voice of an orator. In fact, we have found these transient reductions in intrinsic activity in many parts of the brain to be closely related to the *significance* of sensory signals. For example, paired light flashes presented at regular intervals evoke responses in certain regions of visual cortex and not in others, but if the presentations are irregular or if the subject is instructed to make an operant response to

the flashes, the previously unresponsive region may show a clear attenuation of background activity for about 200 msec. This is often followed by a coherent after-rhythm, sometimes lasting several seconds. The effect is as though a rather irregular oscillation is suddenly damped and then allowed to start up again so that the first few swings fall in phase over many trials. The importance of these effects in relation to language is that they appear only when the subject is instructed or encouraged to make some relevant response, and one of the most effective classes of such responses is speech. This is particularly evident when the utterance is a truly linguistic one, that is, when the word or phrase involves a decision by the subject and the choice of a descriptor.

Using the combined patterns of evoked responses, activity suppression, and coherent after-rhythms, one can distinguish between the trivial aspects of speech—utterance of a simple stereotyped word such as a talking

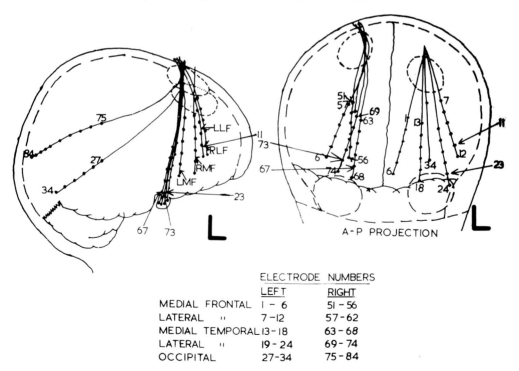

ELECTRODE NUMBERS		
	LEFT	RIGHT
MEDIAL FRONTAL	1 – 6	51 – 56
LATERAL "	7 –12	57 - 62
MEDIAL TEMPORAL	13 – 18	63 – 68
LATERAL "	19 - 24	69 - 74
OCCIPITAL	27 - 34	75 - 84

Fig. 38. X-ray diagram of patient with temporal-lobe epilepsy and sheaves of electrodes implanted in frontal, temporal, and occipital regions.

bird might make—and the serious aspects which involve semantic communication.

The occipital cortex is not the only region whose rhythmic activity is related to behavior. The temporal lobes also display these effects but often in an apparently inverse relation. Recording simultaneously from frontal and temporal cortex we have often seen frontal evoked responses to meaningless sensory stimuli but these dwindle with habituation and the temporal lobe is unaffected. However, when the subject is given a task to perform in relation to the stimuli, to count them or perform a selective operant or verbal response, the frontal evoked responses are amplified and at the same time a rhythm at 6-7 Hz appears in the anterior temporal lobe (probably the hippocampus). Similar rhythms have been seen during conditioning in the cat[3] and are nearly always present in the rabbit but are less common in man. Our impression is that this is because in man the temporal structures are relatively inaccessible and particularly involved with semantic transactions, so that to see these rhythms one must first have electrodes in the right part of a normal temporal lobe and then provide a situation in which the subject is engaged in a semantic problem of some kind.

One of the functions of the temporo-frontal circuit seems to be to maintain an estimate of conditional significance. Electrical stimulation of these systems in a conscious patient rarely evokes any coherent utterance but there is sometimes some sort of time slip. For example, if a patient is asked to count or read and a stimulus is applied to the temporal lobe for a few seconds, he will pause: 1, 2, 3, 4, 5 . . . 6, 7, 8 and so on; and if you asked why he stopped, he will deny stopping. He seems quite conscious and observant but for the stimulus period no time passed for him. This is obviously related to the *déja vu* experience which most people have had at some time. This effect is not usually obtained by stimulation of a diseased temporal lobe.

The relation of temporal lobe function to that of other brain regions can be seen most clearly in conditioning experiments. Both conditional warning stimuli and unconditional imperative ones evoke responses over wide regions of the frontal cortex and initially also in the anterior temporal structures. However, as the association proceeds and the conditional response is established, the frontal lobe develops a contingent negative variation, which submerges the response to the imperative signals. At this stage also the temporal lobe no longer responds to the imperative signals, only to the conditional ones. The temporal mechanisms are not concerned with the imperative responses or actions but only with the establishment of consistent estimates of significance and time. Perhaps we should remember that the ambiguity of the word "temporal" is no accident. The ancients sometimes used the pulsations of the *temporal* artery to measure time, hence its name, and below it may be one of the brain clocks that give the arrow of time its sad direction. In order to perform this function these mechanisms are liberated by storage in the frontal cortex of contingency calculation from involvement with details of immediate action. In states of anxiety, however, this freedom is

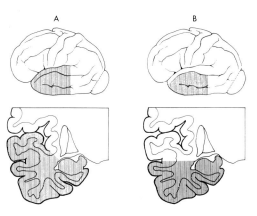

Fig. 39. Outline of typical anterior temporal lobectomies. Approximately two thirds of the patients studied with the delayed auditory feedback technic had sparing of the superior temporal gyrus (B). The other one third had excisions involving all three temporal gyri (A).

lost and the temporal lobe is found to be responding to all classes of stimuli with corresponding confusion of thought and action.

CHAIRMAN MILLIKAN: Dr. Chase, will you continue the discussion, please?

DR. CHASE: I am going to contribute to the discussion on functions of the temporal lobes by reporting some of the research being done at the Johns Hopkins University School of Medicine on psychological and sensory-perceptual deficits resulting from cerebral lesions in man.*

During the past year, we have studied 23 patients with temporal lobe lesions. They are quite comparable to the patients in the Montreal series, insofar as most all of them have long-standing temporal-lobe epilepsy, with sufficient evidence for a restricted focus of abnormal electrical activity to have warranted surgical treatment. The ages of subjects and their intelligence quotients are also comparable in the two series. The surgical procedures used, however, vary in the two series.

Approximately two thirds of the patients in the Hopkins series have had sparing of the superior temporal gyrus (STG) (Fig. 39, B).

*The research reported in this paper is being conducted as part of a collaborative research project on the effects of cerebral lesions on perception and behavior in man at The Johns Hopkins University School of Medicine. This project is under the general direction of Dr. A. Earl Walker and Dr. Dietrich P. Blumer (Division of Neurological Surgery and Department of Psychiatry and Behavioral Sciences). Other investigators who have contributed to the work reported in this discussion are: Mr. John K. Cullen, Jr., Mr. Keith O. Kalmbach, Dr. Rachel E. Stark, Dr. Grace Yeni-Komshian, Mr. David J. Mishelevich, Mr. Gerald W. Wilkins, Mr. James R. Merikangas and Mr. Peter H. Rheinstein (Neurocommunications Laboratory, Department of Psychiatry and Behavioral Sciences); Dr. Charles I. Berlin and Dr. Bruce W. Konigsmark (Division of Otology and Laryngology). This work is supported, in part, by contract PH-43-65-637 with The National Institute of Child Health and Human Development, National Institutes of Health; Grant RD-1899-S from the Vocational Rehabilitation Administration, The Freda R. Caspersen Trust, The Epilepsy Foundation, and USPHS General Clinical Research Center Grant No. 5-MO-IFR-35.

This applies both to the patients subjected to right anterior temporal lobectomy (right temporal lesion group) and to the patients subjected to right anterior temporal lobectomy (right temporal lesion group) and to the patients subjected to left anterior temporal lobectomy (left temporal lesion group). None of our patients have had excision of Heschl's gyrus. Varying amounts of rostral hippocampus and hippocampal gyrus and amygdala have been excised in almost all our patients. Excisions are usually carried posteriorly approximately 6 cm. from the temporal pole. In the Montreal series, ablation of superior temporal gyrus is almost always carried out (Fig. 39, A).

Our patients were examined at varying periods of time from the time of operation. Some were tested within a few months after operation, but most had been operated several years prior to testing.

Pure tone audiometry failed to demonstrate significant impairment of pure tone hearing acuity in any of our patients. A few patients had slight impairment of hearing acuity for high-frequency tones. Speech reception thresholds were found to be normal.

The Eisenson aphasia test was administered to all patients and all the responses were within normal limits, with the exception of those given by the only patient in our series with a lesion involving posterior temporal lobe on the left required for the surgical treatment of a tumor. Dr. Milner kindly provided us with her tapes of the Seashore test of musical talents, and I am happy to be able to repay that courtesy by confirming all her findings obtained with these tests,[278] the most striking, by far, being the deficit in tonal memory for the right temporal-lesion patients.

We also confirm the findings of other investigators who have documented a speech discrimination deficit for words presented to the ear contralateral to the temporal-lobe lesion.[34,188] Our speech discrimination tests included phonetically balanced words presented to the two ears simultaneously[27] and spondaic words presented to the two ears simultaneously.[193] In both tests patients identified fewer of the words presented to the ear contralateral to the lesion. The magnitude of this laterality effect was not appreciably affected as a function of whether the patient's lesion involved the right or left temporal lobe.

The new technics that we have applied to the study of acoustic information processing in this patient population specifically concern the temporal decoding of linguistic and nonlinguistic acoustic signals. I do not know of any way to decide on *a priori* grounds what category of temporal information processing the brain might be performing. We can conjecture about this. When one looks at data such as those Dr. Efron has presented,[100] it is tempting to consider that sequential order detection might be one kind of temporal processing. I am in sympathy with the procedure of applying specific technics that require a particular kind of temporal decoding, observing patterns of performance requiring processing of signals that have been formatted differently in time, and drawing inferences about the specific categories of temporal decoding that might be functioning in the biological system.

With these several considerations in mind, we have applied the technic of delaying auditory feedback to the study of our patients with unilateral temporal lobe lesions. Delayed auditory feedback testing has been undertaken with 23 patients. The sex distribution

and age characteristics of the patients are shown on Table 14.

Twelve of the patients had left temporal lesions, and 11 had right temporal lesions. Approximately two thirds of each group had sparing of the superior temporal gyrus (STG+) (Table 15).

Delayed auditory feedback is obtained by simultaneous activation of the record and playback heads of a tape recorder. The speech signal passes from the record head to the playback head, from which point it is picked up and returned to the subject's ears through earphones. The time delay is a function of the tape speed and the distance between the two heads. We have, of course, been using unilateral presentation of the delayed auditory feedback signal (200 msec. delay) while presenting the other ear with masking white noise. Each ear is tested separately in this fashion.

Delayed auditory feedback of speech, whether presented to one ear or both ears at once, results in profound changes in the motor patterning of speech.[417] Figure 40 shows oscillograms of four subjects repeating the phoneme /b/ in groups of three. On the left side of the figure you can see the time-amplitude patterning of these speech samples recorded under conditions of undelayed auditory feedback, and on the right side of the figure you can see the effects of delayed auditory feedback on speech performance.

TABLE 14.

	Control Subjects	Experimental Subjects
Total	22	23
Male	14	17
Female	8	6
Age range (yrs.)	16-55	16-55
Mean age (yrs.)	30.8	37.4

Sex and age of subjects studied with the delayed auditory feedback technic.

TABLE 15.

I.	Total number of patients	23
II.	Left temporal lesions	12
	STG (+)	8
	STG (−)	4
III.	Right temporal lesions	11
	STG (+)	7
	STG (−)	4

Classification according to side and extent of surgical lesions of patients studied with the delayed auditory feedback technic.

There is an increase in sound pressure levels, an increase in phonation times, repetitive errors (repetition of the /b/ four times instead of three), and in the case of subject #4, a complete disorganization of the temporal patterning of speech.

Since these are the changes we observe in almost all normal subjects speaking under delayed auditory feedback, we assume that these changes are a function of normal temporal processing of the temporally distorted auditory feedback. It is probable that the delayed auditory feedback results in a decorrelation in the time domain of a critical subset of the total pattern of sensory feedback being utilized for the organization and control of ongoing speech motor activity.

When we examined the effects of unilateral presentation of delayed auditory feedback to patients with unilateral temporal lobe lesions, the most striking finding was an asymmetry in the effect of the delayed feedback on speech as a function of the ear to which the delayed feedback was presented. When the delayed feedback was presented to the ear contralateral to the temporal-lobe lesion, there was less disturbance of the motor organization of speech than when the delayed feedback was presented to the ear on the side of the temporal-lobe lesion. This was observed for patients with both right and left temporal-lobe lesions, to much the same degree.

Subjects read 50-word passages under conditions of unilateral presentation of delayed auditory feedback, with masking white noise presented to the nontest ear. The test was begun by having the patient read one of the passages under normal reading conditions. He then read another passage with delayed auditory feedback presented to one ear. Another control reading was then obtained under normal reading conditions, followed by delayed auditory feedback to the other ear. Different reading passages were used for each of these four conditions. The entire sequence was then repeated, but this time the order of unilateral delayed auditory feedback presentations was reversed. In a few cases,

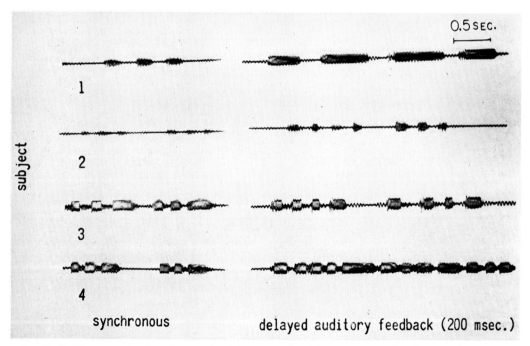

Fig. 40. Oscillograms showing the speech of four normal subjects repeating the phoneme /b/ in groups of three under conditions of undelayed (synchronous) and delayed auditory feedback (200 msec.).

subjects read passages for two or six pairs of test conditions, instead of the standard four pairs of test conditions outlined here. The same reading passages used previously were used again, and in fixed order. Every other subject in the series had his initial unilateral presentation of delayed auditory feedback to the right ear. The other subjects had initial unilateral presentation of delayed auditory feedback to the left ear.

All readings were tape recorded; the tape recordings were played into a Grayson-Stadler Speech Time Analyzer. This instrument registers a count every tenth second. The count is positive if the root mean square voltage of the speech signal is above a predetermined threshold value at the time of sampling, or negative if the root mean square voltage of the speech signal is below the predetermined threshold value at the time of sampling. The threshold voltage value is determined empirically by playing a control reading sample (obtained with undelayed auditory feedback) into the Speech Time Analyzer and adjusting the threshold so as to give a ratio of 50/50, plus/minus counts for the entire control passage sample. The subsequent reading of a passage under delayed auditory feedback is comparably scored, using the threshold voltage value obtained with the control passage.

The histogram (Fig. 41) shows speech changes resulting from delayed auditory feedback for both the patient population and the control population. The basic measure of speech disturbance used was the ratio of plus counts under delayed auditory feedback over the total of plus and minus counts under delayed auditory feedback. This measure comprehends both the increases in time and increases in amplitude that result from delayed auditory feedback of speech. Scores

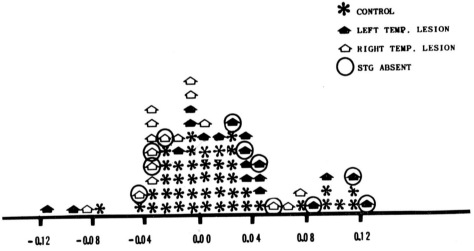

Fig. 41. Histogram showing speech changes resulting from delayed auditory feedback for patients with anterior temporal lobe lesions and normal subjects. The measure of speech disturbance is the ratio of plus counts under delayed auditory feedback over the total of plus and minus counts under delayed auditory feedback (see text). This measurement comprehends both increases in time and increases in amplitude that result in speech under delayed auditory feedback. Scores obtained under conditions of unilateral delayed auditory feedback to the right ear have been subtracted from scores resulting from unilateral presentation of delayed auditory feedback to the left ear. Therefore, all the positive scores indicate greater disturbance of speech on unilateral delayed auditory feedback presentation to the left ear. All negative scores indicate greater disturbance of speech on unilateral delayed auditory feedback presentation to the right ear.

obtained under conditions of unilateral delayed auditory feedback to the right ear have been subtracted from scores resulting from unilateral presentation of delayed auditory feedback to the left ear. Therefore, all the positive scores (those scores shown to the right of 0.00) indicate greater disturbance of speech on unilateral delayed auditory feedback presentation to the left ear.

It may be noted that most of the scores obtained from patients with left temporal-lobe lesions are found to the right of 0.00, thus indicating greater speech disturbance when delayed auditory feedback is presented to the left ear, or the ear on the side of the lesion. This laterality effect tends to be more marked for those patients with left temporal-lobe lesions involving the superior temporal gyrus (circled solid arrows). The negative scores (shown to the left of 0.00) indicate that speech motor activity was more disturbed under conditions of unilateral presentation of delayed auditory feedback to the right ear. It may be observed that most of the scores obtained from patients with right temporal-lobe lesions (white arrows), are to be found to the left of 0.00, thus indicating that greater disturbance of speech motor activity results from unilateral presentation of delayed auditory feedback to the right ear, or the ear on the side of the lesion. Thus both right and left temporal-lobe patients demonstrate greater disturbance of speech motor activity when delayed auditory feedback is presented to the ear on the side of the lesion. This laterality effect is somewhat more marked for the patients with left temporal-lobe lesions than for the patients with right temporal lobe lesions; and for the left temporal lobe group, the subpopulation with absence of the superior temporal gyrus shows the greatest differences in speech disturbance as a function of the ear receiving the delayed speech signal.

These differences in the effect of unilateral presentation of delayed auditory feedback as a function of side of lesion, and sparing or excision of superior temporal gyrus, are not large, however, and the major generaliza-tion that suggests itself upon examination of the data in Figure 41 is that unilateral presentation of delayed auditory feedback is less disruptive of speech motor activity when presented to the ear opposite an anterior temporal lobe lesion that it is when presented to the ear on the side of the lesion, for both right and left temporal-lobe lesion patients.

We plan to continue the study of unilateral delayed auditory feedback effects on the speech of patients with unilateral anterior temporal-lobe lesions. If the laterality effect shown in the data I have reviewed here continues to be demonstrated, we shall explore the possible mechanisms of this effect in greater detail. One major question of concern to us is whether the laterality effect is contingent upon utilization of linguistic material. Would comparable asymmetries be apparent if the unilateral delayed auditory feedback could not be recognized as intelligible speech? In order to study this question, we plan to invert the speech signal in the frequency domain (single sideband technic[377]), in order to remove intelligibility, while preserving the gross temporal architecture of the running stream of speech. The frequency-inverted speech signal would be presented in the same manner as intelligible speech signals in the experiments reviewed above. When this is done with normal subjects, we observe the same qualitative changes in speech motor activity under conditions of delayed feedback as we observe when unaltered speech signals are used.

DR. FALCONER: I would like to comment on some of the points raised by Dr. Milner in her paper, particularly as regards these auditory learning defects, auditory memory deficits, following removal of the anterior part of the left temporal lobe.

In the Guy's Maudsley Neurosurgical Unit in London we have a large number of cases of temporal lobectomy, with resections comparable to those done in Montreal, but always including the hippocampal structures. The indications are similar to those in Montreal.

I think the two series can, therefore, be compared.

My colleague, Dr. Victor Meyer,[272a] found that, after removal of the anterior part of the left temporal lobe, there was always an auditory learning deficit. Dr. Meyer, following on the work of Dr. Milner, confirmed this by similar kinds of tests of paired associates, delayed auditory recall stories, and he also went further and, after a year, repeated the tests and the abnormality was still there. He then made the assumption, which has proved to be false, that the defect was permanent.

This affected, for a while, the flow of cases we were getting for operation for temporal-lobe epilepsy, because some of our colleagues felt that, after operation, patients had an ordinary learning deficit with which they might be handicapped. I could illustrate to you some ways in which it did handicap patients.

One patient, for example, who was a telephonist engaged in long distance telephone routing, found he had to write down the numbers of the telephones he had to route and, after a while, he gave up that occupation, even though he was fit-free.

Another patient who was a travel agent, fluent in English, French, and Arabic, whenever he came to me jotted down everything I said with pencil and paper, and in this way he seemed to memorize what had been said. However, if he did not have his pencil and paper, he did not memorize it.

As the years went by, we found, in following up these patients, that this defect seemed to disappear. So my colleague, Mr. Colin Blakemore, has recently reviewed all the cases, including 95 per cent of the cases that Dr. Meyer had studied, and found that this defect almost invariably disappears after three years. It disappears more quickly in those patients who are rendered seizure-free than those who still have continuing seizures. Just what the compensation is, I do not know. But to give you an example, one of our most striking examples is a young business executive in a textile firm who was fluent in English and French. It was his job to go through France and through the North African Countries on behalf of his firm, taking orders for the firm's textiles. He used to jot notes down with pencil and paper, and thus could compensate for this auditory learning deficit. As the years went by, the need for pencil and paper disappeared. Not only did it disappear, but he began to learn Spanish by means of gramophone records. He now is fluent in Spanish as well as in French and English, and fluent in Spanish to the point that he can hold long telephone conversations with business people in Spanish without recourse to notes. Therefore, I would like to think that this defect that Dr. Milner put on the left hand side disappears after, say, three years in many instances and usually completely in five. The mechanism by which it disappears we do not know.

DR. HIRSH: I have been sitting, going around in a circle, trying to answer for myself the question of whether this lobe is indeed the temporal lobe or the verbal lobe. I think it is quite clear that, since I did not hear you mention any difficulty with individual word recognition—I think I heard you say before that there was none—that the microtime I was speaking of seems not to be affected with these lesions, as long as they do not interfere with the primary projection regions. Again, I do not know the neuroanatomy enough to know whether or not the gyrus that remains in most of the patients is comparable to what my physiological friends call A_1 in the cat, where they do most of the recording from auditory input information. Then, I am not sure that temporal and verbal are very different, in that I think original language learning is entirely auditory, is entirely processed in time.

There are two other kinds of information that I think should be brought in here. To take just one example, some of the nonsense syllable repetition exercises that were described show that, when people are presented with printed nonsense syllables in a long serial list, and they are supposed to reproduce the list, when they make errors, the particular errors that occur are more representative of acoustic confusions than of printed letter confusions. This has been interpreted by some—and I think I would tend to accept the interpretation—that this relatively short verbal memory or storage is essentially an auditory one, and perhaps so because it is so close to the speech area, just forward, on the left side.

In this very connection, I do not think that, trying to distinguish verbal component from temporal component, Dick Chase, you quite put it to the test with turning the spectrum upside down, because again, as I mentioned, the perception of speech depends in part on spectral cues but, in large part, on nonspectral cues, the way in which things change in time, which I think is synonymous with your phrase "temporal architecture." So just by turning the spectrum around but yet conserving the temporal feature, you have not yet thrown away all intelligibility. Your auditory-motor system might still be operating within a linguistic framework.

I am delighted to hear the coincidence of these results from Dr. Milner about short-term memory for verbal material, whether that material gets presented to the ear or the eye.

CHAIRMAN MILLIKAN: Dr. Chase, do you have an answer?

DR. CHASE: I share your point completely, Dr. Hirsh. I do not think it makes sense to attempt to take time away from the receptive aspects of linguistic behavior. Obviously, speech possesses a hierarchy of temporal organizations. The question of major concern to us, however, is whether the brain mechanisms involved in temporal decoding of speech are, in some measure, not specific to the decoding of linguistic-acoustic signals. I think that this question should be vigorously explored.

Let me make one other point, Dr. Millikan. When we speak about the temporal ordering of experience, we might use this as a touchstone for calling attention to a fact that is well known to clinicians: patients with temporal-lobe lesions present, as a prominent clinical feature, profound disturbances of behavior. The perceptual deficits that Dr. Milner and others have spoken of can, of course, be documented in this patient population. However, unlike aphasic patients, patients with anterior temporal-lobe lesions do not present themselves for medical attention because of difficulties in handling verbal or spatial organization. They have difficulties with the police; they have difficulties with teachers, parents, and siblings. They have molar disturbances of behavior.

I think it presents a challenge to consider whether some of the brain mechanisms underlying specific cognitive and perceptual deficits might also underlie some of the more molar disturbances of behavior which are, in fact, the more prominent features of clinical syndromes involving the temporal lobe.

DR. RICHARD L. MASLAND: I am very much interested in this question raised by Dr. Hirsh as to whether the temporal lobe is the temporal lobe or the verbal lobe. Dr. Milner's data appear to suggest that the left temporal lobe is the verbal lobe and the right temporal lobe is the temporal lobe. There is, however, an apparent conflict between her data and those of Dr. Efron. Dr. Milner's data suggest that injury of the right temporal lobe impairs memory for rhythm. Is that correct?

DR. MILNER: Melodies.

DR. MASLAND: Dr. Efron's data indicate that lesions in the left hemisphere impair appreciation of time intervals.

DR. EFRON: I should insert a major reservation. Dr. Milner's patients were not aphasic, and those that had the defect I described all were aphasic.

DR. MASLAND: They were left temporal lobe.

DR. EFRON: But selected by virtue of having aphasia, not by virtue of having a left temporal lobe.

DR. MASLAND: But your patients with the right hemisphere lesions did not show this impairment, and Dr. Milner has shown impairment of recall of patterns of sound from injury to the right temporal lobe.

The question that occurs to me is, is there a possibility that Dr. Milner's results stemmed from the fact that her test represented an interhemispheric task? I would like to raise the question as to the nature of the response that she required of these patients. Did they have to give a verbal or written response relative to what they had experienced with their right hemisphere?

I am disturbed by the data from the patients who have had the callosum sectioned. These observations raise the question as to whether individuals who were given a task requiring the right hemisphere, were being asked to respond with the left. This may have complicated the task for the individual with the right hemisphere removed.

CHAIRMAN MILLIKAN: Dr. Milner, would you respond to that question?

DR. MILNER: First, I must point out that there is little or no disturbance in the discrimination of simple rhythms after right temporal lobectomy. The auditory-discrimination defect appears most clearly on the Seashore Tonal Memory test, in which a short sequence of notes is played twice in rapid succession, after which the subject has to decide which note was changed in pitch at the second playing. This analysis of melodic patterns is impaired by right temporal lobectomy, although simple pitch discrimination seems not to be affected by the lesion.[278] Such tonal-pattern discriminations are quite unlike the tasks used by Dr. Efron, and, therefore, I do not think that our results are necessarily in conflict.

With regard to the nature of the response required on the Tonal Memory test, this is admittedly verbal. The subject has to say, or write down, the number (corresponding to the position in the sequence of four or five notes) of the note which had changed. None of our patients, not even the dysphasic ones, had difficulty in counting from one to five, and I doubt very much that the verbal response was complicating the task for the

right temporal group, since the corpus callosum was intact.

Further evidence of impaired appreciation of melodies after right temporal lobectomy comes from a recent study by Shankweiler[357] who tested memory for traditional tunes. The subject listened to a few bars and was then required to continue the tune by humming, and also, if he could, to name it. After right temporal lobectomy, patients obtain abnormally low scores on both these measures, although if they can hum the tune they can usually name it. After left temporal lobectomy, there is a selective impairment of naming, consistent with the low scores on other verbal memory tasks, but humming scores are much higher and are significantly better than those obtained by the right temporal group. For these various reasons, we think that discrimination and recognition of melodic patterns is more dependent upon the right temporal lobe than the left. I am, of course, very happy to learn that Dr. Chase has confirmed our findings for the Seashore Tonal Memory test.

DR. PURPURA: I wanted to comment on some of Dr. Walter's findings and ask a question. I made reference before to some studies of thalamic stimulation with effects on speech behavior. It has been shown that there are massive connections between ventral anterior nuclei of the thalamus and orbitofrontal regions of cortex. It is also known that there are connections between the orbitofrontal regions and amygdala and amygdala to hippocampus. I was wondering if you have noted in your thalamic studies any evidence for the production of jargon aphasia with stimulation of dorsomedial nuclei or other structures with powerful connections to the cortical regions which exhibit the C.N.V.'s.

DR. GREY WALTER: We have had no autopsies on our patients, so we are never quite sure which part of the temporal lobe we are in, except from the x-ray relationships which, of course, would be plus or minus a centimeter.

The effects we have seen with stimulation of temporal lobe, particularly in patients with no clinical signs of epilepsy, tend to be utterances of an uncharacteristic type which might be taken as evidence of psychotic or paranoid delusion, if recorded by a psychiatrist. They are often well organized and usually forgotten by the patient. These utterances are sometimes accompanied by aggressive actions directed at whoever is nearest. The region involved is probably slightly above the amygdaloid region in man. Recording from multiple electrodes in temporal and frontal lobes shows a striking disturbance of the orbital-frontal lobe electrical rhythms as well as in the temporal ones. This looks like a very restricted temporal-lobe seizure. This suggests that we are interfering with a very complex system in such a way as to evoke a systematic pattern of behavior, including stereotyped language and gesture and even physical attack resembling a paranoid outburst in a patient with no history of such tendencies.

DR. EFRON: I would like to answer Dr. Masland's question with a proposal for further work. I think the query which is bothering him nobody can answer until Dr. Milner or Dr. Chase repeat the same kind of studies which I did in patients with temporal-lobe lesions on either side, but with their patients with temporal-lobe lesions—*without* aphasia. That is the crucial point—*without* aphasia. All the patients that I used had an aphasia. I was looking for people who had lesions in the dominant temporal lobe. Looking around the wards, in the institution in which I work, for patients with lesions in the dominant temporal lobe, I selected patients with aphasia. It turned out they had this major sequencing defect. I did not have available to me the rather remarkable collection of patients with temporal-lobe lesions but without aphasia which Dr. Milner, Dr. Falconer, and Dr. Chase have. If one had that kind of patient, the type of temporal sequence analysis that I have done—and Dr. Holmes and Dr. Edwards have now done—would

enable us to answer the question. We cannot be certain at present if the defect in sequencing occurs only with dominant temporal-lobe lesions which produce aphasia.

DR. MILNER: Certainly the Montreal patients were unlike the severely dysphasic patients studied by Dr. Efron. Some were, however, mildly dysphasic in the early postoperative period, although not in follow-up study.

DR. ROSENBLITH: I do not know whether this is the time for this somewhat methodological remark. I am impressed with the fact that we have had questions that have been essentially of a terminological nature and have reflected the underlying concern of all of us here that we do not understand the anatomical circuitry; there is the point Dr. Grey Walter made that you can take a part out of the circuit but you must be careful as to what you observe from the remainder of the evidence. We do not have a system diagram for the kind of ways in which the various responses are being generated, in other words, if there should be a way of testing the dumb or the wise hemisphere. I think it was clear to me from Dr. Sperry's very elegant presentation that you clearly have to understand not only the information processing as it goes in but also the executive acts as they come out, and under the control of which hemisphere it is, before you can say what you can conclude from the kind of diagram you have been talking about.

I think the repeated questions as to what is the anatomy and whether this is the temporal lobe or the verbal lobe are really only stating we do not have what a systems engineer would call a systems diagram. Maybe we cannot produce it today or during this Conference, but at least we should know what the potentialities are, perhaps, for two parallel ways of getting the same kind of response. Maybe we should try to parcel out some of the difficulties that arise when you ask questions from a temporal lobe about time.

DR. GIAN FRANCO ROSSI: I would like to add a word to Dr. Purpura's remarks on a subcortical participation in the mechanism of speech. I think Dr. Myers and Dr. Geschwind commented upon it, taking a negative position. I agree with Dr. Geschwind on the fact that, in the classical neurological literature, there is not sufficient evidence for a subcortical relevant participation in language mechanisms. However, it seems to me that some interesting findings have been obtained following thalamic lesions in stereotaxic surgery. Dr. Purpura mentioned the effect of thalamic stimulation on language and Dr. Grey Walter too, mentioned it—and pointed out how selective such an effect may be, and strictly related to the stimulated thalamic nucleus.

If I remember correctly, at the recent International Symposium on Stereoencephalotomy, in Copenhagen, Dr. Krayenbühl described disturbances of speech, not only following thalamic stimulation, but also following thalamic lesion.

Finally, Dalle Ore and his associates, of Verona, have recently analyzed a large amount of material on thalamic stimulations and lesions and have provided a good indication for the existence of thalamic influence on speech. Therefore, I think that the evidence of a participation of the thalamus— or more generally of subcortical structures —to language mechanisms is not lacking; perhaps, what is lacking is an indication of a lateralization or, if you prefer, of "dominance" at subcortical level.

DR. MYERS: The thalamus is not usually described as having relation to language function. Penfield and Roberts,[309] in their book on speech and brain mechanisms, made only scant reference to a possible association between damage to the thalamus and disorder of speech. However, language disturbances may be seen with lesions of the thalamus, as, for example, with intrinsic tumors. However, the disorders exhibited may not be described as disorders of speech since the defects tend to be so diffuse and so severe they are more likely described as confusional states or as dementia. Particularly interesting in this regard is the case of Schulman who exhibited severe diffuse drop-out of nerve cells in the thalamus bilaterally associated with progressive dementia and impoverishment of speech along with other changes.

Aphasic disturbances are most commonly seen with vascular lesions involving the cortex or white matter of the hemisphere. In contrast to the frequency of such hemisphere lesions, sizeable vascular lesions involving the thalamus in isolation are rare. A part of the failure to associate language disturbances with lesions of the thalamus may be this infrequency of occurrence of isolated involvement of the thalamus by severe vascular disease or, for that matter, by other disease processes such as tumors or inflammations.

Dr. Grey Walter earlier in this Conference described arrest of speech with electrical stimulation in the human thalamus. Speech disruption with thalamus stimulation has been described by other workers as well. These new data also suggest an involvement of the thalamus in the manifestations of speech. Clearly more study needs to be carried out on this important, as yet unresolved, question of thalamus and speech function.

DR. GREY WALTER: I want to ask Dr. Chase about the application of delayed auditory feedback. We played around with this for a while some years ago, when it first came out, with normal subjects. We found that the effect of delayed auditory feedback on the rhythm and coherence of speech was a function of age among other factors. Elderly people who perhaps tended to talk too much anyway and never listened to what anybody was saying were relatively unaffected by the delayed auditory feedback, whereas younger people were affected, as you say. In your particular population, you say they were excellently matched for age and sex, but I think the average age is quite low because very few elderly people come to operation this way. I wondered if you had compared the results in normal old people. This might give us an idea of the functions of the temporal lobes as they decline, the temporal lobes, as we all know, being rather marginal in blood supply.

CHAIRMAN MILLIKAN: Would you reply?

DR. CHASE: This is the first time this observation has ever been called to my attention. I am glad to have it called to my attention. I have never had an opportunity to observe the effects of delayed auditory feedback on the speech of elderly subjects.

I can, however, contribute some information at the other end of the age spectrum, because I have had an opportunity to observe the effects of delayed auditory feedback on the speech of a population of normal children ranging in age from two to twelve years. In this population there is little question about the fact that the very young children show much less disturbance of speech motor activity under delayed auditory feedback than the older children.[64]

DR. GESCHWIND: Most of the patients that I have seen with speech disturbance after thalamic surgery for parkinsonism were not aphasic but either were mute or else demonstrated a marked diminution in rate and volume of speech, but showed no abnormalities in the language so produced. There may be cases who were clearly aphasic but I have not yet seen or read of any. I would stress that I would not deny the possibility of transient aphasias from thalamic lesions, just as we know that there is one cortical site from which transient but not permanent aphasias can result. Schwab[347] reported on the cases operated by himself and Foerster with lesions in the frontal parasagittal region which abuts on the supplementary motor cortex. In 14 out of 21 cases with excisions in this region aphasia occurred transiently. More recently Penfield and Roberts[309] have discussed similar cases, as have Alajouanine et al.[8] and Petit-Dutaillis.[313] I do not know what the significance of this region is for speech. We should not overlook these transient syndromes and concentrate only on those lesions which produce permanent effects since such transient syndromes almost certainly point to physiologically important mechanisms.

CHAIRMAN MILLIKAN: We will continue with Dr. Hécaen, discussing "Brain Mechanisms Suggested by Studies of Parietal Lobes."

Brain Mechanisms Suggested by Studies of Parietal Lobes

HENRY HÉCAEN

Centre Neurochirurgical Ste. Anne
Paris, France

We shall consider here only the posterior region of the parietal lobe and exclude the area of somatosensory representation, although damage to the lower part of the latter region may be a partial determinant of motor aphasia and even, according to Luria,[249] of one particular kind of aphasia, so-called afferent motor aphasia. However, together with damage to the posterior part of the parietal lobe, we must consider also the parieto-temporo-occipital junction mainly centered around the supramarginal gyrus and the angular gyrus. We shall try to summarize what is known about symptoms associated with damage in this zone, be it in the minor or in the major hemisphere. Then we shall try to utilize these results to understand better the part played by damage of this area of the cortex in language disorders.

Although dominance of the left hemisphere has been accepted from the very beginning of anatomoclinical study of the language disorders, it is only recently that hemispheric asymmetry in this posterior junction has been considered possible for functions other than language. This difference of symptoms depending upon which hemisphere is damaged has become more and more established in recent years, but it has not yet received general recognition. Thus, before looking into anatomoclinical information obtained

The research upon which the study is based was carried out by the R.C.P. No. 41 C.N.R.S., with the aid of Institut National de Santé et de la Recherche Médicale.

from a study of left hemisphere damage, we must outline the general features of the main functional disorders occasioned by damage to the posterior junction of the right minor hemisphere.

Symptomatology of Lesions of the Right Posterior Junction. This includes somatognosic, praxic, and visuognosic aspects.

Somatognosia. The earliest studies concerning knowledge of the body and its disorders showed that these disorders present very different aspects according to whether the lesion is situated in one or the other hemisphere. If the minor hemisphere is damaged, somatognosic disorders generally affect the contralateral half of the body, for example, denial of hemiplegia; unawareness or even rejection of this same half of the body; and a feeling of strangeness for the whole side, for one limb, or for one of its segments. Subsequent clinical study has fully confirmed the indications provided by these initial case reports. The part played by parietal damage is quite evident here, since the relative frequency of such disorders is almost as high in isolated parietal damage as in massive parieto-occipital lesions.

It is only fair to point out that these quantitative data have not convinced everyone, especially with respect to the concept that there is a different representation of the knowledge of the body according to the hemisphere. For example, Denny-Brown and Chambers[85] believe that the higher frequency of such disorders in right lesions as compared with left lesions is not due to a special hemispheric functional organization but rather to the subjects' different reactions to tests. For Weinstein et al.[400] the predominance of left-side anosognosia is due mainly to an artifact of the examination. The higher frequency of anosognosia shown by patients with right hemisphere damage may be attributed to the fact that, even though it may exist, anosognosia cannot be conceptualized in confabulatory form or by a highly metaphorical gesture such as the pantomime of massive neglect of one side of the body by the aphasic patient with a left hemisphere lesion. In such a patient, incomprehensible jargon, verbal stereotypy, and silence replace the "anosognosia" as expressed by verbal or gestural metaphors in patients with right hemisphere lesions.

Praxis. Damage of the left parietal lobe was at first held responsible for praxic disorders.[231] However, when new types of praxic disorders were discovered, it was proved that right parietal-lobe damage was quite capable of determining such disorders. Thus, in 1944 Paterson and Zangwill[304] showed that with right lesions there are visuoconstructive disorders. Dyspraxia for dressing was similarly connected with lesions of this hemisphere.

Moreover, it became increasingly apparent that constructive disorders were more frequent and more severe in lesions of the minor hemisphere than in those of the major one, while some authors contended that there were qualitative differences in these disorders according to the hemisphere damaged. Again Denny-Brown and Chambers[85] have opposed such a conception and hold that in lesions of either hemisphere constructive difficulties are due to amorphosynthesis, but that on the left side the failure is, in addition, due to the propositional nature of the task. It is to be noted that in this case the frequency of constructive disorders should be higher for lesions of the dominant hemisphere than in right lesions yet all observers agree that the contrary is true. However, Costa and Vaughan,[76] using the method of test inter-

correlation, have shown that in right lesions there is a uniform deficit on all perceptive tests, whether these include a constructive task or not, whereas in left lesions the "perceptual" tests are not intercorrelated. Thus, in right lesions constructive disorders must be considered as part of a larger pattern of visuospatial deficit.

Piercy and Smyth,[319] using Raven's Progressive Matrices, have shown that the scores of subjects with right lesions on this perceptual test were higher than those of subjects with left lesions. Moreover, on this test the subjects with right lesions could be divided into two groups: apraxic and nonapraxic. But they insisted on the fact that the same test also shows a distinction between apraxics and nonapraxics in left lesions. The seriousness of the constructive apraxia was more marked in right than in left lesions. These authors hold the opinion that the degree of failure on the perceptive test was related to the intensity of the constructive disorder on whatever side the lesion may be. This was, therefore, not in favor of a qualitative difference of apraxic disturbances according to the hemisphere. Thus, the question is still subject to discussion.

Recently Dubois et al.,[92] studying the language of subjects with right hemisphere damage, have shown a double relation: on the one hand, between perseveration phenomena as expressed in the grammatical tests and iterative writing disorders and, on the other hand, between constructive apraxia and written arithmetic. Moreover, considering the relations existing between constructive apraxia and perseveration, on the one hand, and dyscalculia and dysgraphia on the other hand, it could be concluded that two different factors intervene simultaneously. These two sets of relations, although isolated, seemed to correspond in the series to parietal or parieto-occipital lesions, while other types of relationships, independent of the former, seemed to correspond to a different localization (verified cases are too few to permit a firm conclusion).

These facts allow us to interpret Piercy and his collaborators' observations of the greater number of strokes in right lesion apraxic drawing as compared with the drawing of subjects with left lesions in terms of a perseveration factor expressed in one particular field. The bond between constructive disorders and a special type of dyscalculia (figures poorly placed, neglect of the left side) allows us to consider that the factor underlying these disorders may be linked with a disturbance of spatial organization, this being quite particular since there is no relation with topographical disturbance.

As for dressing apraxia, which Denny-Brown considers as a mere result of amorphosynthesis, it is definitely more frequent in right lesions than in left ones (21.8 per cent as against 3.9 per cent in our series). But since it is almost always associated with constructive apraxia, which is itself four times more frequent, there may be, as Piercy points out, what Teuber calls an order of fragility. The few cases of this form encountered without constructive apraxia may be due to another deficit, in particular, hemiasomatognosia.

Disorders of the Apprehension of Spatial Data. Even if the lesional origin of these disorders seems to be more occipital than parietal, they are too bound up with the preceding ones not to be mentioned here. Their polysensorial character must likewise be pointed out and particularly the proprioceptive-visual integration, so as not to minimize the part played by a zone particularly important for this intersensorial relation. These disorders of spatial data seem to be on various levels: the lowest is unilateral spatial agnosia, when neglect of one side of the space concerns particularly the visual domain. But they may also involve somatosensory, oculomotor, and somatomotor aspects and, at times, even auditory functions. The relation of this agnosia to unilateral disorders of somatognosia cannot be denied. We have encountered it in 55 of 413 cases with retrorolandic lesions, 51 times in right lesions, four times

in left lesions; in these latter cases, three subjects were left-handed. Moreover, the study of clinical associations in the group of subjects with unilateral spatial agnosia, compared with the group which had none, showed its close relation to four types of disorders; sensory relation of the body to space, use of space, lowering of intellectual vigilance, and a negative correlation with language disorder. We therefore cannot accept the conclusions of Battersby et al.[19] that spatial disorders are not significantly more frequent with right lesions.

The other spatial disorders, such as disturbances in topographical concepts and loss of topographical memory, also seem to be connected with right lesions but perhaps less strikingly so. Thus, the first mentioned was found 40 times in 399 cases of retrorolandic lesions: 29 right lesions, eight left lesions (including four left-handed subjects), and three bilateral lesions. The second was found 15 times in 398 cases: nine right lesions, two left, and four bilateral. As for the context of the clinical associations of these disorders, it is similar to that of unilateral spatial agnosia but of slightly less importance.

The findings of Semmes et al.[352] in their test for finding a route from maps presented visually and haptically are not in accord with ours. Indeed, although a parietal lesion may be at the origin of difficulties in this test, no hemispheric prevalence could be shown.

Agnosia for Faces. Out of the 22 cases of facial agnosia in our series, a right lesion was predominant in 16 cases; the lesions were bilateral in four cases, and in two cases the lesion was in the left hemisphere. When cases were verified, there was always damage of the parieto-temporo-occipital junction. The clinical context was very much the same as that of spatial agnosia, although the sensory disorders no longer concerned the vestibular and visual domains; oculomotor disorders and lowering of intellectual vigilance were no longer connected with gnosic disorders. A negative correlation with aphasia persisted.

Spatial Dyslexia, Dysgraphia, and Dyscal-

culia. Even if alexia and agraphia in right lesions are not the same as in left lesions (that is, bearing upon the comprehension or transcription of the graphic code), there are, however, disturbances in writing or reading which come from perceptual difficulties with the spatial arrangement of letters and sentences. *Spatial dyslexia* is characterized not only by neglect of the left side of a text and sometimes of one or more words (or, more rarely, of part of a word) but also by inability to distinguish letters and words which overlap each other and by difficulty in passing from one line to another. This spatial dyslexia is, moreover, more frequent in occipital than parietal lesions when the lesion is of an isolated lobe. However, it is more frequent and marked in global lesions of the junction when there is a mass effect.

Spatial dysgraphia is not exceptional since we have found 19 cases (15.7 per cent) out of 121 right lesions. The features of this dysgraphia totally separate it from the agraphia of left hemisphere disease. Aside from particularly severe cases where the patient can only iterate simple, generally curved forms, three principal types of spatial dysgraphia may be found: writing on the right-hand side of the page; inability to write in a straight line (diagonal or wavy writing); and iterations involving mainly the vertical strokes (m, n, i, v) and, more rarely, letters or words. These alterations usually do not destroy the actual structure of the word, which remains legible. The grammatical structure of sentences is never altered.

We have already mentioned the close relation of this agraphia to perseveration phenomena found in grammatical tests and also its relation to constructive apraxia and dyscalculia. The very features of this dysgraphia make us think that it is a question of perseveration disturbing the graphism as a spatial realization rather than as a code. Here again parietal damage seems to be of prime importance and occipital damage of rather less significance.

Now let us consider *dyscalculia* in right hemisphere lesions. Three types of disturbance can be distinguished: acalculia caused by figure or number alexia, anarithmetia (loss of the ability to carry out arithmetical operations); and spatial dyscalculia (inability to carry out the operations due to faulty placing of figures or neglect of part of the figures while the principles of the operations are preserved). The distribution of these three types of disturbance in our groups of patients was found to be as follows:

Spatial dyscalculia
35 cases out of 148 right lesions
4 cases out of 195 left lesions
Figure alexia
1 case out of 148 right lesions
57 cases out of 195 left lesions
Anarithmetia
10 cases out of 149 right lesions
44 cases out of 195 left lesions

These results show that spatial dyscalculia seems specific to posterior damage of the right hemisphere. This confirms the analysis of the clinical context, the elements of which correspond to those of spatial agnosia and constructive apraxia through right lesions. From the point of view of intrahemispheric localization, isolated parietal lesions are more frequent in these disturbances than occipital and temporal lesions, but they are especially caused by large parieto-occipital and parieto-temporo-occipital lesions. However, this relative polarization in the parietal lobe must be borne in mind considering the polarization of spatial dyslexia in the occipital lobe.

Praxic and Gnosic Symptoms in Damage to the Left Parietal Lobe. Let us now analyze the praxic and gnosic symptoms of damage to the left parietal lobe before considering the role played by these lesions in verbal and writing disorders.

Somatognosia. Disorders in knowledge of the body here concern both sides of the body, whether it be a local disorder (finger agnosia) or a general one (autotopagnosia). Left hemisphere damage doubtless plays a part. Our figures for right-handed subjects are as follows: right lesions, 2.99 per cent; left lesions,

19.01 per cent. The region causing the most severe impairment is that including the supra-marginal gyrus and the angular gyrus.

The problem is actually more complex: finger agnosia would seem to be only an element of Gerstmann's syndrome when it is associated with agraphia, acalculia, and indistinction between left and right. However, Benton[24] is opposed to this conception. He has studied intertest correlations, bearing on the elements of the syndrome and of other parietal capacities (for example, constructive apraxia), in 100 subjects with brain damage. The correlations were not greater between the four Gerstmann elements than between these elements and the three others not attributed to Gerstmann's syndrome. Moreover, Benton sees no direct relation between finger schema and the dominant hemisphere. For him the great importance of these lesions is due only to relations which exist between this hemisphere and symbolic processes, language disorders representing an essential component of finger agnosia. In this respect, it should be noted that in his series finger localization had the highest correlation with left-right orientation. However, Benton's opinion has not been universally accepted. Thus Kinsbourne and Warrington,[203] utilizing nonverbal tests, report that their cases demonstrated a specific difficulty in relating fingers to each other in correct spatial sequence.

From a careful study of the conditions of the deficit, Ettlinger[107] is inclined to favor Stengel's[371] opinion that finger agnosia is part of a disorder of spatial orientation ("the inability of the patient to relate in space objects which form part of an organized whole, to each other and to himself according to rules acquired by experience"). We thus come back to the concept of a basic disorder depending upon a certain anatomical localization, the posterior parietal region, which gives it a spatial tonality, advanced by Lange[216] and Janota[186] among others and in a very global way by Conrad,[73] who defined it as a disturbance "of the faculty of grasping

a whole in its part." Ehrenwald,[103] while admitting this basic disorder, thought that the specificity of the syndrome could depend only on the combined presence of another disorder: disorganization of the body scheme.

It should be added that a comparative study of the frequencies of somatognosic disorders in right and left lesions according to the topography and extent of the lesion showed a different organization according to the hemisphere. The prevalence of the parietal lesion, so definite in hemiasomatognosia (right lesion), diminished for finger agnosia (left lesion), the frequency of this disorder in temporal and even in occipital lesions being appreciable. In addition, the mass effect was even heavier for finger agnosia than for hemiasomatognosia; this may be attributed, in our opinion, to the importance of temporal and occipital factors (that is, in functional terms, to visual and verbal factors). With somatognostic disturbances in left lesions the kinesthetic factor is always important but in a less exclusive way than with disorders of the body scheme in right lesions.

Praxis. Ideomotor and ideational apraxia seem to be always connected with left hemisphere lesions when damage is lateralized. Moreover, in our series they seem to be more frequent in parietal lesions and, to a slightly lesser degree, in parieto-occipital lesions than in isolated temporal lesions or parieto-temporal lesions. They are much less frequent in massive parieto-temporo-occipital lesions, which thus excludes the mass effect. The frequency of constructive apraxia in left lesions according to localization reveals analogies with those of apraxia by right lesion, but the mass effect is here less marked.

Acalculia. We have already seen that acalculia is part of Gerstmann's syndrome, its connection with finger agnosia being possibly artificial. Number alexia is naturally a characteristic of left lesions. In our series its frequency was especially high in temporo-occipital lesions in association with verbal alexia. However, it differs from the former in terms of its relative frequency in isolated parietal lesions.

As for anarithmetia, its frequency curve in the same series clearly shows parietal prevalence which is only slightly accentuated by mass effects. Certainly since all difficulties in written arithmetic are grouped under the name of anarithmetia, we have a definitely heterogeneous group with respect to basic mechanisms. It suffices to point out that the frequency of anarithmetia is still high in isolated temporal lesions (40.5 per cent), in order not to minimize the importance of language disorders. However, the inversion of the frequencies of aphasia and anarithmetia for parietal and temporal lesions must be mentioned.

Visual Agnosia. Here the part played by the parietal lobe seems slight in lesions of the dominant hemisphere, in which occipital and temporo-occipital lesions are likely to produce object, picture, and color agnosia. As for spatial agnosia, its low frequency in left lesions cannot lead to any firm conclusion. However, it may be pointed out that it is highest in temporo-occipital lesions (15.4 per cent), exceeding spatial agnosia in parieto-occipital lesions (11.1 per cent), which is not in consonance with the observations of right lesions.

Aphasia. And now we come to aphasia in parietal damage. The part played in aphasia by posterior parietal damage has been recognized for a long time. As early as 1880 Dejerine[83] emphasized the importance of damage of the angular gyrus in alexia with agraphia, while later[82] he distinguished this type of alexia from pure word-blindness due to more posterior damage (lingual gyrus). In the "zone of language" that he defined, at the height of anatomoclinical efforts of the associationist age, the posterior part was made up of the angular gyrus representing the center of visual images of words.

Although Marie[257] considered that this region was part of the Wernicke zone, he did not accord any special role to it in the production of particular clinical aspects. Later

with Foix[258] he had to concede that there was aphasia of the angular gyrus with alexia predominating. Again Foix,[119] from his work on vascular pathology, described the symptoms of softening of the various terminal branches of the sylvian artery; parieto-angular gyrus softening (moderate aphasia of Wernicke with alexia predominating, ideomotor apraxia, and hemianopsia); temporo-angular gyrus softening (aphasia of Wernicke, ideatory, apraxia, and hemianopsia).

Amnesic aphasia was, of course, generally attributed to posterior lesions of the language area. Goldstein[143] although considering that it derived from a disorder of abstraction, thought that, when the damage was localized, its origin was in the parieto-temporal region. However, he thought only in terms of partial damage of this region since otherwise there would be disorder of the instrumentalities of language. Many authors including Hoff,[172] without necessarily accepting Goldstein's thesis, also localize the damage giving rise to amnesic aphasia in the angular gyrus.

Recent work on the lesional localization of aphasic symptoms also shows the importance of parietal injury. For example, studying aphasic patients injured during the war, Schiller[344] emphasized the importance of perseveration phenomena, of an expression disorder like stuttering, and of word and sentence distortion. Conrad[74] noted sensory aphasia after upper parietal and temporal damage. Bay[20] likewise considers that the region giving rise to sensory aphasia is mainly temporo-parietal. Russell and Espir[340] also conclude that the angular and supramarginal gyri are part of the "speech area"; any injury of this area occasions "central aphasia," that is, the form of aphasia in which all language mechanisms are defective.

Finally, Penfield and Roberts,[309] using the stimulation method, found that aphasic responses can be obtained from several zones: Broca's area, the supplementary motor area, the posterior temporal zone, and the posterior parietal zone; these two latter areas can be considered either separately or combined.

The most important area for language realization is the posterior temporo-parietal area composed of the posterior part of the temporal lobe and of the supramarginal and angular gyri.

The importance of the parietal region is also manifest in one of our series of cases of varying nature. Out of 162 cases showing left retrorolandic damage with sensory aphasia but not alexia, it can be seen that their frequency in parieto-temporal damage is 80 per cent but only 73 per cent in the case of isolated temporal damage. Even isolated parietal damage produces aphasia in 57 per cent of the cases.

We also have studied the intensity of the various aphasic symptoms according to the site and extent of lesions in 214 cases of left hemispheric damage. In isolated parietal lesions the average intensity of different disorders remains relatively low except for agraphia and lower than the intensity noted in isolated temporal lesions. However, comparison of the frequency of various symptoms in damage to both lobes at once shows that it is higher in parietotemporal lesions for verbal comprehension, repetition, and writing.

In comparisons of groups with and without damage to the parietal lobe, this lobe is seen to play some part in all aspects of language disorders considered. However, it is unquestionably positive only for agraphia. Although the frequency remains high for naming disorders, verbal comprehension, repetition, and reading, it is lower than in temporal damage.

The role of the posterior parietal zone in language mechanisms is thus securely established by anatomopathological data. However, do these symptoms have any special features? Several findings already mentioned seem to show that "parietal" aphasia is especially characterized in verbal amnesia, alexic disorders, and agraphia predominate in the setting of moderate sensory aphasia. There are likewise often expressive difficulties called parietal stuttering.

Dejerine[82] believed that damage to the supramarginal gyrus produces sensory aphasia, while damage to the angular gyrus produces alexia-agraphia. Foix[119] agreed with this and noted that, in addition, when there was suprasylvian damage to the supramarginal gyrus, there were also expressive difficulties not bearing upon simple sounds. He thought that this might be somewhat like ideomotor apraxia. As for amnesic aphasia, this is so often encountered in all types of brain injury in different loci that it is difficult to localize. This aphasic syndrome is frequently associated with bilateral asomatognosia, anarithmetia and figure alexia, and ideomotor and constructive apraxia. Whether these symptoms depend on a factor they have in common with language disorders or whether they are due only to the fact that the anatomical bases are close to each other is an open question.

There remains the problem of particular types of aphasia depending upon parietal damage. These syndromes should occur alone when damage is limited and be characterized by a more global aphasic syndrome when damage is more widespread. This had led us to study the problems of semantic aphasic, conduction aphasia, and agraphia.

(a) Semantic aphasia. Head[148] describes semantic aphasia as the inability to recognize the complete sense of words and sentences beyond the direct verbal sense, combined with the inability to grasp the sense of complex pictures and to recognize spatial positions and relations. Head attributed this to damage to the posterior parietal region.

Although many authors think that semantic aphasia is in fact only aphasia occurring on an intellectually weakened background, Luria[249] thinks it depends upon posterior parietal and parieto-occipital damage invading the language zone. Damage in this region would seem to render the subject incapable of "simultaneous synthesis." As far as language is concerned, such a disorder would be manifest as lack of comprehension of the logico-grammatical forms of language. There may be successful communication of events but not of relations. The abstract sentence can no longer be broken up into isolated elements, nor can it be built up again from isolated elements because of the loss of "complex simultaneous synthesis."

It is no longer, as in the other types of aphasia, the phonetic code of the language which cannot be used, but the semantic code. Thus, in Luria's opinion, although this aphasia does not come from a fundamental disorder in the Gestalt sense, it does nevertheless show the alteration of a particular cerebral mechanism, responsible for the function of "simultaneous and spatial synthesis," which is expressed principally in the visual spatial and kinesthetic domains, but which may interfere with language because of the extent of damage. This explains why semantic aphasia is associated with visuospatial disorders, constructive apraxia, acalculia, and finger agnosia. Luria thus agrees with the authors who, as we have seen for Gerstmann's syndrome, state that there is a basic disorder which is manifest in one or another domain according to the extent of damage, but which is always unitary in nature.

The notion of a functional zone which directs, coordinates, and controls several activities is therefore evident in a number of studies. The main difficulty seems to be rather in Luria's description of parietal aphasia. We do not think that parietal damage brings about alterations in the semantic code. When such alterations do appear, there seems to be a more general, more "intellectual" deficit depending not upon focal damage but, rather, upon diffuse or at least upon more extensive damage.

(b) Conduction aphasia. In our opinion this clinical form is much more typical of parietal damage. It was postulated by Wernicke[408] and gradually recognized at least as a complex of symptoms defined essentially by a positive feature (difficulty or inability in repetition tasks) and a negative feature (the absence of verbal comprehension disorders). Other features are literal and verbal paraphasia (recognized as such by the subject), writing and spelling disorders, and reading

disorders. It is a rare syndrome but there are now enough reported cases to make it sure that it occurs in this form without associated elements. There are often cases of aphasia which are very similar to conduction aphasia but which cannot be unequivocally identified as such because of comprehension difficulties.

Wernicke[408] thought that conduction aphasia resulted from damage of the insula by rupture of communication between the center of motor images of the word and the center of auditory verbal images, but this has not been verified by anatomoclinical cases. However, posterior parietal damage is constantly found. Temporal damage is also frequent, although slight and limited to the posterior part of T 1 - T 2. For Kleist[206] and Hoeft[171] the second transverse gyrus is responsible. Goldstein[143] and Conrad[74] maintained that this form existed as such and emphasized the importance of the time factor in it. Many other authors, however, have thought that it is a mere sequel of sensory aphasia or an association of sensory aphasia and motor aphasia.

It must in fact be considered as aphasia of the first articulation, namely, of the unit as defined on the level of the moneme, or the phrase, and of the sentence. The phonematic programming is, however, not impaired here as the phonic errors in emission depend on the word or phrase programming without any difficulty in the phonematic motor realization, as in the phonic programming aphasia.

Conduction aphasia does not depend on the channel used. Both written and spoken language are disturbed. Writing difficulties are more marked since there is transcoding. Reading aloud is severely disturbed, and written orders are carried out with great difficulty. This type of aphasia is a disorganization in the execution of the encoding program. Errors in spontaneous language are produced in the spoken chain at the places where there are sudden variations in the quantity of information. Length and variation of the quantity of information make disturbance greater in repetition than in spontaneous language. Repetition of items with meaning constantly shows fewer errors than meaningless items (different quantities of information), but errors progress according to the length of the word. In sentence repetition stumbling occurs particularly at the beginning of a new sentence because of the improbability of one sentence considering the preceding one. Thus, repetition tests encourage the appearance of this disorder, but repetition cannot be considered as linguistically autonomous and one cannot speak of repetition aphasia since there is parallel disturbance in all forms of encoding.

Despite its frequent association with amnesic aphasia, conduction aphasia is fundamentally different because of certain features, namely, the presence of phonic approximations in naming and especially the different behavior in the test of "opposites." Failures are exactly inverse in the two groups according to whether semantic opposites or morphological opposites are involved. The subject with amnesic aphasia fails the former test, which is easy for subjects with conduction aphasia, who, in turn, are incapable of finding morphological opposites, which are easy for subjects suffering from amnesic aphasia. At all phases of regression of the various disorders, the structural relation between them remains.

It would seem, therefore, that conduction aphasia represents an autonomous form of disorganization belonging to the class of expressive aphasia quite distinct from phonic programming aphasia (motor disturbance) and that it cannot be considered as a regression phase of sensory aphasia with which it has no structural relation. It represents an expressive aphasia which is to motor aphasia what, in the gestural field, ideomotor apraxia is to melokinetic apraxia. Such a relation is supported by the prevalence of posterior parietal damage in this form, despite constant association of temporal damage.

Kleist[206] suggested it might be "ideokinetic apraxia of sound formation," while others have thought that it was a disorder of the parietal junction involving verbal execution[204] or the capacity of concentrating attention on articulated sounds. But these authors still postulated a certain amount of associated sensory aphasia to explain the syndrome, while Hilpert[166] believed it was merely not being able to arouse kinesthetic engrams by sound and optical impressions. This "ataxic" disorder is in the field of parietal function. The neurolinguistic analysis of three very pure cases by Dubois et al.[92] confirms the specific feature of this language disorganization. It is also defined by several features which give it the character of sentence programming aphasia. It may be added that the analysis of three new cases of this type of aphasia have allowed us to confirm the preliminary observations.

(c) Parietal agraphia. Although there is nearly always a writing disorder, whatever the type of aphasia and wherever the damage within the speech area, quantitative and qualitative differences exist in these different types of agraphia. The role of parietal damage seems particularly important. Parietal agraphia has been recognized for a long time, its apraxic aspect being more or less important according to the author. The importance of parietal damage (supramarginal gyrus and angular gyrus) is also shown by our study of 214 cases of verified left hemispheric damage of varying etiology, the majority being cases of tumor and trauma. We have tried to quantify the disorders of the various modalities of language on a scale from 0 (absence of disorder) to 4 (complete loss of the modality). We must specify that we have considered only alterations of spontaneous writing or dictation but not of copying. For each of the topographical varieties of damage (site and extent), we have considered only an index of disorganization: the addition of the points for each case corresponding to each localization has been divided by the total number of observations with respect to this localization.

In the case of damage to a single lobe, the index of writing disorders is fairly high only for the temporal lobe (1.35) and the parietal lobe (1.13); when both these lobes are damaged, parieto-temporal (2), parieto-occipital (2), and frontoparietal damage (1.88) give the highest indices. In extensive parieto-temporo-occipital damage the index is as high as 3.66. Secondarily, in this same series we have compared the degree of disorder of two groups, namely, with isolated or nonisolated damage of this lobe as against no damage of this same lobe. The importance of the parietal factor is here distinctly manifest (2.11 as against 0.73), while elsewhere the temporal factor alone could be considered (1.78 as against 0.74).

The same analysis has been done on a series of unilateral hemispheric lesions similar to the former series but where not all the cases are verified. Here the different frequencies of the various clinical symptoms of the group with agraphia have been compared with those of the group without agraphia. It was found that four clinical groupings are especially associated with writing disorders: language disorganization (sensory aphasia and alexia); anarithmetia and figure alexia; apraxia, asomatognosia, somatosensory disorders and, perhaps, spatial agnosia; and finally intellectual deterioration. Thus, we have a clinical picture of a group of associations with their recognized origin in parietal damage. Of course, studies of this kind, where the qualitative aspects of the various types of agraphia are not dissociated, can only give approximations, such as the importance of parietal damage and the frequency of a group of clinical associations including praxic, asomatognosic, and somatosensory syndromes.

In order to better characterize agraphia in left parietal injury, we have reviewed our cases where damage of this lobe is accompanied by agraphia. It first appeared that, apart from acalculia, there was no constant association with Gerstmann's syndrome. The various types of apraxia and even constructive apraxia were in fact not constantly met in conjunction with agraphia although this was frequently the case. Association with spoken language disorders seems peculiar to this type of agraphia. But although the degree of agraphia is generally related to the degree of spoken language disorders, it is not necessarily so and there are some cases in which there is total agraphia but hardly any aphasia or alexia. It should be mentioned, however, that the praxic feature of the graphic disorder is then the most prominent.

Parietal agraphia is different from the writing disorders in sensory or motor aphasia in that it may not be considered as merely another aspect of spoken language disorders. The first thing to be noted is that there is often difficulty in tracing graphemes correctly (distortion, inversion of forms). The use of lettered bricks improves writing but without completely cutting out errors. In this respect, we must mention that we have not seen the special aspect of agraphia reported by Kinsbourne and Warrington[203] in Gerstmann's syndrome, namely, correct choice of letters to make a word but errors in combining these. Spelling faults are numerous and often considerable. There are also a great many iterations.

With a moderate degree of disorder the construction of a short sentence, despite considerable paragraphia, is relatively good and, in any case, there is no agrammatism as in the writing of motor aphasics. In contrast to sensory aphasia, the meaning of the message can also be recognized. Moreover, it should be noted that the patient often tries to help himself by pronouncing aloud what he wants to write down. There always seem to be faults in copying. There are the same distortions of graphemes, the same types of paragraphia, although to a lesser degree, as in dictated or spontaneous writing, whether there be alexia or not. As a rule, the patient can write only isolated figures or small numbers whether they be dictated or copied. Spelling is always affected.

The writing of one of our patients was quite typical of this parietal agraphia. He was of good sociocultural level and showed a

syndrome of right-left confusion, finger agnosia, and anarithmetia but without either
apraxia, alexia, or language disorders except
for some difficulty in finding opposites. His
spontaneous writing showed paragraphia
without syntactic disorders: "Je suis tombée
malade denmiche (dimanche) matin en reve-
nant du marché je ne suis pas, arrevené
(arrivé) à découper un cannaid (canard)
j'ai voulu coudré j'ai n'ai pas pu," while
there were numerous trials and much
crossing out. Again, dictation showed this
kind of paragraphia while respecting sentences ("collegies" for "collegues," "deve-
mui" for "devenue," "professeur" for "professeur," "sceencees" for "sciences," "soli-
tiatie" for "solidarité"). Such paragraphia,
though less frequent, was found in copying:
"digraises" for "disgraces," "leuir" for
"lieu," "assi" for "aussi," "mionde" for
"monde." "With lettered blocks dictated
words were spelled better; however, we found
"constitunion" for "constitution," "Mon-
archce" for "monarchie;" spelling was likewise very faulty (Charité: Chrite; Horloge:
Horge; regle: rege; Docteur: Doc).

Thus, in comparison with anterior and
temporal damage, writing disorders of parietal origin are distinguished by certain features: difficulty in making graphemes, relative conservation of the syntactic structure
of sentences, and combined disorders of all
writing modalities (spontaneous, to dictation,
copying). And it must be emphasized that,
despite the apraxic features of this type of
agraphia, it cannot be considered as dependent solely upon psychomotor difficulties.
There are always spelling disorders and, although writing may be improved by the use
of lettered blocks, they do not disappear.
Finally, oral language disorders, especially
amnesic aphasia, are almost constant.

Nor can parietal agraphia be considered
as merely the expressive element of a global
disorder of written language, since reading
disorders are not necessarily associated.
Alexia-agraphia is a frequent syndrome in
posterior-parietal damage (angular gyrus)
but this again is not a constant association.
Disorder in copying is not, therefore, completely and inevitably a disorder of visual
reception. It may moreover be noticed in our
anatomical studies that the degree of agraphia
and alexia is reversed according to whether
the damage is parieto-occipital or temporo-
occipital (agraphia = 2 and alexia = 1.6
in parieto-occipital damage as against 1.1 and
2.1, respectively, in temporo-occipital injury).

Integrity of the graphic encoding program
with gestural difficulties totally responsible
for the writing difficulties cannot therefore
be assumed even when there is a disorder of
the motor realization of the form of letters.
This disorder implies praxic disturbances
which are also often manifest in other fields,
especially construction. It is, in fact, a disorder involving the graphic encoding and
affecting both articulations of written language: graphemes, the motor scheme of which
is disturbed, and the organization of these
graphemes into graphic morphemes. The main
disorder may be considered as a disturbance
in the programming of the graphic message,
both in gestural execution and in the organization of code structures principally on the
level of the morpheme, the control which
provides the correspondence between phonic
and graphic structures having disappeared.

Summing up, it may be said that such writing disturbances consist in anarchical functioning of an activity which has acquired relative autonomy from spoken language and even
from reading, since copying is no longer
correctly executed. Symmetrical damage to
the right hemisphere, as we have seen, will
not interfere with phonic-graphic coordination but will disorganize the spatial aspect
of writing.

Are the inferences we have drawn here
from the study of our cases of agraphia in
posterior parietal damage of more general
value? Can this study, if such a disorder be
considered with reference to the disappearance of language as an organizer, give us
information about the mechanisms which
might account for disturbance in a certain

number of activities resulting from damage to the same cortical region? Faced with this series of symptoms brought about by posterior parietal damage, we have to raise again the age-old question: does this region represent a mosaic of functional zones of limited size or, on the other hand, does the destruction of this zone produce a fundamental disorder which is manifested in various fields? In the latter case, either our observational methods may be responsible for the predominance of symptoms of one particular sort or the basic disorder may show up more prominently in a given field because of a topographical extension of damage towards a territory more closely associated with a projection zone.

The discussion, which has opposed the moderate Gestaltists to the extreme localizationists on the subject of the dissociation of the aspects of Gerstmann's syndrome, is still open today. Of course, it no longer seems possible to think of a multiplicity of connecting centers but, rather, of a zone with a unique function but whose various connections would help us to understand how different extents of damage can produce different pathological pictures.

Observations in pathology favor the notion of control and organization bilaterally, but in the left hemisphere because of relations existing with the zone of language, it has a different and more general function. In the dominant hemisphere, integration of the sensitivo-sensory data must be executed in relation with, and through the mediation of, linguistic activities. Knowledge of parts of the body, of space, must be organized verbally in order to provide elements necessary for arithmetical, graphic, gestural, general, or constructive activity. Posterior parietal damage prevents the plan of the sequence to be accomplished. The liaison of the various kinds of apraxia, of acalculia, and of the syndrome of Gerstmann with language disorders seems to show that linguistic disturbance is predominant in the programming disorder that can be recognized in the study of conduction aphasia, "parietal" agraphia,

or ideomotor or ideatory apraxia. Considering the multiple type of symptom in lesions of this posterior parietal zone, it can hardly be a functional loss, while the global or partial character of the injury and differences in its propagation which involve the suppression of one or another afferent stream (kinesthetic, optical, vestibular, audio-verbal) may account for a single disorder, namely, a programming disorder expressed in various fields.

When damage is more particularly parietal, gesture and writing, knowledge of the body, and arithmetic seem more especially affected. Occipital extension brings about disorders in the recognition of pictures, letters, colors, and symbols. Temporal extension produces aphasia, which acquires the features of sensory aphasia as there is greater involvement of this lobe. Thus, the parietal lobe, and more especially its parts leading to the temporal and occipital lobes, seem to be a zone of polysensory integration for both hemispheres. The vestibular, visual, and proprioceptive afferents seem to combine to give forms on a higher level. But in the left hemisphere, it is as if language intervenes to control these primary integrations by imposing categorical principles on the data. Indeed, in the right hemisphere we have seen that damage of this zone gives symptoms in the same domains although they may differ in topography, intensity, or quality.

It is tempting to see only quantitative differences between the constructive performances of subjects with left or right damage. This concept is supported by Piercy and Smyth.[319] Yet certain features make us think that there may be a qualitative variation or at least that the disorganization of constructive activity does not have the same underlying functional disturbance. In right damage the disorder of sensorimotor elements is shown in the handling of spatial data, while on the left a programming difficulty may be suspected, such as is expressed in ideomotor apraxia and especially in ideatory apraxia.

If we consider somatognosic disorders, the difference likewise bears both upon the qualitative and the topographical aspect. Damage on the right gives contralateral neglect closely dependent upon nonintegration of the various streams of sensory information with one or another modality predominating according to the type of symptom. On the left the somatognosic disorder affects both sides of the body; here we have a disorder of naming or designation or, again, of differentiation of fingers or of parts of the body which are not ignored except in some exceptional cases which also have general intellectual disorders. Agraphia and acalculia are closely associated with finger agnosia; agraphia and amnesic aphasia are frequently associated. Writing and arithmetic disorders also appear in damage of the parietal lobe on either side, but in different forms: spatial disorders on the right, and disorders in the use of the graphic code, in recognition of the numerical code, or loss of the principle of arithmetical operations on the left.

Must we consider, then, that the right lobe is a weakened image of the left dominant lobe? This may be conceded for linguistic activities (agraphia, alexia), but the fact must be emphasized that it is the spatial arranging of signs that is disturbed. It must also be noted that a phenomenon as general as perseveration is particularly manifest in writing after right brain damage and gives the graphic disorder a peculiar character, increasing and exteriorizing the spatial disorder. In right occipital injury, reading troubles are also of a particular type while there is no disturbance in decoding of the written code.

Our results in a study of language realization in right hemispheric damage lead us to formulate some hypotheses on hemispheric dominance. Representations of language in the minor hemisphere seem to be a weakened image of those in the dominant hemisphere, but there seems to be symmetry only for the oral motor realization while writing and reading seem to be represented on the right only by their disposition in space.

Finally, the temporal lobe, which, when injured on the left, produces alterations of the reception of language, seems to play a very minor part, and perhaps no part at all, in the function of language when there is corresponding injury on the right.

It must also be remarked that functional asymmetry revealed by pathology seems, despite the absence of anatomical and physiological differences, to correspond to a different functional organization according to the hemisphere. Here we must bear in mind the conclusions of Semmes et al.[351] on somatosensory representation in the two hemispheres based upon the results of their quantitative examinations of brain-damaged patients. In the right hemisphere there is more diffuse representation, univocal sensitive quality, and contralateral representation in relation to the half of the body; in the left hemisphere there is focalization, separated aspects of sensibility, and a representation that may concern both sides of the body. Another argument favoring a different organization in the two hemispheres may be drawn from the anatomoclinical verification carried out with Angelergues[155] on 280 cases of verified unilateral retrorolandic damage. The findings of this study lead to the notion of left functional systemization with three relatively specific structural types (although they may interact with another): language itself centered in the temporal lobe; arithmetic, praxia, and somatognosia requiring verbal programming centered in the parietal lobe; visual symbolic functions (probably closely bound up with verbalization processes) centered in the occipital lobe. In contrast, in the right hemisphere functional organization seems to be both looser and more polyvalent and to concern a nonverbalized form of relations between the body and space; this functional organization has a substrate consisting of the whole of the parieto-temporo-occipital circonvolutions, where there seem to be two partially differentiated poles: one is parietal for arithmetic and somatognosia, the other is occipital for a certain type of visual recognition.

Does this different organization lead us to think that symmetrical zones of the two hemispheres have different functions or that they have different aspects of the same function? As indicated above, I favor the second hypothesis, at the same time admitting that right brain injury disorganizes the spatial reference of various activities while left injury causes disturbances of the systems of signs, codes, and categorizing activity. Thus we believe that an organizing role of verbal mediation in activities of the major hemisphere must be postulated.

We may also consider the hypothesis that there are topographically limited "zones of control" superimposed upon more global mechanisms which insure exercise of the language function, despite the greater or lesser extent of damage. These zones of control necessary for the use of language intervene also in other functions, as suggested by the predominance of damage to the parieto-temporo-occipital junctions in the different practognosic symptoms. The language programming subordinated to the angular gyrus and the supramarginal gyrus would seem at the same time to have a categorizing effect on gestural, somatognosic, and topographical performances. It also seems to permit the use of other codes such as the numerical sign code. Other zones of control which have their seat in temporo-occipital zones seem to insure this categorizing role for visual perception (letters, colors, objects).

In contrast, in the right hemisphere the sensorial data are integrated into zones less focalized than on the left because of the absence of direct liaison with verbalizing processes. Hence, the functions of these zones are confined to the representation of sensory events in their primary somatotopic integration (half-body and half-space), to the achievement of union with motricity, and to immediate recognition of the individuality of the elements of categories which are still present, thanks to the persistent organizing

action of verbalization on action and on perception.

(The following references, not directly alluded to in the text of Dr. Hécaen's presentation, contain further details of his procedures and findings.[151,156-158,256,318]

CHAIRMAN MILLIKAN: Dr. Benton, will you open the discussion?

DR. BENTON: Dr. Hécaen has presented a comprehensive survey of the clinical symptomatology of the posterior regions of the right and left hemisphere. Based upon his own extensive studies and a thoughtful review of the pertinent literature, it is a most impressive contribution. To do justice to the whole of it would require far more time than has been allotted for this discussion and, hence, it seems wise to focus on selected aspects of his detailed analysis. The topics that I should like to consider are, first, the possible meaning of some of the differences in performance observed in patients with right and left hemisphere lesion and then, more briefly, the question of the role of language as a determinant, or at least a correlate, of various parietal performances of an ostensibly perceptual or perceptuomotor nature. I have in mind such activities as visuoconstructive performances (that is, constructional praxis), writing, identification of body parts, and right-left orientation. Dr. Hécaen has considered both of these questions during the course of his presentation.

To take visuoconstructive disabilities ("constructional apraxia") as an example: he has pointed out that visuoconstructive disabilities are both more frequent and more severe in patients with right hemisphere disease than in those with left hemisphere disease. I can certainly substantiate his conclusions from my own observations. For example, in an investigation of the copying of abstract designs in patients with unilateral lesions,[25] I found defective performance in 23 per cent of "right hemisphere" patients as compared to 14 per cent of "left hemisphere" patients, a ratio of about 1.6 to 1. Studying the performances of brain-damaged patients on a three-dimensional block construction task, I found defective performance in 32 per cent of the "right hemisphere" group but in only 14 per cent of the "left hemisphere" group, a ratio of about 2.3 to 1.[26]

When attention is restricted to the occurrence of severely defective performances, the differences are rather more striking. I found grossly defective copying performance in 11 per cent of my patients with right hemisphere disease but in none of my patients with left hemisphere lesions (which is not to say that they may not be encountered on rare occasion). In our study of three-dimensional constructional praxis, grossly defective performances were shown by 16 per cent of the patients with right hemisphere disease but by only 5 per cent of those with left hemisphere disease. Thus, failure on this level by patients with left hemisphere disease is met with only on relatively rare occasions. Moreover, when a patient with left hemisphere disease shows gross defect on constructional tasks, one finds almost invariably that he also shows a considerable degree of general mental impairment, and this is not necessarily so in the case of the right hemisphere patients. In addition, the patient with left hemisphere disease who shows a severe constructional disability is also likely to manifest some degree of ideational or ideomotor apraxia while, as Dr. Hécaen has pointed out, these types of apraxia are practically nonexistent in right-handed patients with disease confined to the right hemisphere.

Many patients with right hemisphere disease show qualitatively peculiar constructions that reflect a neglect of the left half of space. Others may show the so-called "closing in" phenomenon, in which the patient fails to distinguish the model presented to him from his own construction and he utilizes the presented model in his construction. It is a matter of empirical fact that patients with left hemisphere disease rarely show a corresponding neglect of the right half of *their* constructions. By and large, neglect of the

contralateral half of space is a "right hemisphere" phenomenon.

The constructional disabilities shown by the patient with right hemisphere disease can be conceptualized fairly successfully in terms of impairment in the perception of spatial relations, this impairment being accompanied by (perhaps determined by) unilateral visual neglect. This conception is supported by the findings that these patients also prove to be defective in the performance of purely perceptual tasks (such as complex form discrimination) as well as in their performance on perceptuomotor tasks.

But what shall we say about the constructional disabilities shown by patients with left hemisphere disease? They are less frequent and less severe than in patients with right hemisphere lesions but they are not rare. We deal here with more than a few exceptional cases. There is no such thing as "crossed constructional apraxia" in analogy with "crossed aphasia" in right-handed patients. Do we deal here then with a basic visuospatial capacity which is mediated by both hemispheres? If so, why the difference in incidence and severity? As Dr. Hécaen has remarked, given the assumption that the abilities underlying visuoconstructive performances are mediated equally well by each of the hemispheres, one would expect an even higher frequency of observed defect in patients with left hemisphere disease, as compared to those with disease of the opposite hemisphere, because of the complication of thinking and language disorders in the left hemisphere group. But, of course, the reverse relationship is actually observed.

A number of solutions of the problem have been proposed. The most simple asserts that the observed differences between right and left hemisphere cases in respect to prevalence of perceptual and perceptuomotor disabilities is an artifact of case selection and that the right hemisphere plays no special role whatever in the mediation of these performances. The poorer performances of patients with right hemisphere disease are due to the circumstance that their lesions are larger than those of patients with left hemisphere disease *whom we select for examination*. Time does not permit discussion of the pros and cons of this argument which has been advanced by some neurologists. My feeling is that at the present time there is no strong empirical evidence for or against the interpretation. In any case, it is rejected by most students with strong involvement in this problem (including, as we have seen, Dr. Hécaen himself) and solutions of a more positive nature have been advanced.

One of these is that, while both hemispheres play the same qualitative role in mediating these perceptual and constructional performances, the contribution of the right hemisphere is more important from a quantitative standpoint. That is to say, the abilities underlying these activities are, as Piercy, Hécaen, and Ajuriaguerra[318] expressed it some years ago, "bilaterally but unequally represented" in the hemispheres. This hypothesis has a number of merits. It explains why these deficits should be more frequent and more severe in patients with right hemisphere damage, and, at the same time, it accounts for the awkward fact that impairment of at least moderate degree is not rare in patients with lesions of the left hemisphere. Now, on this view, there should *not* be qualitative differences in the performances of the two groups of patients, except perhaps as these may be a function of differences in overall performance level. (This last point has been rather neglected in analyses of the problem.) Nor should there be differences in the correlates of defective performances resulting from lesions in either hemisphere.

But there are empirical indications—rather scanty, to be sure—that, in fact, there are qualitative differences in the performances of the two hemispheric groups and that defects in performance have different correlates in these groups. It has been reported, for example, that it is characteristic of left hemisphere patients to draw better from a model than in response to verbal instructions; in

contrast, the two types of drawings tend to be equally poor in the right hemisphere cases. The drawings of patients with right hemisphere disease have been described as being complex and disorganized with the inclusion of many strokes or elements, while those of the left hemisphere cases are simple and primitive and include fewer elements. As we have heard, Dr. Hécaen interprets this difference as reflecting the operation of a perseverative factor in the performances of the patients with right hemisphere disease. Arrigoni and De Renzi[14] note that some of their patients with left hemisphere disease drew a cube as a simple square, while none of their patients with right hemisphere damage did this. Comparing the copying performances of patients with right and left hemisphere lesions, I found that the right hemisphere group tended to make relatively more distortion and omission errors, while the left hemisphere group tended to make relatively more displacement errors of a minor nature.

Turning to the question of the correlates of defective constructional performances in the two groups of patients, Dr. Hécaen has alluded to the study of Costa and Vaughan,[76] the findings of which suggested that there are higher intercorrelations among perceptual and perceptuomotor performances in patients with right hemisphere lesions than in those with lesions of the left hemisphere. I would comment only that these results should be considered as merely suggestive and that more searching inquiry is indicated. The number of subjects in this interesting study was too small to permit stable intercorrelational analysis, many elderly patients were included, and there was EEG evidence of bilateral dysfunction in some patients, particularly in the right hemisphere group.

In any case, these observations on possible qualitative differences in performance and possible differences in the correlates have led to the conception that in right hemisphere cases the visuoconstructional impairment is, as Dr. Hécaen has said, "part of a larger pattern of visuospatial deficit." On the other hand, in the left hemisphere cases impaired performance is due to a defect either in the execution or in the conceptualization of the task. In passing, it is interesting to recall that the recent emphasis on the "executive" nature of constructional defects in patients with left hemisphere lesion goes right back to the original formulation of Kleist,[206] who conceived of constructional apraxia as an inability to translate an adequate perception into appropriate motor action and who placed the responsible lesion in the posterior *left* hemisphere.

Thus, we have the concept that "constructional apraxia" in patients with left hemisphere disease is a kind of ideomotor apraxia, perhaps simply an attenuated form of ideomotor apraxia. And this brings us to the specific question of the role of language functions in these constructional performances. It goes without saying that by "language functions" we mean all that older authors used to call "internal language"—the use of symbols in thinking, not only symbolic formulation and expression but also symbolic understanding. Does the patient with left hemisphere disease have difficulty with perceptuomotor tasks because he cannot bring verbal-analytic processes to bear on their solution —to help in his analysis of the task and in guiding his movements? Dr. Hécaen's discussion of the parietal origin of Head's semantic aphasia is very much to the point in this respect. As we know, Head's concept that this is a type of aphasia has not been universally accepted. However, I think there would be general agreement that, in whatever category the phenomenon is placed, it represents a disturbance in thinking and especially in verbal thinking. Thus, when it occurs in the absence of overt instrumental language disorders, it would seem to be equivalent to what is often called "latent," "subclinical," or "minimal" aphasia,[315] that is, disturbances in higher level language functions such as grasp of complex propositions, memory for verbal material, verbal associative fluency, and verbal learning. If this betokens a deficit in verbal thinking, what is the relationship between the deficit (so often observed in ostensibly "nonaphasic" patients with left hemisphere disease) and perceptuomotor impairment? An overall positive association between general mental impairment and visuoconstructive deficit has been shown in a number of studies. Moreover, in our own investigations we have found that in patients with left hemisphere disease there is a closer relationship between the occurrence of constructional apraxia and decline in verbal intelligence (as evidenced by a significant discrepancy between the observed and the expected WAIS Verbal Scale IQ scores of a patient) than there is in patients with right hemisphere disease. But whether one has the right to interpret this relationship as causal in nature and whether it signifies the intervention of language processes in visuoconstructive performance remain unanswered questions.

CHAIRMAN MILLIKAN: Are there questions or discussion or comments?

DR. GAZZANIGA: We have demonstrated that our patients have the ability to perform a visual constructional task, that is, to draw a picture of a cube, for example, from the right but not from the left hemisphere, even though the left hemisphere proved able to distinguish verbally between correct and incorrect reproduction of such problems. It appeared to us, keeping in mind the studies on language presented, that each disconnected hemisphere is capable of comprehending the nature of the stimulus, but only the left is able to express language while only the right is able to construct these visual problems. Therefore, the results of these studies favor the view that lateral specialization exists but that it lies more in the motor executive or expressive sphere than in the sensory perceptual components of any performance.

DR. GESCHWIND: The left hemisphere could not do it? It just failed totally?

DR. GAZZANIGA: Yes.

DR. GESCHWIND: That was different from

our patient. In fact, his left hemisphere could perform constructional tasks.

DR. JON EISENSON: I would like to talk briefly on a paper of mine[104] which seems to have been forgotten—I forgot it too, and did not bring it with me. The paper touches on the matter of right brain damage and its relationship to higher verbal intellectual functioning. In my study, patients with right cerebral damage were compared with non-damaged, presumably normal controls in tasks calling for language comprehension and production on a relatively high propositional level. The subjects had to complete multiple choice and open-end sentences and to define words in "free" definitions as well as in multiple-choice written presentations. The levels of difficulty ranged from about that expected of an average 12 year old to about the level of the superior college graduate. Many of the items were highly abstract. Some of the sentences, for example, could be correctly completed, as in the Minkus items of the Stanford-Binet, only with an appropriate abstract word.

My findings indicate that the right brain-damaged patients showed definite decrement compared with controls who had no central nervous system involvements. A rather important exception were the women. I found that the women did not seem to show the same amount of linguistic and intellectual impairment following cerebral involvement as did men of comparable age. It took more than a cerebral lesion in the right hemisphere to get a woman to have any significantly measurable difficulty in productive language or in her comprehension of language. The men showed definite decrement. They also showed difficulty of word definitions, especially for abstract words. There were even differences in their definitions of concrete words. If we were to give quantitative scores for qualitative differences in definitions of the vocabulary on the Stanford-Binet items and the Wechsler, or higher scores for abstract definitions than for concrete ones, the right brain damaged persons would score lower

because they produced fewer abstract definitions than did the non-damaged persons. The males with right cerebral involvement tended to give a great many ego-oriented definitions. So, when asked "What is a gown?" we were likely to get "A gown is something my wife wears or wants me to buy for her and I won't." There was a marked tendency for an increased number of definitions of that type. They were acceptable definitions but not very good ones in regard to generalization of meaning.

DR. BENTON: I would like to comment on Dr. Eisenson's study. I think the findings can be reasonably interpreted as reflecting a blunting of intellect in the brain-damaged patient. I think the crucial comparison which needs to be made is between the right hemisphere patients and nonaphasic left hemisphere patients. When one does this, as Brenda Milner and others have done, one finds that the nonaphasic left hemisphere patient is more impaired than the right hemisphere patient. I do not think we can argue about the findings.

DR. EISENSON: This may be so. The other possibility is that to be abstract linguistically, we must use all the brain cells we have in both hemispheres. This may be another way of saying what Dr. Benton has already observed.

CHAIRMAN MILLIKAN: Other questions or comments?

DR. H. C. LANSDELL: I would like to raise an issue which has been assumed in much of this type of work—I think Dr. Hécaen made reference to it—that there are no known structural hemisphere differences. There is a little-known paper of Di Chiro[88] in which he reported on the venous phase of arteriograms; he was able to show that the vein of Labbe in the hemisphere for speech was noticeably larger than the veins of Trolard. He found the reverse in the other hemisphere: the veins of Trolard seemed to be larger than the vein of Labbe. His results were not right-left differences; they were related to whether or not the speech was in the right or the left hemisphere. That is to say, right hemisphere speech cases had the predominant vein of Labbe in their right hemisphere.

I am glad Dr. Eisenson mentioned the sex differences, because I made[217] a speculation suggesting that there are some left-right differences in the brain which become clear if you look at the sex of the patients. I analyzed Conel's work on four year old children[71] and purported to reinterpret his data to show that in the hand area there was greater myelinization in one hemisphere than the other, depending upon the sex of the subjects. He had concluded that there were no left-right differences. I suggested that if he split them according to male and female, he would find the males were one way and the females the other. I indicated that this might not be a chance relationship, because the left-right differences in two-point thresholds do differ between little girls and boys.[134]

Now I continue to look for this type of data, of course. I feel Connolly's[72] work is rather interesting: he showed that the left hemisphere was longer than the right hemisphere. He also went on to show that, incidentally, it was the reverse in women; but he neglected to discuss this reversal when he went on to generalize about the differences in the hemispheres. He was predisposed to see the longer left hemisphere as a result of the presence of speech. I would want to emphasize that there were differences he had ignored, depending upon the sex of the subjects. I also attempted[217] to interpret some of Matsubara's[262] work on arteriograms showing that in girls the Trolard tended to be predominant in one hemisphere and in adolescent boys it was the reverse. I admit this is all very speculative, but there are sex differences in language, and there may be some hemisphere differences that could be related to this. I would emphasize that the paper von Bonin delivered at the conference in Baltimore[39] was certainly astute in criticizing previous attempts to find hemisphere differences; but it is not necessarily so hopeless a problem.

I have indicated in some of our research[221] that you can get sex differences in left-right differences, particularly in noncognitive material. This should not be discussed here because we are concerned with language. I would like to point out that I find left-right differences more easily in male temporal-lobe cases; the differences are more difficult to discern in female patients. However, I should immediately retreat and say that the statistics of the differences are not very good. In part, it is almost wishful thinking on my part that the differences are reliable in the cognitive sphere. There is one experiment[218] in which I did find reliable differences in verbal ability, comparing pre- versus postoperative scores. The obvious result did occur in the males: the proverbs scores went down after left temporal removal. They did not go down in the female cases. That is the only result where there is a significant difference in the verbal sphere between the two sexes on the left-right phenomena.

DR. GESCHWIND: Dr. Lansdell has brought up the question as to whether the two hemispheres are different. I think that von Bonin[39] was a little too harsh on some of the older studies on this topic. We have had an opportunity to review some of these, in particular the work of Pfeifer,[314] who made a most important study and whose observations must be taken much more seriously than those of Connolly.[72] Pfeifer studied a large number of brains and came to the conclusion that there were gross anatomical differences visible to the naked eye between the left and right supratemporal planes. His descriptions of the supratemporal plane and the anatomical differences between the right and left sides are very detailed, and his paper contains several photographs which are very impressive. The only difficulty with his data was that unfortunately he did not record his statistics in such a way that one could be entirely confident that he was not picking selected cases out of the 50 brains studied.

His work was replicated by Economo and Horn,[97] a work also dismissed by von Bonin.

In a massive study of the cytoarchitecture of the temporal lobe these authors also discussed the question of gross anatomical differences and claimed to confirm Pfeifer's results.

My colleague, Dr. Walter Levitsky, and I have repeated this study. I am happy to tell you that we now have 96 brains, and somewhere in the next few weeks we will have 100 in which we are looking at the supratemporal plane on the right and left. It is our impression at this early stage that we have been able to distinguish some gross anatomical differences (which would not simply be related to sinus or venous drainage or to any of the other factors which lead to some of the minor differences between the hemispheres) between the two supratemporal planes.

The only interpretation of this difference, if it holds up, that I can think of would follow from Pfeifer's assertion that on the left the planum temporale (that is, a small region lying posterior to Heschl's gyrus in the supratemporal plane) is larger. The cytoarchitectonic maps indicate that this region is part of Wernicke's area, which is, of course, a region of auditory association cortex. The greater growth of this region on the left would be related to the pre-eminence of the left Wernicke's area in speech functions. I would stress again the tentativeness of these statements since our work is not yet complete.

DR. FREDERIC L. DARLEY: This is just by way of pointing out that when we re-examine brain differences with regard to sex, we should also take a very careful look at whether the language differences are significant. I think perhaps it is time for us to have a good, critical review of what we know about language differences between the sexes.

Look back at McCarthy's review of language development in Carmichael's *Manual of Child Psychology*[263] and look at what is there on sex differences. When we go back to the studies she reports to see whether there were significant behavioral differences, we find they are usually not significant; they are negligible. In those studies where differences were found, we usually find some explanation for them that has nothing to do with sex but has something to do with case selection, usually differences between the male and female groups with regard to socioeconomic status or intelligence.

Winitz,[415] studying kindergarten children, used a series of a dozen language measures, but on only three were there significant sex differences between boys and girls, the girls exceeding the boys. None of these were on measures generally regarded as of major importance in language development. I certainly am not master of all the literature on sex differences in language, and Dr. Lansdell may have much more information for us. But I think we need to re-examine statements that make us think that girls are linguistically ahead of boys and women are ahead of men.

DR. ETTLINGER: I would like to ask Dr. Hécaen a question: does he have from his own laboratory any systematic evidence which bears on the problem which was briefly raised earlier during the discussion, namely, the issue of defect in performance on language tests in cases of right-sided lesion? We can interpret language tests broadly and apply the fairly stringent criteria proposed by Dr. Benton (or maybe it would after all be permissible and advantageous to apply somewhat less stringent criteria and compare right-sided cases not necessarily with left-sided cases having lesions outside the speech areas but with subcortical cases or posterior fossa cases). I am asking this question because we do not really seem to have solved the problem which was raised by Professor Sperry regarding the successful verbal performance in the commissure cases when verbal inflow reaches the nondominant hemisphere. The question here seems to be, are language systems being used in the right hemisphere by Dr. Sperry's patients and do such systems exist in the intact human subject, or does the nondominant hemisphere make reference to language in the left hemisphere through some commissural pathway? I wonder if Dr. Hécaen can help us in this.

CHAIRMAN MILLIKAN: Would you respond?

DR. HÉCAEN: I can only say that with my language co-workers I have studied language realization in "right" patients. We found some disturbance in the phonologic code only if the lesion was in the parietal area. In contrast, with temporal lesions we found nothing. With parietal and occipital lesions we found, of course, reading and writing disabilities.

DR. PURPURA: I would like to ask Dr. Geschwind if he also plans to study the cyto-architectural differences of the lateral and posterior thalamic nuclei on both sides or whether the study will be limited to cortical regions.

DR. GESCHWIND: This might be a project for the future but is not immediately contemplated.

CHAIRMAN MILLIKAN: Dr. Hécaen, do you have further comments?

DR. HÉCAEN: No.

CHAIRMAN MILLIKAN: After a brief intermission Dr. Rossi will discuss "Experimental Analysis of Cerebral Dominance in Man."

Experimental Analysis of Cerebral Dominance in Man

GIAN FRANCO ROSSI
GUIDO ROSADINI

University of Genoa
Genoa, Italy

OUR TASK IS to discuss the contribution of experimental methods to the study of cerebral dominance in man. The first thing we did after having accepted the kind invitation to take part in this Conference was to look in a good English dictionary to find the exact meaning of "experimental." The answer in the dictionary was that an experiment is "something that is done under careful conditions to find out whether something is true or to discover something new."

Though worrying about our capacity to fulfill the task assigned, we thought it convenient to follow the trace indicated by such a definition. Accordingly we decided to confine ourselves to the presentation and discussion of findings obtained with technics specifically applied to the analysis of cerebral dominance in man. The results of the study of pathological as well as of neurosurgical material were therefore excluded.

So far the two experimental approaches which have been more largely followed and which have been proved capable of giving reliable information are those based upon direct electrical stimulation of the cerebrum and of hemisphere pharmacologic inactivation by injection of a barbiturate into the carotid arteries. The bulk of the results obtained with the first approach are due to Penfield and his associates.[306-309,330] These findings belonging already to classic neurology are well known and do not need to be summarized here. Barbiturate intracarotid injection, a method introduced by Wada in 1949,[394] though performed already in several laboratories[9,11-13, 16,23,47,79,139,181,299,310-312,332,336,337,355,376,378,379, 395,406] has given results which are not so well known and so extensively discussed as the other ones. For this reason and because of our considerable direct experience with this technic, we thought it convenient to center the present report on it. The body of the report will be based on personal results obtained by the application of the method over a period of five years on 126 patients. Part of the results have been already published.[11-13, 311,332]

LIMITS AND POSSIBILITIES OF THE SODIUM AMOBARBITAL TEST

Handedness and speech are the two best known brain functions generally regarded as attributes of hemispheric dominance. A hemispheric specialization is also admitted by the majority of neurologists, though not by all of them,[46,150,152,291,419] for some forms of recognition (gnosic functions) and of formulation and/or execution of a motor plan (praxic functions). The sodium amobarbital intracarotid injection cannot be of any help for the recognition and interpretation of

Supported by the Consiglio Nazionale delle Ricerche (Impresa di Elettrofisiologia) and by the Air Force Office of Scientific Research, European Office of Aerospace Research (OAR) under Contract AF 61(052)-901.

handedness. The limits and the possibilities of the method for the study of speech, gnosic, and praxic functions deserve a brief comment.

Speech may be regarded as the integrated whole of partial performances of several specialized brain districts. Many neuronal aggregates, having their own specific function, participate in the speech mechanisms. The so-called sensory or receptive part of speech is subserved by neurons having a topographical location and functional properties different from those of neurons involved in the motor or expressive mechanisms. Moreover, within the sensory mechanisms one must distinguish between those responsible for reception, understanding, and recall; likewise, the motor mechanisms include articulation, ideation, and so on. A global impairment of sensory as well as motor speech is likely to follow the functional inactivation of a large part of the dominant hemisphere produced by the injection of amobarbital into the corresponding carotid artery. The limits of the method for the analysis of speech mechanisms are therefore obvious.

The recognition and interpretation of gnosic and praxic disturbances require an elaborate neurologic examination. Some information can be gained by observing the behavior of the patient, but one must largely depend on his verbalization. The cooperation of the patient and, above all, time are therefore necessary to test these functions. As we shall see later on, the duration of the hemispheric functional inactivation following intracarotid amobarbital injection is limited to a very few minutes. The general experimental conditions make it very hard for the patient to collaborate with the examiner. Finally, the unavoidable disturbances of speech suppress any possibility of verbal communication when the injection is made on the dominant side. For all these reasons, we do not think the sodium amytal method is suitable for the exploration of gnosic and praxic functions.

It appears, therefore, that what one may ask of the intracarotid amobarbital method is to indicate whether speech, considered as a whole, is exclusively or chiefly represented in one side of the brain (to be considered, therefore, as the dominant one for this function) and which side is it. The validity of the method is supported by the beautiful study of Branch, Milner, and Rasmussen,[47] who compared the results of the intracarotid amobarbital test with those of direct cerebral electrical stimulation and surgical amputations. Furthermore, the method appears to be suitable to reveal functional differences between the two hemispheres independently of a dominance of one over the other. As we shall see, this possibility proved to be quite fruitful for securing evidence about hemispheric specializations hitherto almost unnoticed.

In consideration of the foregoing, our analysis was limited to the following points: (1) lateralization of speech mechanisms and its relation with handedness; and (2) possible existence of hemispheric specializations besides those for speech, gnosic, and praxic functions, and their relation with handedness and speech dominance.

METHOD OF INVESTIGATION AND MATERIAL EXAMINED

The standard examination was made by injecting 100-200 mg. of a 5 per cent solution of amobarbital sodium in 4-5 seconds. In addition, several attempts were made to analyze whether and in what way the results of the test might be influenced by changing the amount of the drug and its dilution and by slowing the speed of injection. No relevant differences were observed, with the exception, of course, of the quantitative relation between amount of the barbiturate (maximum tested: 300 mg.) and effects of the injection. The injection was made percutaneously under local anesthesia, in most cases into the first portion of the internal carotid artery, in the others into the common carotid artery. When bilateral examinations were performed, the right and left sides were usually explored on different days. Anteroposterior and lateral angiograms were made in most cases. The effect of the barbiturate injection on the capacity of the patient to count or answer questions and to keep his arms up in the air, on the knee jerk and plantar reflexes, and on pain sensibility were analyzed. The examination of the patient was protracted for at least ten minutes following the injection. The electroencephalogram was recorded throughout the whole experimental session.

The results of the intracarotid amytal test were considered reliable when (1) no abnormalities were present in the angiogram; (2) a clear-cut motor impairment occurred in the contralateral arm and limb (hemiparesis or hemiparalaysis); (3) slow, high amplitude waves appeared on the ipsilateral EEG recording; and (4) the motor and EEG effects were strictly unilateral.

There were 126 hospitalized subjects studied. In 49 of them the intracarotid amobarbital injection was made bilaterally, in 77 on one side only, for a total of 175 examinations. Forty patients were epileptic; 33 were affected by vascular diseases, 16 by extrapyramidal diseases, 11 by endocranial neoplasms, 12 by psychic disorders, three by vascular malformations, and 11 by various other diseases. The test was used either to determine the side of speech dominance before surgery or for diagnostic purposes, as, for instance, in some epileptic patients.[336,337]

HANDEDNESS AND SPEECH DOMINANCE

Several tests were applied at the beginning of our study to ascertain handedness. However, we soon become convinced that, as stated by Brain,[46] the simple tests were likely to give more reliable information than the elaborate ones. Handedness was therefore established by direct examination and by asking the patient and his relatives which was the hand preferred for carrying out familiar (as, for instance, the use of spoon and scissors, throwing a ball, etc.) as well as less common skilled movements. Some questions on foot and eye preferences were also made.

Out of the total of 126 patients considered for this research, 115 (91.2 per cent) were clearly right-handed and eight (6.4 per cent) left-handed; three patients (2.4 per cent) could not be clearly classified (ambidextrous?).

Speech dominance was considered to be located on the side where intracarotid amobarbital injection produced clear-cut aphasic disturbances. The effect appeared more or less simultaneously with occurrence of contralateral motor disturbances and ipsilateral slow waves in the EEG, almost immediately after the injection. One to three minutes thereafter the patient gradually resumed his ability to count and answer questions, though showing for some more minutes typical perseveration or paraphasia. As stated above, when speaking of the limits of the amytal test, we did not exert particular care in trying to analyze the type of the provoked aphasia. It is our impression, however, that, in the great majority of subjects, the impairment of the motor mechanisms of speech prevailed over that of the sensory mechanisms.

The patients utilizable for an analysis of dominance for speech totalled 84. In the other 42 subjects speech dominance could not be determined either because vascular malformation (as, for instance, arteriovenous aneurysms) or thrombosis altered cerebral circulation and, consequently, the distribution of the injected barbiturate, or because bilateral distribution of the drug occurred even independently of vascular abnormalities, or because the amount of the drug injected was too small to produce sufficient inactivation. Aphasia occurred in 91.6 per cent of the cases following left-side amobarbital injections (left dominance) and in 5.9 per cent following right-side injections (right dominance). In two cases (2.5 per cent) amobarbital produced the typical contralateral hemiparesis upon injection into the right as well as the left carotid artery; however, in one subject both injections failed to produce aphasic disturbances; in the other one, short lasting but clear-cut aphasia followed both left and right side injections.

The relations between lateralization of hand dominance and speech dominance were found to be as follows (Table 16): Right-

TABLE 16.

Speech Dominance	Hand Dominance			
	Left	Right	Bilateral	
Left	73 (98.6%)	2 (28.6%)	2 (66.7%)	77
Right	—	5 (71.4%)	—	5
Bilateral	1 (1.4%)	—	1 (33.3%)	2
	74 (100%)	7 (100%)	3 (100%)	84

Relationship between lateralization of hand dominance and speech dominance in 84 subjects given intracarotid amobarbital sodium injections.

handers: left speech dominance in 98.6 per cent of the subjects, right speech dominance in no cases, and bilateral representation of speech in 1.4 per cent of the cases. Left-handers: right speech dominance in 71.4 per cent and left speech dominance in 28.6 per cent. In the three patients considered to be ambidextrous the major hemisphere for speech was the left one in two cases; bilateral representation of speech was found in the other one.

The low number of left-handed and ambidextrous subjects makes the value of our contribution to the study of the relation between handedness and speech dominance very poor. Nonetheless, the following remarks can be made:

(1) Our findings add further support to the widely accepted view of the possible independence of handedness and speech dominance.

(2) Quite independently of their questionable statistical value, our findings appear at least sufficient to confirm that speech can be represented on the right hemisphere in left-handed persons. The percentage of right speech dominance in our left-handed patients appears to be considerably higher than that reported by other authors on the basis of the analysis of pathological material (see for instance[46,150,152,309,419]) and of the results of the amytal test itself.[47]

(3) Right dominance was never found in the 74 right-handers utilized for this analysis. This seems to confirm the diffuse opinion of the very rare occurrence of an ipsilateral representation of speech in right-handed people. In this respect, our results differ from those obtained with the same method by Branch, Milner, and Rasmussen,[47] who observed a right speech dominance in 10 per cent of their right-handed patients. However, these authors admit that their right-handers belonged to a particularly selected group, and, therefore, their findings probably do not reflect the handedness-speech dominance relation of the normal right-handed population.

(4) The occurrence, as well as the absence, of aphasic disturbances in the same subject upon left and right amobarbital injection indicates that there may be bilateral representation of speech in adults.

HEMISPHERIC SPECIALIZATION FOR MOOD AND EMOTION

In 1959 Terzian and Cecotto[379] noticed the occurrence of emotional reactions in patients undergoing intracartoid amobarbital injection. The most interesting aspect of their observations was that the emotional reaction had different characters according to the side of the injection: a "depressive-catastrophic" reaction followed the barbiturization of the dominant hemisphere, and a "euphoric-maniacal" reaction followed the barbiturization of the nondominant side. These observations were confirmed, to a large extent, by our results.[12,13,311,332]

Out of the total of 175 intracarotid amobarbital tests made in our Institute, emotional reactions occurred 73 times (42 per cent of the cases). Excluding the subjects with abnormal brain circulation and cases in which bilateral distribution of the barbiturate occurred, as well as cases in which doses of the drug too low to produce hemiparesis were used, this percentage increases to 53.7 per cent. Both types of emotional reaction described by Terzian and Cecotta were observed. The depressive type is characterized by a sad attitude of the patient and by his tendency to pessimism; the patient complains of almost everything: his health and the health of his family, his financial conditions, his work, and so on; he is convinced he will soon die and his family will go to ruin; he often starts weeping. The euphoric reaction is characterized at first by a relaxed attitude and then by the extremely optimistic view he takes of everything, by his smiling and making jokes, and by his breaking into actual laughter. In our experience the depressive reaction reaches an intensity rarely observed in the euphoric reaction. Both emotional states may have a duration of several minutes. After their disappearance, the patient, questioned on the cause of his peculiar behavior, is not capable of giving an explanation.

The appearance of motor, sensory, and speech disturbances is strictly related in time to the amobarbital injection. The time of appearance of the emotional reaction is variable; usually it becomes manifest later. This is particularly evident for the depressive reaction, which appears only when the motor, sensory, and speech disturbances are disappearing or have already disappeared. Furthermore, in 14 cases typical and clear-cut depressive or euphoric emotional reactions were produced with doses of amobarbital much lower than those capable of giving even a mild impairment of motor and sensory

functions and of language. Accordingly, no slow waves were present on the EEG, which showed normal rhythms or ipsilateral fast, low amplitude activity.

The sign of the emotional reaction (depression or euphoria) was related to the side of amobarbital injection in the majority of cases (Table 17). Taking into consideration only the patients whose mood was affected by intracarotid amobarbital, left-side injection produced depression in 62 per cent and euphoria in 38 per cent; right-side injection was followed by depression in 16 per cent and by euphoria in 75 per cent, and in four subjects (9 per cent) the right-side injection produced an emotional reaction difficult to define, containing manifestations of both depression and euphoria. In five subjects the same type of emotional reaction (in all of them euphoria) was given by right- as well as by left-side injection.

The relations between type of emotional effect and hand dominance shown in Table 18, were found to be depression following barbiturization of the dominant hemisphere, 68 per cent; of the nondominant hemisphere, 15 per cent; euphoria following barbiturization of the dominant brain, 32 per cent; of the nondominant one, 75 per cent. In 10 per cent of the subjects both depressive and euphoric signs followed barbiturate injection on the nondominant side. The amytal test

TABLE 17.

Emotional Reaction	Side of Injection		
	Left	Right	
Depression	18 (62%)	7 (16%)	25
Euphoria	11 (38%)	33 (75%)	44
Depression and euphoria	—	4 (9%)	4
	29 (100%)	44 (100%)	73

Relationship between side of intracarotid amobarbital sodium injection and type of emotional reaction in 73 subjects.

TABLE 18.

Hand Dominance

Emotional Reaction	Dominant	Non-dominant	Bilateral Representation	
Depression	19 (68%)	6 (15%)	—	25
Euphoria	9 (32%)	31 (75%)	4 (100%)	44
Depression and euphoria	—	4 (10%)	—	4
	28 (100%)	41 (100%)	4 (100%)	73

Relationship between lateralization of hand dominance and type of emotional reaction following intracarotid amobarbital sodium injection in 73 subjects.

was applied four times in the three patients classified as ambidextrous; euphoric reactions were always obtained.

TABLE 19.

Speech Dominance

Emotional Reaction	Dominant	Non-dominant	Bilateral Represen-tation	
Depression	15 (60%)	5 (15%)	—	20
Euphoria	10 (40%)	26 (76%)	4 (100%)	40
Depression and euphoria	—	3 (9%)	—	3
	25 (100%)	34 (100%)	4 (100%)	63

Relationship between lateralization of speech dominance and type of emotional reaction following intracarotid amobarbital sodium injection in 63 subjects.

The relations between type of emotional effect and speech dominance, shown in Table 19, were depression following barbiturization of the dominant hemisphere, 60 per cent; of the nondominant hemisphere, 15 per cent; euphoria following barbiturization of the dominant hemisphere, 40 per cent; of the nondominant hemisphere, 76 per cent. In 9 per cent of cases (three patients) receiving the barbiturate in the nondominant hemisphere, the strange mixture of depressive and euphoric manifestations mentioned above was observed. Finally, euphoria followed both left and right intracarotid injections in two patients supposed to have bilateral representation of speech.

The nature of the emotional manifestations following intracarotid amytal injection is difficult to interpret. The phenomenon does not appear to be related to the personality of the subject nor to the conditions of the examination; both depression and euphoria can be elicited in the same subject, during the same experimental session, by changing the side of the injection. On account of the relatively long latency of the emotional reaction and the fact that it is accompanied by electroencephalographic rhythms of normal or "activated" type, we think it unlikely that

it is the direct manifestation of cerebral inactivation. The possible appearance of emotional phenomena following injection of doses of amobarbital too low to produce any neurologic deficit supports this view. These findings, together with the inconstancy of the appearance of the emotional reaction and the fact that it is only rarely present following permanent organic brain damage, suggest that the development of the emotional states here described is due to neural mechanisms quite different from those responsible for motor paralysis and aphasia, namely, functional depression.

Summing up, the analysis of this group of findings leads to the following considerations:

(1) Although the intimate nature of the events observed cannot be explained at the present time, it remains a fact that the emotional state provoked by right-side injection was different from that following left-side injection in almost all the cases examined.

(2) We think that this indicates the existence of a hemispheric specialization whose characteristics are difficult to define but that we may provisionally call "emotional specialization" (that is, having to do with emotions).

(3) According to the results of our present analysis, the type of emotional specialization of the right and left hemisphere may be different in different subjects; nonetheless, there is a definite prevalence of depressive reactions following left-side and of euphoric reactions following right-side barbiturization.

(4) Similar remarks can be made for what concerns the relations between handedness and cerebral speech dominance and emotional specialization: depression following barbiturization of the dominant hemisphere and euphoria following the barbiturization of the nondominant one. We should not forget, however, that different from what appeared from the results of Terzian and Cecotto[379] and of our own previous research,[311,332] such a relation is valid in the majority but by no means in all cases.

The Question of a Hemispheric Dominance for Consciousness

Quite recently Serafetinides, Hoare, and Driver,[356] having used the intracarotid amobarbital test in 22 patients, stated that "loss of consciousness followed the termination of the injection almost invariably when the hemisphere dominant for speech was injected. On the other hand, similar loss of consciousness following injection of the nondominant hemisphere was rare, and of comparatively short duration." Accordingly, the authors suggested that "consciousness is in general linked with the function of the hemisphere dominant for speech." They interpreted unconsciousness following barbiturization of the dominant hemisphere as the consequence of the inactivation of the subcortical arousing system because of the sudden suppression of an important flow of cortico-subcortical impulses taking origin in the dominant cortex.

Transitory confusion or loss of consciousness following injection of amobarbital on the dominant side was mentioned in almost all the papers dealing with the intracarotid amytal test,[139,309-312,332,336,376,379,395] and specifically discussed by Terzian[378] and Alema and Rosadini[11] before the publication of the article by Serafetinides and co-workers. However, probably on account of its inconstance, its very short duration (5-10 sec.), and its possible appearance even following injection in the nondominant side, it was not given particular consideration.

For several years we have been interested in the neural mechanisms responsible for the changes of consciousness,[334,335] and the hypothesis put forth by Serafetinides and co-workers was indeed an attractive one. We decided, therefore, to analyze our material with the precise aim of checking whether reliable signs of a role of the dominant hemisphere in consciousness mechanisms might be found. We thought that to this purpose it was necessary to have at least one objective sign of the patient's degree of awareness. The general conditions of the examination and, above all, the fact that the suspected unconsciousness was likely to occur when the patient was completely aphasic, obviously complicated an evaluation based on the usual neurologic criteria. Several patients were therefore instructed to work a switch held in the hand ipsilateral to the intracarotid injection any time they heard a certain sound or saw a flash of light. Stimulus and response were recorded on the electroencephalogram.[10,11]

Figure 42 illustrates the results obtained in a typical experiment. The subject fails to work the switch at the very appearance of aphasia and contralateral hemiparesis but soon resumes his ability to perform; only a slight increase in the latency of the response can be observed. This result was considered as an indication that consciousness was not suppressed. This test was applied 17 times in 12 subjects, eight times on the left and nine on the right side. In no case was impairment of performance outlasting five seconds observed.

Independently of the results obtained with the particular examination just described, out of the total of 175 intracarotid injections performed, consciousness was clearly suppressed five times and probably suppressed ten times. In the five cases having clear-cut loss of consciousness, a bilateral distribution of the injected barbiturate was shown to have occurred (as revealed by the bilateral motor deficit and by the bilateral changes of the EEG); in all five cases the angiograms disclosed a contralateral thrombosis of the internal carotid artery, which was obviously responsible for the bilateral distribution of the injected amobarbital. In the subjects in whom a clouding of consciousness was suspected, though not clearly demonstrated, the amobarbital was injected on the left (dominant) side in five cases and on the right (nondominant) side in the other five.

To sum up, our results do not confirm the hypothesis of a prevalent participation of the dominant hemisphere in the mechanisms of consciousness.

CONCLUDING REMARKS

We gave to our report a very limited purpose, namely, the analytical presentation of the results of an experimental study of brain dominance in man. We had to discuss, first, whether an experimental approach to a problem of such complexity was possible, considering the enormous limitations that experimentation has when applied to man. The reply to this question is definitely positive. The information which can be obtained by the application of the intracarotid amo-

barbital method may be considerable. So far not much has been done to improve the method introduced by Wada several years ago. The conditions of the experiment and the analysis of the findings are still too rough. The technic needs to be, and can be, refined to become more fruitful and allow one to go more deeply into the nature of the phenomena under examination. Nonetheless, the results so far obtained are already sufficient to provide material which can be profitably utilized for analyzing the mechanisms of brain dominance.

The single groups of results presented in this report have been already commented

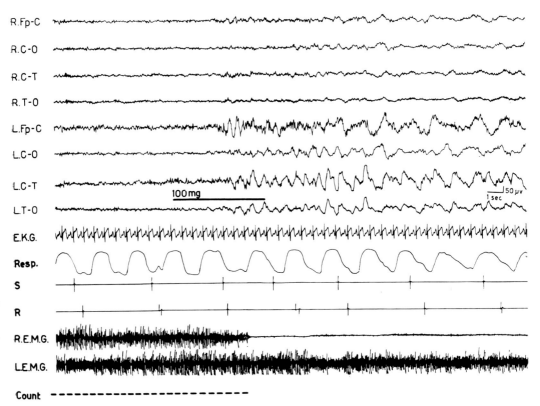

Fig. 42. Electroencephalogram of patient instructed to work a switch held in hand ipsilateral to the intracarotid injection any time he heard a certain sound or saw a flash of light. R.: right; L.: left electroencephalographic recording from Fp-C: frontopolar-central, C-O: central-occipital, C-T: central-temporal, T-O: temporal-occipital regions. E.K.G.: electrocardiogram. Resp.: pneumogram. S.: signal (tone). R., response of the subject. R.E.M.G. and L.E.M.G. electromyogram recorded from the right and left deltoid muscle. Count: subject is counting numbers. Injection of 100 mg. of amobarbital sodium into the left internal carotid artery marked by the horizontal bar.

on in the corresponding sections. We shall confine ourselves now to a brief comment on a particular aspect of brain dominance raised by the finding of what we have called "emotional specialization."

The term "dominance" expresses the idea of unequal capacities of the two hemispheres in a quantitative sense: the dominant hemisphere is that which governs, which controls, the other, the nondominant one. The same conception is at the basis of the other commonly used terms: "major" and "minor" hemispheres. In other words, for the function considered (for instance, speech), the dominant hemisphere "does the work,"[298] while the nondominant one is silent or capable of only rudimental activity. Actually, as far as speech is concerned, this is what seems to appear in the great majority of healthy adult men and is supported by the results of the intracarotid amobarbital test. Whether a similar type of interhemispheric relationship holds for some gnosic and praxic functions is not yet clarified. However, a dominant role of the right hemisphere in this field is generally admitted.[46,150,152,291,419] Summing up, the tendency is to ascribe to each hemisphere in the great majority of adult subjects a specialization in a particular field in which the other hemisphere has nothing to do, or performs only an ancillary or supplementary activity.

The emotional reactions which have been shown to follow intracarotid amobarbital injection add further support to the existence of hemispheric specialization. However, both hemispheres appear to play a role in the same functional field in the same subject. In our experience, this appears only very rarely for language; at any rate, even when both hemispheres appear to take active part in the language mechanisms, no sign of a qualitative difference between them is apparent. As far as emotional specialization is concerned, the result of the barbiturization of the two hemispheres is of different quality and not merely effect and no-effect, as in the case of speech specialization. As stated before, we do not know the nature of the neural mechanisms underlying the emotional reactions produced by intracarotid amobarbital, and we are fully aware of the great limitation that this factor poses to the discussion of these findings. However, the hemispheric specialization for mood and emotion appears to be independent of a dominance of one hemisphere over the other. If the suggested existence of hemispheric emotional specialization is accepted, the hypothesis can be made that there are functional domains in which the two hemispheres play qualitatively different roles, as opposed to the quantitatively different ones postulated for speech function. Furthermore, it appears that the specialization of the two hemispheres in the emotional sphere is of opposite sign: depressive reaction upon barbiturization of one hemisphere versus euphoric reaction upon barbiturization of the other.

To conclude, the analysis of the results of this experimental approach to the study of hemispheric specialization in man leads to the following considerations:

(1) There are cerebral functions for which only one of the two hemispheres seems to be responsible; the other one does not appear to take any relevant part in them.

(2) There are cerebral functions in which both hemispheres may participate, each one having its own role, opposite in sign to that of the other one.

We are thus confronted with the following problem: Shall we accept the existence of two different types of hemispheric specialization, or shall we try to explain all forms of hemispheric specialization in only one way? The question might provide a good starting point for a discussion among the participants in the Conference.

CHAIRMAN MILLIKAN: Dr. Morrell, will you open the discussion?

DR. MORRELL: I am really not sure I should have been chosen for this. I should take my cue from Dr. Pollack and say that I came prepared to discuss our own experiences with parietal amytal, but I would rather emphasize another point.

First I would like to say that these extraordinary results of Dr. Rossi are certainly worth investigation. We have not observed them, but our technic has been different, and I must say we certainly were not looking for them; at least we did not observe them any more than might be accounted for by the emotional reaction of the patient who finds himself or herself unable to speak.

What I would like to do in opening this discussion on the topic of "Experimental Analysis of Cerebral Dominance in Man" is to suggest that there are some other approaches one may take to experimental analysis of this problem, and to illustrate from our own studies some tentative approaches that we have made. This work comes from a larger-scale study dealing with computer analysis of evoked potentials and which is concerned with the question of whether or not evoked potentials convey some information or are correlated with the information content of the signal which evokes them. This work was done in collaboration with my wife, Dr. Norma Morrell, and Dr. Herman Bushkey.

The question of cerebral dominance can be looked at in another way. If one records evoked responses through the scalp by averaging technics and makes the proposition that the cortex which is activated—which is actively doing something—will be desynchronized or relatively desynchronized, then the response to random clicks might be expected to be different on the two sides, if the activated cortex were unilateral. In this procedure no response is required, the subject sitting comfortably in a chair and not being required to notice the clicks. We found that the response to the two sides was reasonably symmetrical. We did an independent replication of this experiment; it was gone through twice. This is the situation when the subject is not required to respond to the clicks presented in the environment.

Then the subject was required to listen to

a text being read to him. To make sure that he was listening to the text, at intervals the name of some funny animal would be thrown up, and he would be required to remember that name. He was presumably attendant to this language—if I may use the term—task, in the second group. We found that in two sets of averages of 100 each there was a difference between the amplitude of the evoked response on the left side and that on the right. The clicks, incidentally, were still being presented in a random schedule throughout this.

In the immediately succeeding experiment, the subject was required to count the clicks that were presented. Under those circumstances a different change occurred in the side-to-side relationships of the evoked potential wave and shapes, a change in which the left-sided response became much more prominent and had a slightly different relationship. This change was reliable from test to test.

Following this, the control series was again presented and the situation reverted to bilateral symmetry again.

We have used another procedure to see whether or not differences in the responses over the respective motor areas are different when the subject is responding with his right hand as opposed to when he responds with the left hand. The two sets of averages superimpose closely but not quite exactly. As a matter of fact, when the C-3 and C-4 derivation is taken, and these two electrodes are put into the two sides of the differential amplifier, a different wave shape is observed which, as a matter of fact, in this particular case turned out to represent positivity.

A different wave shape is seen in an experiment in which the subject is required to respond with the right hand to a click and with the left hand to a light. These two stimuli are presented in random order or alternating. In the random order situation the difference obtained represents response of the C-3–C-4 derivation to click with the right hand, indicating relative positivity to the right, and to light with the left hand, which potentially showed the reverse, consistently. Again, there were replications of the experiment.

One observation I must admit I do not fully understand yet. The difference noted was more prominent in the alternating situation, that is, the situation in which the subject could predict which signal was coming next, the light or the click. The difference in wave shape was much more prominent than when the click and light were presented randomly. Certain events proved to be the click; I am not sure about the light.

One of the things we have found consistently in the right-handed people we have examined is that when we force them to use the left hand, there is also a more pronounced change in evoked potential in the right hemisphere than the contrary condition.

CHAIRMAN MILLIKAN: Dr. Milner.

DR. MILNER: I enjoyed Dr. Rossi's paper. In Montreal Dr. Charles Branch and I have been greatly interested in the reports from Italy suggesting an affective specialization of the hemispheres, as indicated by the sharply contrasting mood changes elicited by left and right carotid-amytal injections. We had often seen mood changes, but they did not seem to us to bear any consistent relationship to the side of the injection, but rather to reflect the temperament of the individual patient. Thus, jovial patients tended to become markedly euphoric, whereas placid ones showed little affective change; depressive, catastrophic reactions were extremely rare. Nevertheless, stimulated by the Italian findings, we set out to record the direction and intensity of mood change after left and right-sided injection more systematically than heretofore. As will be seen, the results of this quantitative study confirmed our earlier impressions and were thus quite different from those obtained by Dr. Rossi.

What Dr. Branch and I did was to rate each patient's mood after the injection on a five-point scale, as "very euphoric," "slightly euphoric," "unchanged," "slightly depressed," or "very depressed," the standard of comparison being his mood before the injection was made. All patients were subjected to both right- and left-sided injections, the injections being made on different days. A standard dose of 200 mg. of 10 per cent sodium-amytal solution is injected over three seconds into the common carotid artery of one side, with the patient counting aloud slowly, legs flexed, arms raised, and fingers moving;[47] this dose is, of course, much larger than that used by Dr. Rossi and his associates.

We have just analyzed the results for 104 consecutively tested patients on whom such mood ratings had been systematically made. Forty patients (39 per cent) showed, as far as we could judge, identical mood changes after both left- and right-handed injection. Of the remainder, 39 (37 per cent) appeared to be more cheerful after left- than after right-carotid injection, and 25 (24 per cent) appeared to be more cheerful after right-sided injection. Nearly all changes were in the direction of euphoria only five depressive reactions being elicited, three from injection of the dominant and two from the nondominant hemisphere. Thus, we have no evidence linking depressive reactions to left-sided injections and euphoria, or elation, to right-sided ones.

On the other hand, on the question of loss of contact, or "loss of consciousness," such data as we have are in complete agreement with Dr. Rossi's observations, although we do not have his elegant technic. In brief, we find no evidence relating loss of consciousness after unilateral amytal injection to one or other hemisphere. Immediately after the injection is made, we stimulate the patient quite vigorously, both verbally and tactually, to ensure that he responds to our requests if at all possible. If the patient is silent, we make sure that he can squeeze the examiner's hand and move his toes on the noninjected side to command. We also have him demonstrate the use of objects, such as a comb or a toothbrush, which he may be unable to name. When a patient can comply with such requests, we would not consider his unconscious, although he may be mute. Nevertheless, in a certain proportion of cases we lose contact with the patient completely for a while and cannot get him to cooperate.

Loss of contact of one minute or more is a relatively rare occurrence; in 140 consecutive injections, we have observed it only 14 times, six times from the dominant hemisphere for speech and eight times from the nondominant. In all 14 cases the side of injection was contralateral to the side of the brain lesion, which, moreover, was apt to be a severe one. These observations seemed quite reasonable to us, since in such cases the patient was deprived by the drug of his one normally functioning hemisphere and was left with one badly damaged hemisphere. In addition, we have recorded 12 instances of brief loss of contact, all clearing in less than a minute. This effect was unrelated to the side of the lesion and occurred nine times after injection into the dominant hemisphere and three times after injection into the nondominant. This disparity is of no lateralizing significance, in view of the small proportion of cases involved.

Finally, since this Conference is concerned primarily with language, I would like to describe briefly some recent findings in patients appearing to have bilateral speech representation. In our original series of 123 patients in whom intracarotid amytal speech testing had been carried out, there were ten patients in whom some speech disturbance was produced by both left- and right-carotid injection and who were therefore classed as having bilateral speech representation.[47] Since then we have had another eight instances, making a total of 18 out of 212 consecutively studied cases. The phenomenon is clearly related to handedness, occurring in 17 of the 117 left-handed or ambidextrous patients but in only one of 95 right-handers ($X^2 = 12.26$, p $<.001$).

We do not think that this occasional finding of dysphasia after both left- and right-

sided injections can be dismissed as an artifact of unintentional spill-over of the drug to the contralateral uninjected hemisphere, for the neurological signs are clearly unilateral and the speech disturbance characteristically mild from *both* injections, despite a normal degree of hemiparesis. Moreover, we occasionally see qualitative differences in the dysphasia produced by left- and right-sided injections, a finding which could hardly be explained by spread of the drug to the other hemisphere.

We are, of course, only able to test speech rather crudely in the short time available, though we test it in various ways. We have the subject name a number of common objects presented in rapid succession, and have him repeat habitual sequences, such as counting forwards and backwards and saying the days of the week, forward and back. Misnaming (including perseveration and substitution), mistakes in serial order of days or numbers, and jargon are taken as evidence of dysphasia. Left-carotid injection in the typical right-handed patient is followed by mistakes in both naming and serial order, whereas right-carotid injection disturbs neither. However, in nine of the 18 patients considered to have bilateral speech representation, an interesting and totally unexpected dissociation between defects of naming and defects of serial order was observed. Seven patients made mistakes of serial order only after right-sided injection, and they made mistakes in naming but no mistakes in serial order after left-sided injection; two patients showed the reverse pattern.

The validity of this qualitative distinction between the effects of left- and right-carotid injection has been confirmed in some of our postoperative findings, the most striking case being that of a 15 year old left-handed girl, case J. Du., with an epileptogenic lesion of the right parietal lobe. On carotid-amytal speech testing, we obtained errors of serial order from the right-sided injection and errors of naming from the left. Dr. Theodore Rasmussen then made a radical removal of the right parietal cortex, invading the traditional parieto-temporal speech zone. During the first few hours after operation her speech was entirely normal, but within 24 hours she was making the same mistakes in repeating sequences as she had done after right-carotid injection. Both oral and written spelling (another verbal sequential activity) were also severely impaired, but she made no mistakes in naming objects. The speech difficulty developed together with weakness of the left arm, and receded with it.[283] Illustrations of this kind suggest to us that when verbal functions are bilaterally represented, the participation of the two hemispheres may, in some cases, be qualitatively different.

DR. HIRSH: Dr. Milner, I would like to ask if there were in some of your verbal memory tests ones in which a speech response was not required.

DR. MILNER: In the recurring, visual-verbal test modelled on the continuous recognition task of Kimura,[201] a verbal response of "yes" or "no" is usually required, but this is not obligatory. We have had aphasic patients with dominant frontal-lobe lesions do this test well, merely making gestures with the hand to indicate "yes" or "no." Free verbal recall tests, of course, require elaborate verbal output.

DR. HIRSH: Could you confirm the notion of dominance relative to this verbal memory? You take a person who is left-sided for speech. In this kind of memory task when the injection concerns the left hemisphere, does he fail?

DR. MILNER: Yes, patients with injections into the dominant, left hemisphere do not recall sentences they were able to repeat before the injection nor new ones given to them under the influence of the drug, although they can usually recognize them when tested a few minutes later. These are patients without any appreciable damage to the opposite, right temporal region.

DR. HIRSH: Thank you.

DR. JOE R. BROWN: Before commenting, I would like to ask Dr. Rossi if I understood correctly that one patient did not develop any aphasic response from injection of either side?

DR. ROSSI: Yes.

DR. BROWN: I postulated this possibility in a personal conversation with Dr. Rasmussen, and he said he had not ever seen it. I wonder if this particular patient was controlled so that you knew there was actually an EEG change in the hemisphere injected, and whether there were neurologic signs, so that you knew that the hemisphere was actually inactivated.

DR. ROSSI: Yes. This was indeed a particularly interesting case. It was a girl, 20 years old, suffering from epilepsy which could not be clearly classified, electroencephalographically characterized by diffuse, bilateral spike and spike and wave discharges. Pneumoencephalography and bilateral angiography were negative. The results of the amytal test were considered reliable because we could observe, following both left- and right-side injections, a clear-cut occurrence of contralateral paresis, actually paralysis, and a typical slowing of the electroencephalographic rhythms limited to the ipsilateral hemisphere. The cerebral hemispheres were certainly put out of function. Nonetheless, we could not observe speech disturbances. She stopped counting for a very few seconds (no more than 10 sec.) but resumed immediately the ability to count. This is, in our opinion, a negative response. We do not consider a suppression of counting limited to a very few seconds as an indication that speech mechanisms have been affected by the amobarbital injection.

DR. GREY WALTER: Dr. Rossi said in his last sentence that counting or failure to count is not a very good test of speech dominance. Many patients with continuous slow activity in the brain and, certainly, loss of contact may still count perfectly well but cannot talk. They count like a parrot talks. This seems to be more like the talking bird. I would doubt that the ability to count a series of digits is very much evidence of the full utilization of the so-called speech centers.

DR. LANSDELL: First I should comment that it is obvious that because Dr. Rossi's case was a female, he got no disruption.

Two years ago[220] we reported on the nature of what we called the dysnomic effects in the carotid amytal test. We felt there was a relationship between the object-naming errors and the nature of the initial phonemes in the nouns which should be used to name the objects. The initial phonemes tended to be more familiar, or more frequent in the language, when errors were incurred. We interpreted this to mean that there was possibly a failure of inhibition to select among the familiar phonemes.

I would like to report that my wife recently attempted[222] to extend these observations on naming in a study of 30 fairly intelligent normal people by putting them under the stress of speed. She used a film strip portraying 72 objects, and the pictures of the objects were transilluminated onto a screen about 7 by 5 inches. There is one other feature I should mention about the experiment. Every second frame was a picture of the word "and." The purpose of these "ands" was to "recycle" the verbal activity after the disruption of an error. The frame rate was one frame every 0.45 seconds. The errors that these normal people made did not correlate with the initial phoneme characteristic of the nouns. However, one result was similar in implication to the original research: the substitutions these normal people made had higher frequency phonemes than the correct nouns in the initial position.

There were two other results of interest: the number of phonemes in the words to be used in naming the objects was significantly correlated with the number of errors; and the Thorndike-Lorge word frequency measure[385] was also significantly correlated with the errors, that is to say, the high frequency words had fewer errors.

My point here is just to emphasize that it is possible to discern some phonemic aspects of the nature of dysnomic errors even in normal people. I think some day we may have enough cases to check our original result in the carotid amytal test.

DR. MAGOUN: I was interested in asking whether, by a nodding of the head or a sign with the unaffected hand, it is possible to check the ability of a patient to read written words or a text and see whether or not this capacity is preserved at the time when his ability to speak drops out during pharmacological block of the dominant hemisphere? I realize that, upon injecting the carotid, the more posterior parts of the hemisphere may remain unaffected since the posterior cerebral artery, deriving its major vascular supply from the basilar, may preserve normal function in this region.

Because of this, can reading ability be explored also during block of the ability speak induced by direct electrical stimulation of the brain? Moreover, in the latter case, can tests be made of the patient's ability to continue writing? In general, can an effort be made to test ability for reading and writing, as well as for hearing and speaking, in experimental block of speech mechanisms either by pharmacological means or by direct cortical stimulation in your studies?

CHAIRMAN MILLIKAN: Dr. Rossi, will you respond to this question?

DR. ROSSI: I think I said in the last part of our report that we fully realize that the intracarotid amobarbital method as it has been used so far, at least by us, is still too rough; it can certainly be improved.

I quite agree that examining the capacity of counting, and looking for the suppression of counting, is not the best way to analyze language mechanisms. In some subjects we utilized counting, but whenever it was possible, in those subjects who proved to be willing to collaborate and capable of doing so, we utilized not counting but answering questions. The questions, verbal questions, were presented to the patient before, during, and after the examination. This certainly gives much more information than counting. I do not know what can be done during brain stimulation, but I think it should be possible to work on patients reading questions during the examination. That could perhaps be done even during the amytal test.

DR. MILNER: With regard to reading, we do not attempt anything very elaborate. We do, however, give the patient a series of names of objects to read aloud. Here it is unusual to elicit mistakes, and, even when we do, reading aloud invariably returned to normal before other verbal responses. In fact, we have now learned that when a patient becomes mute after carotid-amytal injection the most effective way of getting him to start to speak is to give him some words to read aloud. In a few cases, we have also presented simple written commands, requiring the patient to point to a particular object in a group of objects, and this also patients were able to do at a time when they were still unable to count or name objects without error. We have attributed the relatively rapid recovery skill after carotid-amytal injection to the preservation of posterior-cerebral-artery function, a point just brought out by Dr. Magoun.

I would like to comment briefly on the possible usefulness of counting and other serial tasks in the demonstration of dysphasia. I agree, of course, that suppression of counting is not in itself sufficient evidence of dominant hemisphere dysfunction. Dr. Wilder Penfield has frequently pointed out that mere speech arrest (as observed, for example, during cortical stimulation or during a clinical seizure) does not suffice as a demonstration of aphasia. For this label to be applied, it is essential that the patient make actual mistakes in speech or writing. However, serial tasks are valuable tools in eliciting such errors. Mistakes in counting forwards or backwards, or in saying the days of the week (as when the patient perseverates, or gets the serial order wrong) are normally part and parcel of the dysphasic picture seen after left-carotid injection in right-handed subjects,

and follow the same time course as disorders of naming. They are also common features of the transient postoperative dysphasia which follows a cortical excision in the dominant hemisphere bordering upon speech areas.

DR. WILLIAM F. CAVENESS: Mr. Chairman, if I may make a more general comment, I would like to go back to a statement made by Dr. Chomsky who said that when man acquired a language, he acquired a system of abstractions. This is exactly what was said by William James. His actual words were that words provided the symbols for the crystallization of complex ideas and, further, that this provided the means of holding several such symbols in consciousness at once and reflecting upon them forward and backward in time. Professor James also said that this was probably the greatest difference between mentation in man and animals.

Marion Hines, Margaret Kinnard, Fred Mettler, and others have pointed out that one of the major differences between the anatomy of the brain of the macaque mulatta and man is the close juxtaposition of the primary motor and sensory areas and the lack of associational areas in between them. Also, they have pointed out how the frontal lobe is scooped out and, similarly, the temporal lobe. Regarding this very generous and diffuse associational area that man has acquired, I would like to pose a philosophical question: Might not that be the area in which to search for Dr. Chomsky's depth of language?

CHAIRMAN MILLIKAN: Are there other comments, questions, or discussion?

DR. MAGOUN: Coming back again to the emotional disturbances which were observed by Drs. Rossi and Milner, may I ask in what region of the cortex was impairment of function a factor in the manifestation of these affective states? I infer that they did not result from block of the speech mechanisms *per se*, since the patients were able to speak during the disturbance. It appeared that the disturbances occurred after the speech mechanisms had recovered from their anesthetic block. Do you have any insight as to what was the state of impairment of the cortex at the time that these hyperactive or depressive changes were at their peak?

CHAIRMAN MILLIKAN: Dr. Rossi.

DR. ROSSI: I am glad Dr. Magoun spoke about the emotional reactions, and, also, of Dr. Milner's remarks. I am sorry but the answer to Dr. Magoun's question, namely, whether we have any evidence pointing to a certain part of the brain, cortical or subcortical, as the most important site for the mechanisms responsible for the development of the emotional reactions observed, is a negative one.

We started two years ago analyzing patients with surgical amputations of different parts of the brain or with gross brain lesions. We wanted to see whether and in which way the emotional reaction developed upon amobarbital intracarotid injection and, if present, whether it was similar to that of comparatively normal people. The results of the study, however, showed that the development of the emotional reaction in these patients occurs more rarely than in the normal patients.[12] As I stressed when I presented our findings, we do not have any indication on the possible neural mechanism underlying these emotional reactions.

What about the fact that in Italy it is possible to observe emotional reactions while this does not seem possible elsewhere? This is, indeed, quite a problem. In some instances, the emotional reactions are dramatic, as you say here in the States. It is something which strikes everyone present in the room where the examination is performed, and this happens for the depressive as well as for the euphoric reaction. It is quite true that in many patients we did not observe any emotional reaction and in others there were only a few signs of them. However, we considered negative all the subjects in which the reaction was doubtful. Dr. Milner asked whether the presence or at least the type of the reaction could not be related to the personality of the patient. We do not think so, because, as I said, the two types of reaction may occur in

the same subject and in the same experimental session, only by changing the side of the injection. Therefore the personality of the subject does not seem to have a relevant role in the phenomenon.

What else can explain the fact that you do not observe these reactions while we do? You usually inject a larger amount of amobarbital than we do. However, our maximum dose was 300 mg., a very large one, and we still had the reaction. The phenomenon does not seem to be dependent on the amount of the drug injected. Differently from what occurs for the motor paralysis or aphasia, the emotional reaction can develop with very low doses of the barbiturate. I am sorry not to be able to give an explanation of such a difference. Perhaps I can invite you to Genoa to see what we call emotional reactions. It is well known that Italian people are particularly emotive. I do not know whether our positive findings are due to the fact that we work on material which is better suited than yours for the study of the phenomena under discussion.

CHAIRMAN MILLIKAN: Do you have another comment?

DR. MILNER: Only that I too am puzzled by this disagreement. Dr. Rossi's findings are very clear and point to the side of injection as a critical factor in determining the quality of the emotional response. Our own results are quite different, and it is difficult to see how a mere increase in drug dosage could account for the disparity. Incidentally, the reason we have emphasized the personality of the particular patient is that we have such similar results for the two hemispheres of the same individual. As for the intensity of the reaction, we have certainly seen extreme euphoria though rarely depression. However, our most euphoric patients seem to be those with frontal-lobe lesions and a chronic uninhibited cheeriness, which the drug enhances.

DR. EVARTS: I would like to comment on the emotional reaction to lysergic acid diethylamide (LSD-25) in normal control subjects in a situation in which we were administering a number of psychological and psychomotor tests. In this situation, in which they were busy with their tests, many subjects displayed little or no emotional reaction to the drug. It is well known, however, that LSD can produce a wide variety of emotional reactions when consumed in a different context.

I would like to suggest that the subject's general orientation, the experimental setup, and the type of motivation that the subject has, could greatly modify something like this. I would think this would be a fairly likely explanation.

DR. HÉCAEN: With relatively few cases, it seems to me I can confirm Dr. Rossi's findings, maybe because it seems to me that euphoria is really to neglect weakness during the injection. There is some relation between the two.

DR. GESCHWIND: I would like to stress slightly the point made by Dr. Hécaen. I do not think it is a rare clinical experience to see the patient with acute left hemiplegia who is unconcerned about it and is even euphoric. As Dr. Hécaen suggests, this is probably related to inattention. There is a curious difference among patients with left hemisphere lesions and aphasia in terms of emotional responses. This makes me wonder slightly about the possibility of the left hemisphere having a single emotional tone. It is striking that in the patient with Broca's aphasia and right hemiplegia the most common emotional response is depression. Even if you reassure such a patient he very often bursts into tears. On the other hand, the classical Wernicke's aphasics with fluent speech, very bad comprehension, and without a hemiplegia are quite different. They are not merely unconcerned but often quite actively euphoric. When people laugh at their errors, they laugh, and they do not seem to be disturbed by what is going on. I suspect that this is quite closely related to their failure to comprehend their own errors. By contrast, another group of patients with fluent, paraphasic speech but without comprehension difficulty

is quite different. This second group of patients generally are quite concerned, know they are making errors, and are generally depressed.

We have always thought that the reason for this is that the Wernicke's aphasic has no way of knowing internally that he has made an error. This group, that is, the Wernicke's aphasics can by contrast to the usual picture of euphoria manifest emotional agitation, as was pointed out by Adolf Meyer many years ago. The way in which they become disturbed is quite interesting. They almost never develop a simple depression but rather show bizarre behavior. They become angry with the people around them, and it often appears that they feel that the others are at fault in not understanding their speech.

Nearly every patient that we have had to transfer to the psychiatric service has had a grossly fluent aphasia. Dr. Rossi's patients, of course, became depressed after the aphasia has cleared, which may present still another problem. Certainly, the more anterior parts of the speech area would be those, one would think, more heavily affected by the amytal and thus depression might be expected more frequently.

DR. MAGOUN: I am reminded, by the elaboration that these affective states had their greatest intensity as the anesthesia was lingering, that, in some types of barbiturate anesthesia in man, there is, with a light dose, an excitatory phase, marked by conspicuous low-voltage, fast discharge in the EEG. I wonder whether Dr. Rossi has ever had the opportunity, at the beginning of his tests, to inject a light dose of anesthesia, which would only induce an excitatory stage in the EEG, and see whether this had any correlation with the appearance of these affective states?

The other question which I think all of us want to ask Dr. Milner relates to the nationalities of the patients at Montreal. Did only the phlegmatic Englishman come to McGill, or were excitable French-Canadians included as well? In general, is there any Nordic-Latin correlation in the situation?

DR. MILNER: About 20 per cent of the patients were French-Canadians, many of them very phlegmatic; a larger number were from the United States. There were two patients of Italian descent and they differed markedly from one another. One was a remarkably placid young girl from Rome, and the other a young man from the United States who, in contrast, showed great emotional lability. He was, in fact, one of the very few patients showing after carotid-amytal injection the rapid shifts of mood from one extreme to the other which Dr. Rossi reported as an occasional finding in his own series.

CHAIRMAN MILLIKAN: Dr. Rossi, will you respond to the question about the excitability of the EEG?

DR. ROSSI: Actually, in our experience these puzzling emotional reactions never develop when the slow waves are recorded in the EEG, or, to put it in other terms, they never develop when the EEG rhythms of the injected hemisphere are of the type recorded during surgical barbiturate anesthesia. It develops only when the EEG is normal or when fast, low-amplitude activity—typical of the low barbiturization—is present. Does that answer your question?

DR. GREY WALTER: I wonder whether anybody has tried this technic with intraventricular injection rather than carotid injection. There are several groups of workers, particularly in Sweden, who have been comparing the effects of intra-arterial and intraventricular injection of various barbiturates and they find striking differences. It just occurred to me that some of the effects, both the discrepancies between Dr. Rossi's and Dr. Milner's results, and some of the anomalies in the results themselves on both sides, might be due to variations in the blood-brain barrier properties of the drug, and this could be cleared up by intraventricular injection on the two sides.

CHAIRMAN MILLIKAN: Have you tried that, Dr. Rossi?

DR. ROSSI: We never have.

CHAIRMAN MILLIKAN: If there are no other comments, we will continue with Dr. Falconer, who will discuss "Brain Mechanisms Suggested by Neurophysiologic Studies."

Brain Mechanisms Suggested by Neurophysiologic Studies

MURRAY A. FALCONER

The Maudsley Hospital
London, England

WE HAVE in the brain two cerebral hemispheres which, in spite of Dr. Geschwind, I think are structurally identically the mirror images one of the other. A student or investigator coming new to the study of neurology might, therefore, presume that the functions of the two cerebral hemispheres are either identical or complementary. Yet we all know, or at least we are taught, that in right-handed persons (dextrals) the left cerebral hemisphere is "dominant" for speech, while in left-handed persons (sinistrals) either hemisphere may be dominant for speech but, again, more often the left hemisphere than the right. A long line of investigators, dating back to Broca and the Daxes, father and son, have established this.[77]

By dominance we mean that the cerebral control of communication by either written or spoken speech appears to reside in the dominant cerebral hemisphere. Some have even gone as far as to imply that the minor cerebral hemisphere, which is usually the right cerebral hemisphere except in some sinistrals, usually plays little or no part in speech functions. Yet Broca himself thought that both cerebral hemispheres played some part in speech, in particular, the faculty of comprehending the connection between words and ideas. Hughlings Jackson, although he accepted Broca's observations and confirmed them by some of his own, felt that both hemispheres were employed in speech and, in his classic paper "On the Nature of the Duality of the Brain,"[184] he stated his view that "the

right cerebral hemisphere is the one for the *most* automatic use of words, and the left the one in which the automatic use of words merges into the voluntary use of words—into speech." In a footnote he instanced a patient, presumably with a right hemiplegia, whom he knew could only say "no" when asked a question. This patient was asked to say "no" before a class but remained speechless. However, when asked the preposterous question, "Are you a hundred years old?" he replied "No." But when then asked to say "no" again, he could not.

I propose, therefore, to outline some observations which my colleagues and I have made which have a bearing on the speech functions of the two hemispheres and which lend some support to Hughlings Jackson's views. In particular, I wish to discuss those speech disturbances that commonly occur in psychomotor seizures of temporal lobe origin and to make a distinction between ictal dysphasia and ictal speech automatisms. This distinction is important because, whereas ictal dysphasic utterances usually are associated with seizures originating in the dominant cerebral hemisphere, ictal speech automatisms may arise with seizures originating in either hemisphere, and possibly slightly more frequently with seizures originating in the minor hemisphere than in the major. Many of these observations have already been published, but I shall draw them together in this paper, especially as there is little mention of ictal

185

speech automatisms in the Anglo-American literature.

First, may I discuss some definitions. Ictal dysphasia, as Serafetinides and I[354] defined it, is an inability on the part of the patient to express himself by the correct words while he is still conscious and without impairment of articulation or hearing. Dysphasic utterances, according to this definition, can occur at the start of a seizure, during a minor seizure if consciousness is not lost, or at the end of a seizure when consciousness is regained. A cardinal feature of ictal dysphasia thus is that it occurs during a period of awareness and is subsequently recalled by the patient. In this way we endeavored to exclude speech arrest and also jargon speech uttered during a period of confusion with disorientation, as we did not know how to differentiate it from mere vocalization.

Ictal speech automatisms we defined as utterances occurring at the beginning of or during an epileptic seizure of identifiable words or phrases which are linguistically correct but for which the patient is subsequently amnesic. We described five subtypes classified as warning, repetitive, irrelevant, emotional, or perplexed, and we excluded jargon. A patient at the beginning of a seizure might say, "Here it comes," "Hold my hand," or something like this; in the course of a seizure one of my patients, who had an aura that there was a man behind her back, would suddenly shout out, "I don't care what you do to me; I don't care what you do!" Subsequently these patients were amnesic for this type of utterance. Although there may be some qualitative differences in relation to the seizure between these various types of utterances, we grouped them all together because they reveal an ability and, indeed, an inclination to talk which is closely related to the ictus.

In this sense we regarded ictal speech automatisms as positive phenomena which, due to amnesia, can only be studied objectively, whereas ictal dysphasia we regarded as a negative phenomenon which, being remembered, can be studied both objectively and subjectively. Lennox[225] quoted John of Gaddesden as having recorded an ictal speech automatism—one of the earliest recorded instances of an ictal speech automatism—when he wrote in 1314: "And sometimes the paroxysm is short . . . then the patient himself stood up, recited the Lord's Prayer, spat once, and threw off the paroxysm."

In Table 20 I want to show you the overall incidence of the ictal speech automatism in 100 consecutive patients originally described by us in 1963.[354] These patients had temporal-lobe epilepsy, similar to those described by Dr. Milner and which met the following three criteria: first, they were all cases in which, before operation, a large space-occupying lesion had been excluded radiologically; second, all cases were resistant to drugs; and, third, they were all cases in which the temporal lobe, which was resected, had shown a spike-discharging focus. In some of them the spike discharge focus was unilateral; in others, bilateral. If it was bilateral, the spike focus had to be markedly dominant on one side before we undertook a resection. These 100 patients were collected between the years 1952 and 1961 and have been reviewed by

TABLE 20.

Type of Speech Disturbance	Left-sided Resections	Right-sided Resections	Totals	
Dysphasia	31*	4†	35	} in 68 patients
Speech automatisms	16	22	38	
No speech disturbance	13	19	32	
Totals	56	44	100	

Preoperative paroxysmal speech disturbance in 100 consecutive patients with temporal lobe epilepsy. (From Serafetinides and Falconer.[354])

*4 patients also had speech automatism.
†1 patient also had speech automatism.

from stimulating the temporal-lobe convexity, but stimulation of the amygdala through an indwelling insulated electrode immediately provoked a seizure during which he repeated his usual repetitive phrase several times. The corticogram at this period showed a recruiting discharge in the amygdala with desynchronization of all other electrodes. Later widespread abnormal activity appeared. The suprasylvian electrodes were not involved until after the ictal automatism had ceased. We then went ahead and resected the anterior 6 cm. of the temporal lobe including the uncus, amygdala, and anterior part of the hippocampus. Histological examination showed a well-marked mesial temporal sclerosis (hippocampal sclerosis plus amygdalar sclerosis). The patient had had only one seizure in the intervening three years, and this occurred 14 months after operation when he suddenly stopped his anticonvulsant tablets while on holiday.

Now I would like to discuss the significance of these ictal speech automatisms. There is general agreement in the literature that ictal dysphasia occurs with seizures originating in the dominant cerebral hemisphere, but few of us have written about ictal speech automatisms. Lennox[225] was one, and he did not attempt to lateralize them. Bingley[29] in 1958 reported having observed the phenomenon in 29 of 74 cases of temporal-lobe epilepsy due to causes other than neoplasms and found that it occurred slightly more often when the EEG focus was in the minor hemisphere than in the major.

Hécaen and Angelergues[154] in 1960 described similar findings. They noted in 32 cases of ictal speech automatism out of 208 epileptic patients that the EEG focus was situated in the right hemisphere in 13, in the left in 11, and in 8 undecided.

There are probably several reasons why ictal speech automatisms have been overlooked. First, they are usually overshadowed by other auras or features of the epileptic attack, and the physician is loath to accept as part of the seizure pattern features which do not fit in with his preconceived notions of the physiology of the brain. Second, the phenomenon to which I have been referring has been noted in the past but described in other terms. Gibbs, Gibbs, and Fuster[135] in 1948 described them as "automatisms" or "confused talking," and Feindel and Penfield[116] referred to them as "inappropriate speech," "irrelevant speech," or "irrelevant rambling speech." Some of my own colleagues who have seen these patients have labeled it as "dysphasia" without realizing that the patient was speaking in an amnesic state.

I would like to come back to the patient I just described because we were able to induce two seizures, one by intravenous Metrazol and the other by the stimulation of the amygdala. There seems to be a clear distinction between the epigastric aura which occurred at the commencement of the attack and the ictal speech automatism which followed within a few seconds, for he remembers the former but not the latter. Also I would like to remind you that the ictal speech automatism occurred at the state while the electrical seizure activity was still confined to the minor hemisphere and perhaps even to the minor temporal lobe.

There is another point of interest about our patient: his ictal speech automatism was in English, his fifth language, and not in Polish, his mother tongue. This is especially interesting because the general view is that, when polyglots become dysphasic, their mother tongue tends to be better preserved than their subsequently acquired languages. The only explanation that seems valid to us is that his initial fits occurred shortly after he came to England and at a stage when he was learning English. Further, most of them occurred while he was working in the company of his English workmates. This suggests to us that cultural factors may have had an influence on the form that his ictal speech automatism took.

Now, we do not know precisely where in the cerebral hemisphere speech arises. In their book on *Speech and Brain Mechanisms*[309]

Penfield and Roberts illustrate the three areas in the major hemisphere in which they think speech may originate: first, the conventional Broca's area, second, the Wernicke's area around the back end of the sylvian fissure, and third, the supplementary motor area (see Fig. 32). These are areas in which, at operation, speech arrest may be obtained by electrical stimulation. In two of these areas, Broca's area and Wernicke's area, lesions may lead to permanent dysphasia, but not in the supplementary motor area.

The myth has grown up that speech is originated in one or the other of these areas, but there is no proof of that. Perhaps in our cases of speech automatism with epilepsy originating in the minor hemisphere, the speech may originate either in these areas or in some other areas, such as the homologous areas in the minor cerebral hemisphere. It may be that, as a result of the ictal speech disturbance, either of these areas on the major and minor hemisphere is free but inhibiting the effects of epilepsy.

We cannot, therefore, decide on this evidence where the speech arose in these ictal speech automatisms, but we can speculate. First, the fact that in temporal-lobe epilepsy ictal dysphasia is almost invariably associated with seizures arising in the dominant temporal lobe suggests that the ictal discharges somehow or other interfere with the functioning of these traditionally accepted speech centers in the same hemisphere. They could not, to the best of our knowledge, influence the other, the minor, hemisphere.

In contrast, the neuronal discharges that occurred during ictal speech automatism, which I again remind you occurs in either hemisphere but slightly more often from the minor hemisphere, seem to leave the traditional speech centers in the major hemisphere undisturbed. It is tempting, therefore, to think that these ictal speech automatisms may perhaps sometimes arise in homologous areas of the minor hemisphere. I would remind you again of Hughlings Jackson's view which he held and wrote in 1874 when he said, "The

right is the half of the brain for the automatic use of words, the left for both the automatic and voluntary use." Perhaps his view is correct, and this flimsy evidence may support it.

CHAIRMAN MILLIKAN: Dr. Grey Walter, will you begin the discussion, please?

DR. GREY WALTER: Mr. Falconer has drawn attention to one of the most important features of our Conference, the relationship between voluntary, conscious behavior, on the one hand, and automatic or reflexive activity, on the other.

I would like to extend this discussion to other regions of the brain and other phenomena, more as a discussion of the general title of this particular session, that is, *"Physiological Mechanisms Underlying Speech,"* rather than of the details of Mr. Falconer's paper.

One comment which is directly relevant to his material is the question of the effect of lesions on polyglots. It so happens that the very first patient whom I saw 35 years ago in whom I was able to locate a brain tumor by EEG was also a Pole. He turned out to have a very large meningioma of the left frontal lobe which I was able to locate to the satisfaction of the surgeon. He was a Polish rabbi and before operation spoke only Polish to us, which we did not understand. But he had previously also spoken Russian, German, Yiddish, Hebrew, and English quite fluently.

The meningioma was removed by Mr. McKissock, and EEG was repeated. I spoke to him first in my very limited Russian, then in more extensive German, and finally in English. His recovery did follow the classical course, or at any rate the more usual one. First, he still only spoke his mother tongue as when he had his meningioma. After removal, he gradually recovered the use, first of Russian, then German, Yiddish, and Hebrew, and finally English. This is the usual sequence and shows there is some hierarchy of acquired habits.

I should like to speak of language rather as a special case of conscious (or perhaps voluntary, as Hughlings Jackson said) systematic, contingent adaptation. If I may define it in this way, I can discuss some of the recent discoveries we have made in relation to brain function in general terms, of which language is a special case which must obey the physiological rules for the management of such behavior.

We can enumerate some of these basic features as follows: (1) Dispersive convergence; (2) idiodromic projection; (3) contingent negative variation (CNV) or expectancy wave (E wave); (4) semantic responses.

These observations are derived from a number of experiments, some with implanted electrodes and some with scalp derivates on normal subjects. In relation to the topic of this session, we are mainly concerned with the superior frontal regions, which I am going to suggest to you are particularly in-

volved not only with language but in general with this process of voluntary, systematic, contingent adaptation.

The paradigm of these experiments consists of unconditional and conditional presentations in sets of 12 or so, with computer averages, and the complete conjugation consists of tests of habituation, association, and association with operant response. Then various games are played with the subject or patient. Many of these games are linguistic, in which the stimulus is not a flash or clock, as indicated here, but the provision of a word or sound or picture. These studies have been made far more interesting by the discovery that we can record and measure responses of the brain to purely semantic signals, that is, signals in which the information rather than the energy is the effective parameter.

Figure 43 illustrates two of the points listed: dispersive convergence of sensory responses in the frontal lobe, which is receiv-

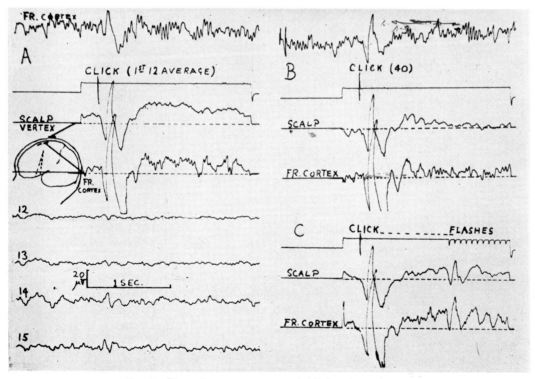

Fig. 43. Dispersive convergence and idiodromic projection.

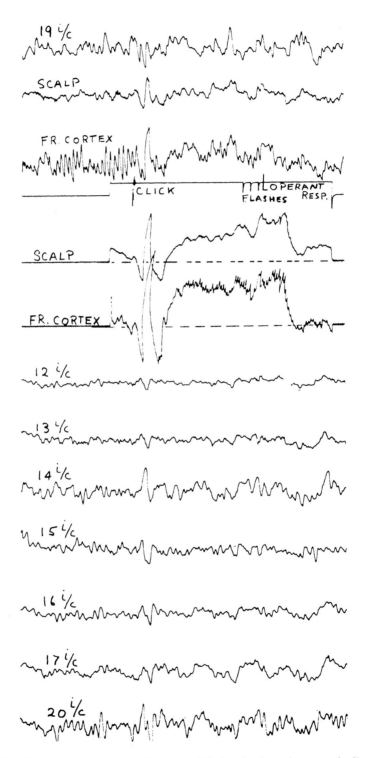

Fig. 44. Responses to associated clicks and flashes (scalp and intracerebral).

ing both auditory and visual information, and idiodromic projection: the signals are carried by private lines so there is no inter-modality occlusion in these nonspecific areas.

There are comparisons of scalp and direct brain recordings, and they also show the effects of habituation which remind us of the importance of the effect Dr. Magoun mentioned. The secondary features of these responses tend to dwindle if such signals are presented monotonously without engagement of the subject.

Figure 44 shows the responses to asso-ciated clicks and flashes when the subject is asked to do something about the flashes. This is of the utmost importance. If the subject is asked to press a button or say a word or take some action or make a decision and thus become engaged in some

way in the response to the second stimulus, a new effect appears. This is the contingent negative variation (CNV) or expectancy wave (E wave) which arises always and only (in relatively normal people) when there is a significant association between a warning stimulus and an imperative one to which the subject is impelled or required to respond.

Notice also, in many frontal regions, re-sponses to the conditional stimulus. Some of the intrinsic rhythms are also modified or temporarily suppressed.

Figure 45 shows records from the scalp in a normal volunteer subject with exactly the same features. The CNV builds up only after the subject has been asked to press a

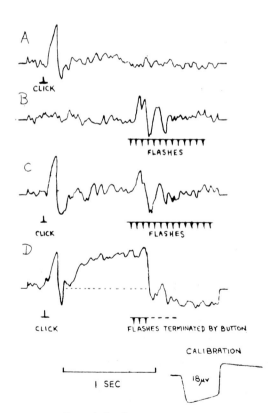

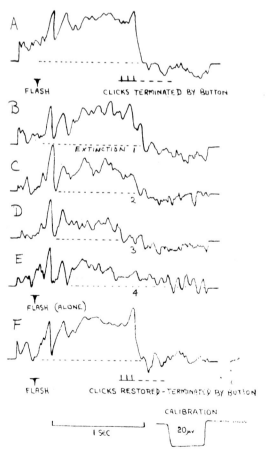

Fig. 45. Record (scalp, normal subject) of build-up of CNV. Figs. 45-47 reprinted from *Nature*.

Fig. 46. Decline of CNV with extinction.

button to stop the flashes. We think it may represent depolarization of the apical dendrites in the superior frontal cortex.

Figure 46 shows the decline of the CNV following withdrawal of the imperative stimulus, in this case with reversal of modality context. In the first "extinction" trials there is true conditional response, but this gradually declines with the CNV and is restored again by representation of the stimulus; the CNV follows, in fact, all the classical laws of Pavlovian conditioning.

Figure 47A shows what happens if the subject decides to be, as we say in England, bloody-minded and not to cooperate by pressing the button. The appearance of the CNV is contingent upon his willingness to press the button. Also (Fig. 47B), if one tells the subject beforehand in words what is going to happen, then the CNV disappears at once, while it took 20 or 30 trials to suppress it when there was no linguistic information. A single word from a trusted colleague is equivalent to 30 direct experiences.

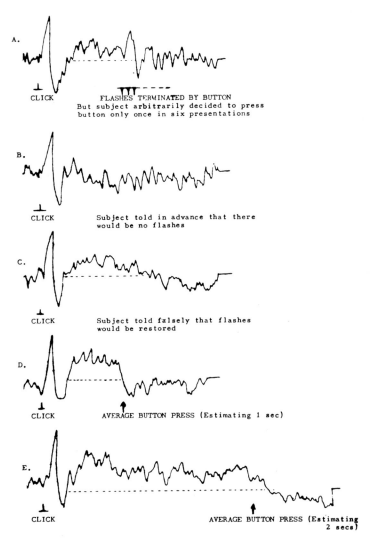

Fig. 47. A. CNV with arbitrary pressing of button by subject. B. Subject told in advance there would be no flashes. C. Subject lied to.

One can titrate the power of a word against the direct experience, as one titrates acid with a base solution. If you lie to the subject (Fig. 47C), in the first few trials he will respond to your suggestion as though the direct experience would verify it, but when he realizes you told a lie, the CNV disappears. You can balance the power of your word against his direct experience and assess the significance of verbal or linguistic signals in terms of the physiological stimuli.

If you dilute the significance of the conditional signals by giving partial reinforcement so that the probability of association falls to 0.5, the CNV will die away, and in the normal subject will mirror the decline in subjective estimate of probability built up by the subject that the conditional signals imply an event to which he must respond.

The rise and decline of the CNV in this sort of situation can be represented in a histogram (Fig. 48). This shows the gradual building up of the CNV over the first 24 trials, its diminution during probability dilution or equivocation and then during extinction. This can be repeated many times in a normal subject.

An important factor here is that we are not dealing with an intensity-related effect. Figure 49A shows the response to a very loud conditional click, with the evoked response, CNV, and the response to the imperative flashes when the subject pressses the button. Figure 49B shows the response when the intensity of the click is reduced almost to threshold. The evoked response is somewhat smaller, but the CNV is exactly the same because the faint clicks contain the same information as the loud ones. Taking this to the obvious extreme, the interruption of a continuous tone produces an "off" response of longer latency, and exactly the same CNV as before (Fig. 49C). This is evidence that the contingent variation is an effect dependent not on intensity or modality but only on significance of subjective information content.

We have also studied the effect of varying the interval between the signals. When this is shorter than 0.5 sec., the CNV does not have time to develop, but it appears sometimes as a series of slow waves over intervals of up to 20 sec. between conditional and imperative signals.

The general features of the CNV and its relation to mental state and response time in this sort of situation suggest that it may be an outward and visible sign of the cortical processes mediating short-term memory.

Since these effects are not related to intensity but to information content of the stimuli, we can use purely semantic stimuli with negligible or even negative energy content. With our rig the computers and projectors can be initiated by speech, either by the experimenter or the subject, and the

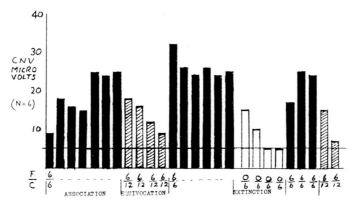

Fig. 48. Histogram of equivocation and extinction.

responses, particularly these long slow negative components, reflect the semantic impact of the words, both as isolated signals and in a conversational context. If the same word is repeated many times, the response dies away, but diverse or varied words or phrases maintain the response. When the signals are long words, in which the meaning, the semantic key, depends on the last syllable or phoneme, the late negative component is particularly pronounced. In effect, the first sounds of the word act as a conditional signal, evoking a response followed by a CNV which lasts until the end of the word. Furthermore, as Kornhuber and Deecke[209] found in relation to voluntary motor acts, when a subject decides to make a spontane-

ous voluntary utterance, his decision is *preceded* for about one second by a similar slow negative wave in the frontal cortex. This effect can be seen clearly only by playing tricks with the computer since the moment of a spontaneous act cannot, by definition, be found beforehand, but the Readiness or Intention Wave can often be seen even in the primary record.

We have studied these waves with radio telemetry also. We can affirm that they precede and accompany every conscious, spontaneous, voluntary decision and action, such as deciding to talk or walk, throwing or catching a ball, starting and stopping a vehicle, as well as in response to arbitrary external signals as in the laboratory.

This suggests that even an apparently chance impulse to act or speak is not a merely metaphorical impulse but a response to an internal signal, operating through the same mechanisms and subject to the same laws as the responses to the artificial physiological stimuli which reveal the statistical adaptive operations of the brain. Of these voluntary systematic contingent adaptations language is a special and perhaps for us the most important case.

CHAIRMAN MILLIKAN: Questions, comments, discussion?

DR. MASLAND: What is the distribution of that wave?

DR. GREY WALTER: It involves the whole of the superior frontal cortex, but in small patches all over, including only about 1 per cent of the available cortical tissue as far as we can estimate by comparing its amplitude with the size of maximal afterdischarges. The reason you see it is that it arises over a large area about the size of your hand. There is sometimes an indication that the CNV sweeps back toward the premotor zone from the frontal poles.

DR. PURPURA: This seems to be at least related to some of the components of D.C. shift one sees with many types of "novelty" activation of midbrain reticular systems and below. You say it is a depolarization phe-

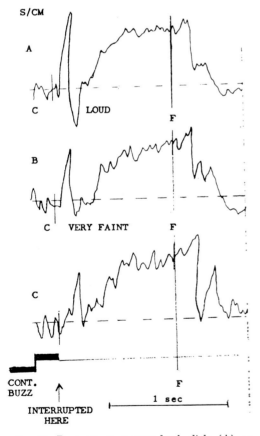

Fig. 49. Response to a very loud click (A), a very faint click (B), and the interruption of a continuous tone (C).

nomenon, involving presumably the apical dendritic system. Have you plotted this intracortically? Does the CNV have a turn-over point? What is its intracortical distribution?

DR. GREY WALTER: We have not used true microelectrodes but the potential field seems to turn over just below the surface and it is for this reason I suggested that it involves the uppermost layer of the dendritic feltwork.

DR. CAVENESS: Would you relate the list on the blackboard to what you said?

DR. GREY WALTER: Yes. You make me feel like Humpty Dumpty. By "dispersive" I mean that the information from the various sensory modalities, eyes, ears and somatosensory structures, is dispersed over frontal cortex so as to occupy only about 1 per cent of the available tissue in any one area, but is also "convergent" in the sense that the information from these sensory sources converges on one and the same cortical area.

The second feature, idiodromic projection, means literally that the sensory sources have private lines to frontal cortex; there is no interaction between these sensory inflows until they get to cortex and therefore there is no intramodality occlusion. It is like trains going on separate tracks; when they reach the platform at the terminus, their passengers mix up, but on the way the trains hopefully do not collide or interfere with one another. This is a very important point in the working of frontal cortex.

Third, Contingent Negative Variation is self-explanatory since the negative potential change at the cortical surface is contingent on association of sensory or internal signals and engagement of the subject. This phrase is bad for translation into French, German, or Russian and so we also call it the Expectancy Wave, which begs a question but gives the meaning.

Fourth, semantic response refers to the observation that the brain responds electrically to stimuli in which the energy is negligible or even negative. In physiologic work one usually deals with bright flashes of light or loud sounds or touches to the skin, but in this situation one can use signals which actually have less energy than the background. In some experiments we can actually measure the amount of selective information in the programs given to the subject, and the response is more or less a linear function of the selective information.

DR. CAVENESS: May I ask Mr. Falconer what the evidence was that this was not the dominant hemisphere.

MR. FALCONER: The Polish patient I described was, first, right-handed. Second, there never had been any dysphasic phases noted. Third, speech arrest was not obtained by stimulating his left temporal lobe at operation. He was not dysphasic after the removal of the nondominant lobe. I admit we did not prove by carotid sodium pentothal he was left-hemisphere dominant, but the other three points we think indicate he was left-hemisphere dominant.

DR. GESCHWIND: Several investigators working on polyglot aphasia in recent years have pointed out that the classical order is the exception rather than the rule. Lambert[213] in Montreal probably has done the most extensive work on this problem. He has found that it is not true as a general rule that the native tongue returns first. A much safer rule, though it is not absolute, either in Lambert's experience or in that of other people is that that language which is best preserved when the patient becomes aphasic is the language which he was using most and knew best just before he became aphasic. It is a common experience, at least among the bilingual French-Canadian population of Montreal, to find that English returns better in many of these people than French.

Even Lambert's solution may not be the final one. Thus, it is common experience that someone who has not spoken a foreign language for several years may require a few days to return to his previous state of fluency. Dr. Davis Howes (unpublished data) therefore decided that it was not reasonable to compare the two languages in polyglot aphasics until the patient was given a few days' practice in the less used language. Under these circumstances he found, by the use of his statistical measures of aphasic language, that the patient was equally proficient or, if you will, equally poor in both languages. On this basis, it is reasonable to suspect that some of the differences previously described in the performances in different languages by polyglots might be spuriously large, resulting from the failure to give the patient adequate practice in one of his languages.

A third factor, and one overlooked in the past, was brought out by Charlton.[60] He found that many polyglots have strong feelings about their languages and on emotional grounds may refuse to speak one language. Thus Charlton found that German refugees in New York may refuse to speak German even when their English is extremely poor, and this refusal may persist even when the patient becomes aphasic.

DR. ROSSI: At the end of our presentation this evening, we suggested that our findings of a development of the emotional reaction following amobarbital injection in each one of the two hemispheres might indicate that both hemispheres participate in the same function, the role of each one of them being opposite to that of the other hemisphere.

Now I would like to comment on the interesting case presented by Mr. Falconer. At the end of the presentation of this case, he raised the problem of the site of origin of the speech automatisms presented by his patient. They seem to have taken origin in the right hemisphere, the nondominant one for speech. Dr. Falconer suggested, if I understood him correctly, that the cortical region, or the brain region, involved was homologous to that of the dominant hemisphere. Is that correct?

MR. FALCONER: Yes.

DR. ROSSI: Let us suppose we have two epileptic patients, one having the epileptic focus in the dominant and the other one in the nondominant hemisphere; both patients show ictal speech manifestations. The ictal phenomenon arising in the nondominant hemisphere

manifests itself as a speech automatism, the ictal phenomenon arising in the dominant hemisphere as an ictal dysphasia. Is that correct? What is the difference between the two types of ictal phenomena? On one side in the case of the ictal manifestations arising in the nondominant hemisphere, we have a positive phenomenon, that is, speech: "I beg your pardon . . . I beg your pardon." In the other case we have a negative effect: we have impairment of speech.

Can we not try to relate this phenomenology to the one we presented today speaking of the emotional reaction, that is, that both hemispheres participate with an opposite role in the same functional field? In the case of the emotional reactions developing upon intracarotid amobarbital injection we see depression following barbiturization of one hemisphere and euphoria following barbiturization of the other. In the case of speech manifestations due to epilepsy, we see dysphasia, that is, impairment of speech, when the disease is in the dominant hemisphere, and ictal speech automatisms, that is, in a way, increase of activity or starting of activity of the language mechanisms when the disease is in the nondominant hemisphere. I do not know whether I have made clear my point.

I am looking to the possibility of finding in the results of this analysis of brain diseases affecting speech or language some support for the hypothesis we made to explain brain specialization on the basis of the effects we observed on emotion following intracarotid amobarbital, namely, that both hemispheres may take an active part in fulfilling a given function, each one having its own role, and that perhaps some brain functions are ascribed to only one hemisphere—considered, therefore, as the "dominant" one—on account of our inability to find out the part played by the other hemisphere.

This is not a question; it is just a comment. I wonder whether it could be discussed because, to me at least, it is an important one.

MR. FALCONER: First, a point of correction. Ictal speech automatisms we regard as positive phenomena, an attempt or an ability to speak, no matter whether they arise in the nondominant or the dominant hemisphere. They are subsequently recalled by the patient, whereas ictal dysphasia, which we regard as a negative phenomenon, occurs during a period of amnesia, is almost always associated with a seizure arising in the dominant hemisphere, and is subsequently forgotten.

I think you expressed what I tried to say when I said that where the speech arises is a matter of speculation. If we say that it arises in one of these traditional areas (Broca's area, Wernicke's area, or the supplementary motor area), the tradition is that it arises in the major hemisphere. Now there are homologous areas to those in the minor hemisphere, and we do not know their function. But, certainly, ictal dysphasia you could conceive as interfering with the traditional speech areas in the major hemisphere by a process of mere extension of the ictal discharges from the temporal lobe. The difficulty about ictal speech automatisms is they can arise in either hemisphere but more often the minor than the major. The difference is a ratio of about 6:5. It is not a very striking difference. In the case of ictal speech automatisms, which are really emotional, as you suggest, they are not remembered afterwards; their precise relation to the ictus we do not know, but they probably bear out the patient's mood during the ictus. It is, to me, not inconceivable that they could stimulate either the traditional areas in the major hemisphere or the homologous areas in the minor hemisphere. In ictal speech automatisms the speech is linguistically correct, whereas in ictal dysphasia the speech is incorrect. Certainly, they are both attempts at speech, but I think ictal speech automatisms lend some support to Jackson's view that, under certain circumstances, speech may arise in the minor hemisphere.

DR. MAGOUN: My questions may conceivably interrelate these two fascinating presentations of Drs. Grey Walter and Falconer, even though the topographic foci of their interests in the brain look distant. May I ask Dr. Grey Walter whether any interrelationship may exist between the surface negative variation of his expectancy wave in the superior frontal cortex and the conspicuous theta rhythm, which also involves variation in the polarity of dendrites, and which Adey[1] records from the animal hippocampus and temporal cortex during the expectancy phase of learned performance. Grey Walter's lyric description of his expectancy wave, as the outward and visible sign of an inward and spiritual memory, raises the further question of its relations to temporal lobe mechanisms which are proposed to be importantly involved in the processing of current information into storage, as memory, as well as in later recall. There are a number of indications that while the hippocampus and temporal lobe may be instrumental in the initial induction of memory, the long-time storage of memory and its availability for retrieval subsequently becomes much more widely distributed in the cortex. Is it in this sense that Dr. Grey Walter conceives of his expectancy wave as an expression of memory?

May I ask Mr. Falconer whether or not he believes that the hippocampus, on which I know he has done much work, is importantly involved in man in the formation of memory of symbolic speech and language, as distinct from that of signals from primary objects? Dr. Neilsen of Los Angeles once asked whether a second system may exist in man for laying down memories of the codes and symbols of speech and language, and one independent of the ancient hippocampal cortex whose phylogenetic age and stereotyped structure would not seem well designed for such a function. All the speech mechanisms that have been discussed at this conference appear to be distributed through the lateral temporal cortex and to extend farther laterally and dorsally into the parietal and frontal lobes, and hence to be quite distant topographically from the inferomedial temporal region which, in lower forms, is proposed to serve information processing and storage.[2]

I would welcome any responses which these questions may evoke concerning the storage of memory of speech and language in the cerebral cortex of man.

CHAIRMAN MILLIKAN: Would you comment?

MR. FALCONER: What you have said, Dr. Magoun, is an interesting speculation and one I had not thought of. As I take it, we all know that structures responsible for the laying down of memory include the hippocampal structures, the mammillary bodies, the connecting systems in the fornix tracts, and the mammillothalamic bundles. Certainly, as Drs. Scoville and Milner showed,[348] interference with the hippocampal structures bilaterally leads to stopping of recording of memory. Similarly, diseased structures involved with the mammillary bodies have the same effect. So that current memory seems to be laid down within those structures—current and recent memories.

With regard to the memories Dr. Penfield elicited by stimulation of the lateral temporal cortex, I think in most instances, he was working within the sylvian fissure, usually just with his electrode protruding into the superior temporal gyrus. Those were, I presume, remote memories he was recording. I do not know how many instances there were that he had, but they were not very great, and Dr. Milner can tell us, but I do not think it was more than five or six patients that he got these memories from. Whether these long-term memories were laid down in the superior temporal gyrus and were then activated into speech, I do not know. That is pure speculation. I cannot go further than that.

CHAIRMAN MILLIKAN: Dr. Walter!

DR. GREY WALTER: To illustrate the question Dr. Magoun asked, Figures 50 and 51 are a record of a patient with a chronic intractable anxiety before and after treatment. This is a polygraphic record from electrodes in the lateral frontal cortex and temporal lobe,

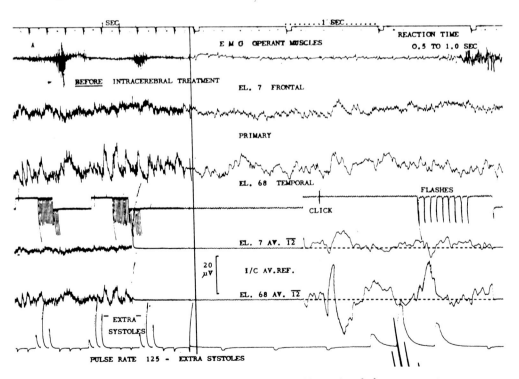

Fig. 50. Record of patient with chronic intractable anxiety before treatment.

probably hippocampus. Before the treatment this patient showed no CNV or expectancy wave, and the temporal lobe showed a large response to both conditional and imperative stimuli. Also the reaction time was long and variable, and the pulse rate was high with frequent extrasystoles. After the polarization of four electrodes in the orbital-frontal cortex, the temporal lobe's attitude to the situation was transformed and a CNV developed; as it developed, the temporal lobe imperative response disappeared. At the same time, the operant response became rapid and regular, the pulse rate fell, and the extrasystoles vanished. This is a rule in all subjects in whom we have been able to make this examination, that when the expectancy wave is well developed in the frontal cortex, the temporal lobe no longer has to worry about imperative stimuli. It concerns itself with the implications of the conditional response. I think this may be connected with the function of the temporal lobe as memory store. The clin-

ical features are also instructive in such cases. The figure is from a patient who had been almost paralyzed by fear for some years, but she had been referred to us as a profound depression because of apparently mute indifference which turned out to be due to profound chronic anxiety. When treated by electrocoagulation of selected supraorbital regions according to the treatment we developed in Bristol, she became fluent and composed and chatted quite freely.

If the temporal lobe is preoccupied with moment-to-moment transactions with direct physical stimuli, it cannot engage in the complicated function of speech. If it is relieved from this job in a situation in which there is a CNV, then it can cope with the speech functions.

Next with regard to the intrinsic rhythms in the brain, we have ample evidence that, in those few people who show the effect, the coherent after-rhythms in the brain occur in those conditions in which a CNV or expect-

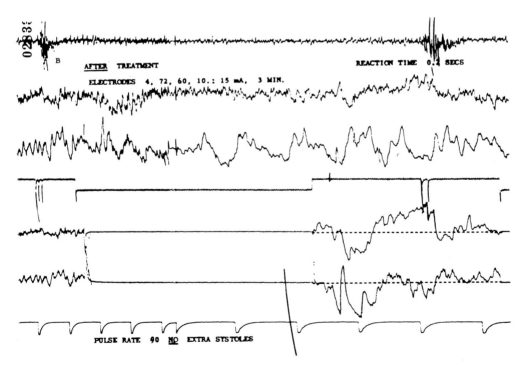

Fig. 51. Record of patient with chronic intractable anxiety after treatment.

ancy wave develops. We have records which show the coherent after-rhythm that Brazier[48] and Barlow[15] described several years ago developing in conditions in which the expectancy waves occur; as the wave subsides with equivocation or distraction, the coherence also diminishes in the occipital cortex. We have one or two cases also in which the hippocampal rhythm also appears in the same conditions in which the expectancy wave occurs. Perhaps this is a sign of how the brain interrogates its memory core when the significance of an association has been established.

DR. MASLAND: I have two different comments. It is incorrect to think of the point where memory is laid down, or the point where speech arises. I do not believe that the chart which Penfield and Roberts have presented was presented by them as depicting the point of origin of speech. I believe it was a chart of the areas where stimulation or destruction interfered with speech. I think these are quite different issues.

In respect to the individual who experienced repetitive action as a result of seizure in the temporal lobe, I wonder if this is not comparable to the individual who experiences a programmed movement of some kind as the result of a focus in the temporal lobe. In this instance, certainly, we do not feel that movement originates in the temporal lobe but, rather, that the activity of the temporal lobe has in some fashion set in motion a train of events which probably involves the entire nervous system and that, in fact, we may be dealing with a mechanism of recall or activation. Such a concept is quite different from the thesis that this particular area of the brain is specifically involved or concerned with the complicated, integrated process which ultimately evolves.

Similarly, in connection with the question of memory, I would feel personally that there is much evidence to suggest that the storage of memory involves probably the entire central nervous system, and that the temporal lobe areas are those areas which are involved with

the processes whereby this alteration of the nervous system takes place, rather than that this is the point within which this trace, whatever it is, is stored.

The other point which intrigues me is the nature of the expectancy wave. I wonder whether this might not have something to do with the time sense. I am intrigued by this gradual build-up of a change of state. I think we are all concerned with the magnificent mechanism which the animals have through which they are aware of the passage of time.

It is possible that some process of this type, taking place gradually over a long period of time, may in fact be the mechanism whereby changes take place which are recognized by the individual as passage of time?

DR. GREY WALTER: Yes, I think Dr. Masland is quite right. When we first observed this effect about four years ago, I was convinced it was some kind of leak from the time base of our oscilloscope; it had the same saw-tooth waveform, with a slope varying according to the time interval between stimuli.

I am tempted to regard this as one of the ways—not necessarily the only way—in which we estimate short-time intervals, of the order of half a second up to half a minute. In fact, in experiments in which all the subject has to do is to estimate time, merely to decide when, say, ten seconds have passed, one can see this wave build-up over ten seconds ±2, and then cut off shortly.

I would suggest the hypothesis that this is one of the time-base systems in the brain, another one being the regular coherent rhythms which are sometimes superimposed. These may be the actual ticking of the clock, of which the cut-off of the CNV is the chime.

CHAIRMAN MILLIKAN: Dr. Falconer, would you comment about the matter of the origination of speech?

MR. FALCONER: Dr. Masland, you are correct. I thought, in my paper, I did say that those areas that were mapped out in Penfield and Roberts' chart are the areas from which they obtained speech arrest, and

Broca's and Wernicke's areas were the areas from which they obtained dysphasic errors that persisted with permanent lesions. However, they did not persist with lesions of the supplementary motor area.

I went on to say that it has become a myth that that is the area from which ideational speech might originate. Certainly, in Penfield and Roberts' book that was the term they used for those areas. We do not know where speech originates, but we know that lesions in those areas, Broca's area and Wernicke's area in the major hemisphere, will produce permanent dysphasia. Where speech originates, I really do not know. I just tried to speculate, that in some circumstances speech might arise within the minor hemisphere.

CHAIRMAN MILLIKAN: Any last comments or questions? We will now have a discussion of "Lacunae and Research Approaches to Them."

Lacunae and Research Approaches to Them. I.

HANS-LUKAS TEUBER

Massachusetts Institute of Technology
Cambridge, Massachusetts

CHAIRMAN MILLIKAN: On this final day of our Conference four individuals have been scheduled to participate in a discussion of "Lacunae and Research Approaches to Them." Dr. R. D. Adams is not here. Dr. Masland kindly consented some days ago to replace Dr. Adams. The format will be to have the individual presentations, each of them to be followed by comments, if you care to make them, or questions. We will first hear from Dr. Teuber.

DR. TEUBER: Mr. Chairman, my mandate, as I understand it, was to listen to this Conference with a vow of silence; to list the lacunae, the gaps in our understanding of brain mechanisms and language; and to think of experiments that might fill these gaps.

There were three themes in our discussions throughout this Conference: we spoke about processing of linguistic input, its central elaboration, and the patterning of output. I submit that these themes are the gaps that have become apparent, the three lacunae in our understanding of language in its relation to the brain. This may sound like an expression of despair, as though we had learned nothing throughout this Conference; but I believe, on the contrary, that much has been gained by pointing at these gaps. In fact, what we heard can form a framework for new investigation.

Lacunae are windows through which one can look at the work that needs to be done. Besides, the windows that were opened appear

to face in the same direction: problems of input, central processing, and output have formal similarity, so that solutions for any of these problems would go a long way towards illuminating the others.

To guide our discussion I have listed three themes, or gaps, together with three sub-headings for each; this gives us nine points which shall be taken up in sequence,

I. Input Processing
   A. Distinctive features and syntactic rules as "innate releasing mechanisms"
   B. Reality of linguistic segments
   C. Possible physiologic mechanisms

II. Central Elaboration
   A. Cross-modal and supra-modal processes
   B. "Transfer" within systems
   C. Relation between hemispheres

III. Problems of Patterning of Output
   A. Active vs. passive movement
   B. Corollary discharge and related postulates
   C. Physiology of voluntary motion

I. INPUT PROCESSING (RECEPTION)

Here we are facing our first lacuna and we must admit that it gapes rather widely: we simply do not know how the listener manages to analyze the stream of speech, structures it into phonemes and morphemes, and comprehends strings of sentences according to syntactic rules. Nor do we seem to know

204

how this understanding of speech, on all levels, is acquired by the normal child; and unless we understand that problem, we cannot even begin to understand what happens when these achievements break down in the aphasic, in the presence of lesions in the brain. The paramount importance of modern linguistics, in this connection, seems to me to lie in the following: the linguists are beginning to specify what it means to have language, to perceive it, and to produce it.

The achievement of the ordinary listener and speaker, in any given language, is staggering.[67,68,185,194] It differs from the problem posed by the imitative capacities of mocking birds, and the precise antiphony of shrikes, by the fact that in man comprehension as well as production of speech entails the use of generative rules which every child discovers for himself, for his mother tongue, during the optimal period for first-language learning, even though no child, and very few adults, can describe these rules. For that matter, many of these rules are only now being discovered by linguists. How then does the child proceed in acquiring phonemes and morphemes and grammatically ordered strings?

This Conference has reinforced my belief that for an answer to this question we cannot turn exclusively to psychophysical experiments nor to conventional theories of learning. Admittedly, the former tell us a good deal about the structure of phonemes, and the latter attempt to deal with any form of learning and thus claim to explain first-language learning like any other. Yet, if we consider what is understood in comprehension of speech, we are forced to turn, I believe, from psychologists to ethologists with their emphasis on unlearned, fixed-action patterns, specific for particular species, and the corresponding innate releasing mechanisms, the IRM's, which represent genetically determined structures in the nervous system, ready to receive certain specific stimulus configurations that call forth particular action patterns. These IRM's thus represent, in a sense,

innate ideas, residing in a given nervous system as a product of evolutionary selection; they are as characteristic for that species as a particular plumage for a bird, or a particular disposition of fins for a fish.

This radically nativistic view of language is not restricted to myself and my immediate colleagues. It has been forcefully propounded by Chomsky[66] and Lenneberg.[224] If it had not become apparent before this Conference, it has become clear during the last few days that linguists are ethologists, working with man as their species for study, and ethologists linguists, working with nonverbalizing species.

The tasks facing every human language user are so complex that some important aspects of language cannot be learned but would have to be innate (a point made by Chomsky). Which particular language will be acquired by any given child still depends on what language he hears spoken around him, but some essential features of language —presumably those considered by current linguists as universal features of language— may well be innate in the strict sense of that term. In this view, each normal child comes equipped with a special apparatus for apprehending phonemes, for compounding them into morphemes, and for segmenting the stream of speech according to some syntax.

The corresponding apparatus in his nervous system is plastic enough to acquire any language, during the critical period, and to acquire any of the possible languages with essentially equal ease. Aphasia, in its varied forms, would then be a breakdown of this central apparatus. Yet such a claim, besides being radical, is empty unless we can define experimentally those features of language acquisition, on phonemic, syntactic and, perhaps, semantic levels, that defy present-day stimulus-response theories of language, and unless we can make at least some conjectures about the central machinery and its physiologic action. We believe that this can be done, at least in outline form, so that this particular lacuna might be filled.

A. *Distinctive Features and Syntactic Rules as Innate Releasing Mechanisms*

Our discussions have underscored what a staggering task it is to understand how we understand language. There is the problem of phonemes and their recognition. Work has been reviewed which shows the wide range of tolerance for a great many variations in those acoustical structures which distinguish one morpheme from the other, combined with an intolerance for certain critical changes which mark the transition from phoneme to phoncme. It further appears that in the normal child many phonemic distinctions are made on the receptive side *before* the child can produce these same distinctions in its own linguistic output.

Actually, much more information is needed on this particular point; we need to explore the order in which phonemic distinctions appear in the child's perception of speech (is it the order based on increasing numbers of distinctive features?) and the order of their appearance (subsequently) on the output side, in the child's own utterances. Pending the acquisition of such data, however, I would like to venture a guess: it may well turn out that certain universal features of human language[145] such as the patterning of phonemes in terms of distinctive features, are innate.

Experiments are now in progress in our departmental laboratories, based on these assumptions; in some of these, normal infants listen to tape recordings of phonemes and also to acoustical patterns that do not represent phonemes in any language. We expect to be able to demonstrate a predisposition for differential response, possibly in the autonomic nervous system, to these two classes of acoustical events. These experiments attempt to do for the earliest stages in speech perception what the ethologists have done for the study of certain key complexes—the eyes and body contour of the owl, as a releaser of mobbing reaction in chaffinches would be one example. It represents a search for innate releasing mechanisms, just as recent work by Fantz, Hershenson, and others tried to demonstrate the existence of certain visual discriminations and preferences in very young infants.[115,136,165]

B. *Reality of Linguistic Segments*

The problem of grammar can be approached in a similar fashion.[31] Human listeners structure the stream of speech not only by selective attention to phonemes and morphemes but through the equally amazing achievement of syntactic analysis, apparently resynthesizing the flow of speech just heard according to standard syntactic rules. The psychological and, hence, physiological reality of this kind of segmentation can be explored quite directly with a variation of Broadbent's technic involving two-channel listening.[212]

In current experiments by Drs. Fodor and Bever in our department,[118,121] a sentence is presented through earphones in one ear, while a click is presented at some arbitrary point within the sentence to the other ear. When Fodor presents the results of this work (and he does it much better than I could here), he says that the experiments are done in order to ask "Why do foreigners talk so fast?" and he quickly answers, "Because we fail to hear the pauses they do not make!" A typical example is the following statement: "In her hope of marrying Jane was optimistic." If the click, entering the other ear, is placed right under "Jane," most listeners will misperceive it as having occurred just before, thus displacing the click towards the major syntactic break.

It can be shown in several ways that this effect is due to the syntactic structure and not to any physical pause or changes of intonation. One simple device is to delete the first two words of the test sentence, by removing "in her" from the tape and substituting the words "but his" at the beginning of the sentence, so that the sentence becomes "but his hope of marrying Jane was optimistic." If the click is again presented, at the same point in time, that is, right under

"Jane," it is now displaced in the opposite direction with a strong tendency to hear it as if it had come after the word "Jane."

In this way we can use the click as a probe for the kind of syntactic structure which the listener imposes on the sentence. In a sentence with ambiguous syntactic structure, the click will travel forward or backward depending on how the sentence was perceived. If the sentence is replaced by a random string of words or by a phrase in a foreign language, the effect vanishes. In more recent studies attempts are being made to find non-verbal indicators for this effect; a mild electric shock is delivered to the listener at some point during the presentation of the sentence and his galvanic skin response recorded. It is still too early to say whether this technic will permit us to monitor the acquisition of syntax by young children or its dissolution in the aphasias.

C. Possible Physiologic Mechanisms

We may do well to admit here, from the outset, that we are still far from being able to fill this particular gap; in fact, it seems extremely difficult to think of experimental attacks in this area. Yet a few things come to mind. If the basis of language learning (and of language loss) is a central neural apparatus preset for acoustical analysis of phonemes and morphemes and strings, we might derive clues for its mode of action from a curious analogy recently pointed out by Clowes and by Sutherland[373]: the analogy between a Chomsky-type grammar, with its hierarchy of structures, and the equally hierarchical order of pattern detectors in the vertebrate visual system, so beautifully elucidated by Hubel and Wiesel[176-178] and by Lettvin and his colleagues.[226]

Neurons in the visual system have long been known to be so connected with photoreceptors and with one another, that each individual neuron looks at a larger or smaller portion of the total visual field. Still more importantly, the receptive field of a given neuron is organized in such a way that, at the retinal levels, its central portion might be excited by light and its periphery inhibited (or conversely). By the simple device of taking a number of such receptor-field structures in a row and interconnecting them, the embryonic visual system builds itself a line detector. For example, a series of roughly circular receptor fields located vertically one above the other, in cat or monkey retina, may discharge convergently into one single cortical neuron in the striate area, whose combined receptor field will thus have an elongated shape with vertical orientation. The row of excitatory center regions will form a slender excitatory ridge surrounded by inhibitory flanks.

For such a unit the appropriate releasing stimulus is neither diffuse light nor a single point of light but a luminous bar in alignment with the vertical excitatory ridge. Rotate the luminous bar out of alignment into oblique positions, and the discharge of this particular neural unit will diminish in proportion to the overlap between the stimulus pattern and the inhibitory flanking regions of the receptive field. This particular unit with its vertically oriented receptive field is therefore a verticality detector, just as other units with obliquely or horizontally oriented excitatory and inhibitory regions represent obliqueness and horizontality detectors, respectively.

Furthermore, by combining the output of several direction-sensitive cells into a higher-order unit, that higher-order unit can be made to respond preferentially to corners, or tongues, so that the simple principles of excitation and inhibition in receptor fields can be used to build up increasingly complex pattern detectors by a hierarchical process. Elsewhere[381] I have said that this process embodies a principle of "cascade specification of input." The actual evidence for these arrangements is particularly strong for the visual cortex of cat and monkey where Hubel and Wiesel can show the clear progression in complexity of receptor-field elements as they proceed from primary visual cortex—area 17

—to the concentrically surrounding cortical bands of areas 18 and 19 in the occipital lobe.

Furthermore, the evidence available so far strongly suggests that these feature-extracting mechanisms on the cortical level are innate, since they are found in newborn kittens as soon as their eyes have opened. Keeping the animal in darkness or diffuse light for sufficiently long periods during their early post-natal development will produce atrophy of this innate receptor-field apparatus. This consequence of sensory deprivation had previously been misinterpreted. Failure of normal pattern perception in dark-reared animals was taken as proof that pattern vision is learned and that the visual sector of the central nervous system acquires its organization through prolonged interaction with patterned stimuli.[393] Apparently varied experience with visual patterns is needed to maintain a mechanism for pattern extraction which is strictly inborn and ready to have its differential activities released by particular patterns.

What has to be acquired may be on a different level: in the course of normal post-natal development higher animals, including man, must find ways to adjust their essentially static receptor-field organization to those apparent displacements and transformations of the environment that are consequences of the organism's own movements— but this is a different matter altogether. What is important here is the hoped-for parallel between the known pattern-extraction machinery in the visual system, and the still unknown arrangements in the auditory nervous system for the patterning of linguistic inputs. The formal analogy, stressed by Dr. Sutherland, between Chomsky-type grammars and the Hubel-Wiesel type of analysis of visual systems may provide a hint about the kind of hierarchical arrangements we might have to look for in those regions of the brain where language input is received and analyzed.

The great difficulty is that a direct physiologic attack on these conjectural mechanisms can only be made in man, since the neural apparatus we postulate would be a species-specific feature of man's brain, a feature probably lacking in the brain of other animals (although Dr. Lilly might wish to have us make an exception for his dolphins). Yet, in spite of this difficulty, we may learn something from the antiphony of the shrike, with its extreme precision (as set forth by Professor Thorpe) and from the speech-imitations by mocking birds. I am forced to agree with Professor Chomsky in stressing how far these forms of sound production differ from language. A Mynah bird or parrot is capable of imitating a jabber of voices, while we cannot. These imitations are, in a sense, too good to represent language: they benefit from the absence of linguistic structures which we ourselves impose on the speech we hear. In other words, I would claim that the mocking bird lacks phonemes, morphemes, and syntax: this is why it fails to generate spontaneous speech but can only mock.

Yet, it may still be possible to learn something from parrots. At the beginning of this century, Kalischer[192] trained parrots to talk, and then performed various selective ablations from their brain. He surely did not produce aphasia in this way but anarthria and dysarthria; yet his approach is worth reviving. There is also considerable promise in the physiologic study of song birds, not only because of the amazing precision in the timing of their antiphonal song, which Thorpe has so beautifully demonstrated, but also because of the intriguing mixture between learned and unlearned elements in many forms of vocal behavior in birds.

Physiologic studies in birds will not yield the essential pattern analyzers for speech but they may take us part of the way, perhaps by elucidating the primary differences between innate and acquired patterns in their receptive and emissive vocal repertoire. The crucial thing to do would be to employ natural stimuli, such as snatches of the bird's own song rather than the usual laboratory stand-by, the noise burst and the oscillator-produced pure tone. Just as the visual system is not built to receive diffuse light or luminous dots, but to extract patterns, so the auditory system of different species is attuned initially to certain sound configurations, such as the frog to its croak, so that the croak becomes the adequate stimulus for doing auditory physiology in frogs. For man, I would predict that distinctive feature-analysis might be shown to proceed on the level of auditory-cortex units with an increasing bias for finding those units in the left rather than right cerebral hemisphere as the individual matures.

II. CENTRAL ELABORATION

At first sight there may seem to be no bigger gap in our understanding than the conundrum posed by the question of central elaboration of speech—the problem of what happens between input and output. Yet you will note that the problem shrinks as our understanding of input and output grows. As long as we deal with oversimplified and biologically inadequate stimuli, central processing will seem to assume major burdens that may actually be carried at lower levels, by the pattern-extracting capacity of the primary pathway, a capacity that may become revealed as soon as the adequate stimulus patterns are presented.

Lines and directions of lines, colors, edges, corners—all these are the normal food for visual systems and, in man, distinctive features and syntactic segments may be the corresponding "elements" of neural processing for speech at the input side. What then remains for "central" processing? Undoubtedly one of the crucial aspects of language, beyond its formal characteristics described by the linguist, is the labeling of objects. Language imposes order on events by permitting their classification, and it provides a tool for representing absent objects and for manipulating them hypothetically "in one's mind."

For all this, it would seem essential that there be some central mechanism for transcending the division between the different senses, for identifying an object felt with an object seen, and both with the object we can name; there should be some form of cross-modal processing resulting in supra-modal, more than sensory, categories, extracted from or imposed upon experience. The problems surrounding the possible relation between words and objects are an essential concern of philosophy. But for those of us who are preoccupied with brain mechanisms in language, it may suffice to look for possible ways in which the central processing of inputs bridges the divisions between senses and leads over into action.

A. *Cross-modal and Supra-modal Processes*

Everyone seemed agreed that language frees us to a large extent from the tyranny of the senses, that it gives us access to concepts that combine information from different sensory modalities and are thus intersensory or suprasensory, but the riddle remains as to how this is achieved.[117] To say that language is needed to "mediate" suprasensory objects requires that we understand how we know in the first place that a thing seen is identical with that same thing felt. The paradox here was posed by the many studies reviewed for us which seemed to indicate nearly complete absence of any transfer from one sense modality to the other, in monkeys, and even under some conditions in man. The evidence is impressive but Dr. Ettlinger did put an upper and lower limit on his conclusion regarding the absence of cross-modal transfer: he suggested that the failure of transfer holds for so-called associate learning but not for certain other forms of learning in animal and man—the more primitive kind of learning which he called perceptual learning, and the kind of learning based on cross-modal matching, where the animal can react to an object alternately perceived through one sense, say sight, and another, such as touch.

Failure of transfer was shown when a monkey had to learn to discriminate test objects within an array, first by palpation alone, and then was tested for transfer of these learned discriminations to a new series of trials in which the same objects had to be discriminated by sight. Apparently an essential condition for failure of transfer is discrimination learning, so that one wonders whether transfer might not appear under conditions where little or no learning seems needed: would a monkey not show identical alarm reactions to a felt snake as he does to a seen snake? In any case, perceptual learning rather than associate learning may be the type of learning relevant to our understanding of first-language acquisition.

Perceptual learning is involved whenever we distinguish more and more subtle differences among phonemes, or when we, as Westerners, begin to appreciate the individuality of facial features among Chinese. It is nonverbal learning, par excellence, but may underlie much of one's early achievement of distinctions among familiar objects and event sequences and thus be prerequisite for subsequent application of linguistic patterns to the events perceived. I am, of course, aware of the tendency, in many quarters, to turn the problem around and to say that linguistic structures produce the possibility of structuring the events around us, but I find the strong forms of this belief incredible, since some structure has to be perceived before names can be applied.

A great deal then of early learning would be perceptual,[137,316] and particularly that of one's mother tongue. In this sense, first-language learning fits much better into what ethologists call imprinting, a very special early form of learning which ethologists claim is firmly anchored in more elementary, preformed dispositions for perceiving certain patterns, but critically dependent on particular inputs gained during early development.

As usually defined, imprinting differs from other forms of learning in a number of respects: it is said to represent learning without differential reward; a kind of learning in which massed practice is paradoxically more effective than spaced practice, and primacy of experience more important than recency;

it is said to be a kind of learning that is practically irreversible (although there is more controversy on this particular point than on the others); lastly, it is learning that appears to be optimal during so-called critical periods after which it can no longer be achieved, or at least not achieved with anything like the original ease. Obviously, all this and particularly the last point, as Dr. Lenneberg has stressed, is just as true for normal first-language acquisition in man as it seems to be true for imprinting as usually described for many subhuman species.

If first-language learning involves perceptual learning, then it might be easier to understand why it becomes so readily attached to multimodal inputs; after all, first-language learning, in the normal child, seems to take place at an age which overlaps with an early phase of intensive perceptual learning of object discriminations, and an enormously rapid development of skilled bodily movement. If we could understand the neurologic mechanisms which underlie these early and critical developments leading to the mastery of language in the normal child, we would have done more than opened a window to look at aphasia: we would have opened a door.

One final point regarding the question of cross-modal and supra-modal learning: if it were generally true that the different senses are hermetically sealed off against each other, it would be extremely difficult to understand the function of those large clusters of cortical and subcortical neurons which seem to respond to more than one kind of sensory input. Dr. Myers presented his beautiful area maps of anatomically coherent cortical fields, but he will agree that the picture gains an additional dimension once we consider the microphysiology of these fields and record from individual neurons. It then turns out that surprisingly large numbers of cortical cells respond to stimulation in two or even three sense modalities. Not all of these can be classified as "nonspecific" in the sense that they are merely signalling generalized arousal.

Their time constants and their time dependency in relation to the sensory input are such that we must accept them as genuinely polysensory neurons. It is perhaps no accident that so many of these are found in the parietal lobes.[191]

B. "Transfer" within Systems

It is nevertheless important for our attempts at understanding the neurology of language that transfer of information under many conditions seems to be at least as difficult within as it is between sensory modalities. Some of the earliest approaches to the pathophysiology of language have invoked various forms of disconnection that would make information storage and recall for linguistic material difficult or impossible. The area defines a lacuna because we still do not know how information in the nervous system is stored or retrieved, hence our groping in dealing with central processing. Some glimpses of what might be involved can be obtained from considering the magnificent observations on effects of commissurotomy, in animal and man, by Professor Sperry and his colleagues, and the clinical observations by Dr. Geschwind.

It was instructive to hear of the most recent developments in this respect: contrary to the early impressions of nearly complete separation of sensory inputs, both animal experiments and observations on man underscore that some information is shared between the divided hemispheres; after all, there is a great deal of connection possible within the brain stem. Conversely, it is becoming increasingly clear that the commissures linking the two cerebral hemispheres fail to provide a perfect and complete replication of trace systems on both sides of the brain. Under any condition, in the split-brain or normal state, what does or does not transfer from one side to the other is clearly dependent on the level of the task and on the level of the response required.

Some of these experiments provide models for an understanding of certain phenomena in those aphasics who show partial comprehension of what is said to them or seemingly perfect comprehension coupled with a lack of capacity to respond. To complement the story rather than to summarize: if we go to the goldfish, as McCleary[265] and his student Ingle[182] have done, we can get beautiful dissociations between eye-to-eye transfer of learning on one level, and failure of transfer on another level, and this in the same animal, without any interruptions of commissures between the optic lobes. Thus, on some tasks the fish may learn to swim forward to avoid an electric shock when a visual pattern is shown to one eye, yet fail to move forward when the same pattern is then shown to the other (untrained) eye. At the same time his heart rate shows a vigorous reaction when the threatening pattern is exhibited to the untrained eye, as though he knew "in his heart" that the pattern was threatening but was unable to act upon this information.

Ingle, continuing these studies in our departmental laboratories, has since shown similar dissociataed effects for transfer within a single retina: the fish is trained to swim forward (and avoid a shock) when a vertical line appears in the anterior half of the field of one eye, and to remain still when an oblique line is presented to the same region within that retina. If the oblique line differs sufficiently in angle from the vertical, the fish will learn the significance of this distinction quickly (remember, in our view he already knows verticals and obliques; he merely has to learn what to do about them); and this simple discrimination transfers from the trained anterior half of the visual field to the untrained posterior half of that same field. Thus, the fish avoids the shock appropriately upon the first confrontation with the critical patterns exhibited to the naive portions of his retina.

However, if the initial discrimination is made more difficult, for example, by making the oblique line only slightly different from vertical, the fish will fail to transfer this discrimination to the posterior part of the field;

when the latter is confronted with the threatening pattern, he does not swim forward as he should, but shows a peculiar change in heart rate, as if "frightened." This is perhaps not so different from one of Dr. Sperry's cases of commissurotomy in man: the lady who reacted emotionally to the embarrassing picture presented to her speechless hemisphere but who could not say how her emotion had been aroused.

These split-brain studies in man make clear that emissive speech may indeed be impossible to produce for a minor hemisphere. It is as if half of the forebrain were mute, at least in those adults whose interhemispheric relations reflect the often-claimed asymmetry for speech. Yet, it is equally important to point out that this asymmetry can be a matter of degree: the most recent work of Sperry and colleagues shows again, and quite definitely, that man's minor hemisphere is not altogether devoid of language. The patients can pick out simple objects from an array, on oral or written commands, although they are unable to say anything about the objects seen or felt through their disconnected minor hemisphere. The minor hemisphere may appear to be mute, but is far from exhibiting global aphasia. How important it would be to know how much of this mutism of the right hemisphere reflects an inherent inferiority of neuronal organization as against differential effects of training, or even effects of prolonged suppression of a latent mechanism on the right by an active mechanism on the left. These questions are old, but they have been sharpened by recent work.

C. Relations between Hemispheres

The lateralization of major aspects of language function to one side of the brain—usually the left—is so well established that we may have been in danger of minimizing the actual or latent contributions by the right hemisphere. Counteracting this trend, this conference has provided an overwhelming array of observations on differential functions of man's hemispheres which put the role of the right hemisphere in a new light. These observations, I believe, mark a major advance in our understanding of hemisphere relations.

Eighteen to 20 years ago nearly everyone would have described the division of labor between the human cerebral hemispheres as an asymmetry in only one direction: the left hemisphere was called dominant, because it was deemed to be like the right except for the addition of one mechanism—that for language (the relation to hand-preference, in this connection, was unclear and remains so, in my opinion, to this day). At that stage it was possible to say that animals below man have two "right" hemispheres, one on each side. What we heard at this meeting shows that this formulation was wrong: the two lateral halves of man's brain stand in a relation to each other which can only be described as reciprocal specialization.

A brilliant confirmation of earlier hunches about this state of affairs (cf. Hebb[149]) comes from the work of Zangwill[303,304,420] and that of Hécaen[153,159] and particularly from the long series of fundamental studies by Milner,[277,279,282,284] which reveal what we like to call a "double dissociation of symptoms": unilateral lesions in the right and left hemispheres of comparable severity produce symptoms in man which differ not only by virtue of the fact that language disorders tend to appear after left-hemisphere lesions, but also because certain spatial tasks, in several sense modalities, are selectively more impaired by lesions on the right.[284] See also Teuber[382] and Weinstein.[401] The several reports at this meeting brought further confirmation of these observations which only a few years ago were still considered quite controversial.

What remains to be done in this respect is to fill a rather obvious lacuna; it is still not quite clear to what extent, and for what behavioral tasks, the reciprocity of right and left hemisphere functions may be said to hold. There are vigorous efforts under way, particularly in the Montreal laboratory, to define the nature of the right-hemisphere syndrome, in terms of function, that is, in terms of underlying process. A full understanding here would require a much deeper grasp than we now possess of the neural mechanisms involved in spatial organization for perception and action. Still the question must be pursued both for its own sake and because it might permit us to look at some aspects of the aphasias after left-hemisphere lesions in a new way. If spatial organization is more vulnerable to right-hemisphere lesions, is the left hemisphere in most of us more important for the maintenance of serial order? Or, to put it less speculatively, what, if any, are the nonlanguage factors in the aphasic syndromes?

It should also be noted that for some of the right-left differences that have been observed, the ultimate explanation may be that similar capacities are represented in dissimilar fashion, right and left. Conceivably the right hemisphere in adult man differs from his left in one respect by exhibiting less focal organization, so that some equally circumscribed lesions, right and left, might produce unequal symptoms for that reason alone.[349,351]

Lastly, we need to approach the problem in developmental terms: it is still not known how early the differentiation between hemispheres arises, whether before birth or soon thereafter, whether predominantly as an effect of genetic factors, or as a result of use. We are all appreciative of the alleged plasticity of the infant brain, but we do not seem to have any strong evidence to suggest that the lateralization of different functions can really be reversed with complete impunity. One obvious task is to perform much more extensive studies than heretofore on childhood hemiplegias, since there is the strong possibility (we have some preliminary data) that right- and left-hemisphere lesions, even in early infancy, produce reciprocally different syndromes, with right hemiplegias being associated with retarded language development and diminished ultimate language competence, while left hemiplegics show spatial and constructional difficulties.

III. Problems of Patterning of Output

Perhaps the biggest single lacuna is represented by our ignorance of the neural bases of speech production. Yet if we admit our ignorance about such fundamentals, we may have set the stage for particularly rapid advances here. Speech is patterned and voluntary—although at this stage in a strenuous conference you may be inclined to doubt both of these premises. The problem of patterning of speech as of any other complex motor activity may well turn out to be analogous to the problem of patterning on the input side so that answers to one of these riddles may provide at least part of the solution for the other.

We have stressed how little we know about the patterning of linguistic input, and have reminded ourselves that the case is different from vision where the type of single-unit analysis pioneered by Hubel and Wiesel, and by Lettvin, permits us to make some first conjectures about the detection of particular figural elements. It was therefore extremely relevant to the topic of this conference that we were given a first glimpse of the microphysiology of the primate motor cortex by Dr. Evarts, in terms reminiscent of the Hubel-Wiesel analysis of the visual system. By contrast, much of our earlier knowledge of the motor cortex was based on macroelectrode studies, often done in anesthetized animals, where massive volleys of impulses could be seen to descend the pyramidal tract upon gross electrical stimulation of the precentral gyrus.

The recent experiments by Evarts disclose a totally different picture: using indwelling microelectrodes in unanesthetized monkeys, he records single-unit activity during simple voluntary movements of the animals' limbs. He thus reveals a remarkable interplay of inhibition and excitation, at the level of single pyramidal cells in the motor cortex.

Actually, many of the units fall silent when a restricted voluntary movement of the contralateral limb occurs.

Some of the participants seem to have been doubtful, at first, how such data might fit into a future neurology of language. I would insist that such observations are essential. We cannot understand the neural basis of speech unless we begin to comprehend how spontaneous and selective movements can be initiated in the central nervous system, how they can be confined to particular configurations of neurons, and how they can be stopped in order to permit the organization, in time, of varying motor patterns that follow upon each other.[223] The gap here between what we need to know and what we can assert as being known is truly enormous, but we are at least beginning to face the fundamental question, the problem of voluntary movement.

A. *Active vs. Passive Movement*

The great obstacle to progress here has been the tacit agreement to rule any discussion of voluntary movement out of court. Admittedly there is little room for active (as against reflex) movements in spinal-cord physiology, and spinal-cord physiology, in turn, has been the model for most theories of learning, with the inevitable result that some crucial factors seem to have been left out. The taboo on any discussion of active rather than reflex movements is understandable because of the metaphysical overtones that cling to the terms "spontaneous" or "voluntary," yet there is now irrefutable behavioral evidence that active movement differs in its consequences from passive motion, and this evidence comes from studies of perceptual learning.

The studies in question are still progressing in the Psychology Laboratories at MIT, under the direction of Held and Hein.[160,161] They began with an exceedingly simple but fundamental observation: normal human observers were given prismatic spectacles to wear so that whatever they saw was systematically distorted: points in perceived space were displaced laterally, and all straight lines seemed curved. If the observer was permitted to walk about actively for one hour, most of these distortions disappeared. If, instead, he was pushed about, over the same path and for the same time, in a wheelchair while wearing the spectacles, he did not adapt. Active movement turned out to be necessary for adaptation to sensory rearrangement.

There now are numerous animal experiments in support of this simple result obtained with normal man. Many of these additional studies involve the rearing of kittens or newborn monkeys under conditions where all their visual experience is obtained while they are either stationary or passively moved. As it turns out, such animals can probably discriminate certain stationary patterns while they are held still but fail to show normal shape and depth perception as soon as they are permitted to move.

Taken together, these experiments support the view that "voluntary" or "active" movement is necessary for the maintenance and even for the origin of normal sensorimotor coordination. Thus, the innate pattern detectors in the sensory systems cannot be sufficient when it comes to perception under conditions of continual change in the relation between the perceiver and his sensory environment. The organism must not only be able to produce movements, and to apprehend patterns, but he must be able to take care of the inevitable interaction between these two sets of activity. He must be able to distinguish those changes in the world which are mere consequences of his self-produced movements, for example, the shifting of contours, as he moves his eyes, from those changes that are consequences of genuine motions in the environment.[380]

B. *The "Corollary Discharge" and Related Postulates*

We believe, therefore, that there must be a distinctive difference in the cerebral mechanisms for spontaneous as against passive or reflex movement. Microelectrode studies of the motor cortex such as those presented here, and similar studies of other cerebral systems, may well give substance to these claims which at this point are still sheer conjecture. What we have postulated over the past eight years is that a voluntary movement (for example, of the eyes) is always characterized by a twofold process: an efferent discharge to the effectors (in the case of eye movements, to the extraocular musculature) and a simultaneous central discharge (the "corollary discharge") to the appropriate sensory systems (here, the visual system) which forewarns them, so to speak, of the impending change. The basic idea was proposed, independently, as early as 1950 by Sperry[368] and by von Holst and Mittelstaedt.[392] Such a mechanism would provide for subjective stability of the world in the course of self-produced movements of the perceiver,[383,384] while simultaneously providing an objective (physiologic) marker for the voluntariness of voluntary movement—assuming that such a central process or "corollary discharge" can be found.

C. Possible Physiologic Mechanisms of Voluntary Movement

Recent developments in the recording of slow potentials from the brain may contribute to a physiologic understanding of active movements and thus ultimately to an understanding of production of speech. Averaging of evoked potentials by small computers has now been extended to show potential shifts which precede rather than follow certain overt activities. Dr. Grey Walter has presented evidence on his discovery of a slow negative shift, the Contingent Negative Variation, which can be recorded from the anterior scalp in normal adults about 200 msec. before the onset of certain acts. Similarly and independently, Kornhuber[208,209] and Vaughan[138] have developed technics for averaging potential shifts in the brain which precede a voluntary movement of hand or foot.

Kornhuber's observation came quite early in the course of these convergent developments, but he had the misfortune of having an assistant erroneously reverse the polarity in the original recordings so that their initial communication had to be retracted. The motor potential ("MP") discovered by Vaughan and Gilden[138] is probably quite similar to the phenomenon studied by Kornhuber, though both seem to differ in certain respects from the Contingent Negative Variation so extensively investigated by Grey Walter. I like to think that some of these curious electrophysiologic antecedents of overt action reflect not just the neural "command" to the musculature but the concomitant presetting of cerebral systems for the expected consequence of the impending action, so that the result can be compared, centrally, with the intent.

It is likely that we may have to look to microelectrode studies before we can sort out those hypothetical components in cerebral activity which precede voluntary movement. Without an understanding of these problems, those involved in the initiation and arrest of movement, in serial order and selective patterning, speech production will remain refractory to neurologic analysis. In any case, whatever direction our search for the physical basis of active movement will take, we shall be forced to look into those processes which occupy what Hirsh called "macrotime"— the periods of at least 100 msec. between the arrival of signals at the cortex and the first appearance of overt motor reactions.

We are bound to flounder among all these gaps in our understanding, but the problems of brain mechanism for language are of such complexity that even partial answers carry disproportionate rewards; they will tell us much more about the brain and about ourselves than continued restriction of arguments to lower-level neural mechanisms. For this reason I found it encouraging that we had a conference where people were bold enough to ask each other questions about the nature of language and about the brain mechanisms involved in it, rather than hold yet another conference on aphasia and its classification.

The study of lower-level mechanism in the nervous system is indispensable for any rational approach to higher levels of function, yet it is also true, as Lashley[223] pointed out, that we must keep before us those aspects of behavior which our physiology will eventually have to explain. Language is central among those higher aspects of behavior; a physiology which has no room for asking questions about language may be wrong in its application to lower mechanisms as well. We were willing to ask our questions regardless of whether there were hopes for an early answer. If we did nothing else but define the extent of our gaps in understanding, we should be satisfied. But I think we did more.

CHAIRMAN MILLIKAN: Are there comments?

DR. HENRY W. BROSIN: I would like to express my admiration for this beautiful summary, both for its depth and its sentiments.

At the risk of being redundant, I would like to repeat a theme given us by Dr. Teuber which, for me, was most impressive, namely the relevance of early learning to abstract thinking. At our first meeting Dr. Thorpe told us that some of his birds do not learn after 14 months, even if they are not in deprived situations. This reminds us of a long series of experiments, particularly those of Riesen from Orange Park,[329] Harlow's monkeys,[147] Bowlby's children,[45] and Rene Spitz' deprived infants,[370] and other series.

Dr. Lilly has emphasized here the enormous cost and personal care required to bring one infant dolphin, with a big brain, to maturity. I won't take the time to stress the parallel to human development since you know that the cost is very great. I believe that as the importance of the subject is realized, we will continue the studies of infant and child development more intensively, as recommended by Darwin in 1872, so that in a decade or two we will know more about the mechanisms which have been discussed here.

I think that the study of early learning in all organisms promises to be most rewarding for our problems in improving the level of abstract thinking. This and related abilities, particularly those we can call the internal controls of behavior in ourselves and in the underprivileged population, both here in the U.S. and abroad, are of the greatest importance to us in learning how to live together.

CHAIRMAN MILLIKAN: Are there other comments? Dr. Magoun, please continue.

Lacunae and Research Approaches to Them. II.

H. W. MAGOUN

University of California at Los Angeles
Los Angeles, California

I SHOULD LIKE to direct my remarks toward the mission-oriented concerns of the Federal Agency that is sponsoring this Conference, which are related both to the preservation of neurological health and to the provision, after neurological disease, of all therapeutic and rehabilitative efforts that can be mobilized. In the area of the subject of this Conference, this latter interest has its focus in what generally is called speech therapy.

Instead of exploring the lacunae that doubtless exist in this area, I should like to propose that a major potential for its improvement lies in the mobilization of all the insights that have been and are continuing to come from a variety of fields of neurological research, in determining how better to influence and manipulate central neural activity so as to maximize the capacity of the cerebral cortex for processing, storing, retrieving, and utilizing information in communication through speech and language. Speech therapy might be expected to gain greatly and improve its effectiveness markedly by gathering and applying all the fragmentary clues that we now possess and seeking further knowledge of each of them toward such a goal. In addition to the improvement of speech therapy that might be expected to result, any broad concepts that could be derived would seem of value also in their applications to the improvement of learning and education generally.

We should begin with the potential relevance of what little is known of the way in which the individual neuron stores, retrieves, and subsequently utilizes information. The great current advances in genetic biochemistry have identified a nucleic acid template for protein and enzyme production, which provides a basic mechanism for reproduction and embryogenesis. There are a number of contemporary neuroscientists who propose that nature has not been profligate enough to have evolved more than a single mechanism for information coding in biology. They postulate a comparable nucleic acid base for encoding and read-out in the nervous system. Learning and memory, in their view, depend upon the specification of neuronal RNA, as a consequence of bombardment by afferent signals from the external world—the more intense and frequent the bombardment, the more rapid and pronounced the specification. Such specified and replicated RNA is proposed, in turn, to provide the template for elaboration of enzyme-like, neuronal transmitter substances, responsible for consequent patterns of neural firing, serving interneuronal transmission of excitation and expressive behavior.[180]

From this point of view, rehabilitative therapy might be considered a kind of applied combination of sensory neurophysiology and neurochemistry which seeks, by manipulating input signals, to specify the nucleic-acid and protein metabolism of residual cortical neural aggregates in a way to improve or restore functions that are impaired or missing following disease. Such therapy should be funda-

217

mentally oriented toward the learning process and specialized only in the respect that it has to deal with learning by a reduced neural substrate, rather than by one whose under-developed potential has not yet become realized fully.

Certainly, we should begin also with exploration of ways of presenting input signals that are involved in communication, particularly those that interrelate stimuli from primary objects with their associated verbal or written symbols, so as to maximize their impact upon the receiving and associational areas of the cerebral cortex. There was some discussion earlier of the means now known to neurophysiology of aggrandizing the amplitude of cortical responses to input signals.

One of these involves the simple increase of intensity of stimulation which, since intensity of activity is coded in any neural channel by an increase in the frequency of its firing, augments excitability by temporal summation. Excitability can be augmented also through spatial summation, by promoting the convergence, within a limited period of time, of signals generated independently at different receptors. In the field of speech therapy the simultaneous presentation of auditory and visual signals can be employed both to promote cross-modal association and to summate excitation at points of convergence. Sensory feedback, in the form of afferent stimulation generated by responses, can also be employed to promote and modulate central excitability. This occurs reflexly whenever proprioceptors are present and is routinely cultivated in speech therapy by providing for sensory feedback over visual channels through the use of a mirror.

There was some discussion earlier, in connection with the dramatic presentations of Drs. Purpura and Grey Walter, of the manner in which graded depolarization of the membranes of ramifying dendrites, short of that generating impulse propagation, can influence the excitability of cortical neurons for discharge. Such a mechanism would appear to underlie the pronounced transcallosal facilitation of cortical activity, described by Bremer,[49] in which excitation of a region of one hemisphere markedly enhances excitability of the homologous region of the opposite hemisphere. Such an observation would certainly appear to have potential application for rehabilitative therapy, as might also observations that direct surface polarization of a cortical region markedly expedites the establishment of conditional reflexes in which the region is involved.[288]

Further consideration may be given here to some more general ways of influencing cortical excitability, which were also briefly discussed earlier. One of these is related to provocation of the orienting reflex and the attentive state, in the genesis of which the novelty of afferent signals is an important feature. In this connection, it is necessary to think of dual routes over which inputs from the senses reach and are able to influence the activity of higher neural levels. One is the classical collection of afferent paths to receiving areas of the cortex, which we learned about in school. This collection, which Pavlov[305] described as his "analyzers," is concerned with the transmission and processing of specific information and with its differentiation and analysis. A second ascending route, distributed through the central core of the neuraxis, with rostral extension into the hemisphere, has a powerful ability to raise or lower the excitability of the cerebral cortex in both generalized and more focal ways. The functions served by these specific and nonspecific cortical input channels are both distinct and supplementary. The specific one conveys the informational content of the afferent message, for its signals are both modality- and locality-related. The nonspecific one, lacking these features, provides instead for behavioral and EEG arousal underlying an orientation and attention to the message.

In addition, excitation of this nonspecific system has been found to exert a powerful facilitatory influence upon specific afferent signals reaching the cortex over the classical sensory paths. As Bremer and Stoupel[50] and

Dumont and Dell[95] have shown, sensory cortical responses double or triple in amplitude during the concomitant stimulation of the nonspecific core system of the brain. The pronounced, but short-lived, facilitation of specific input signals appears identical with that which occurs naturally whenever novel afferent stimuli evoke the orienting reflex.[364,365] In addition to these central events, peripheral changes enable the receptors to gain all possible information about the evocative stimulus, toward which the eyes, head, and body are turned.

These information-promoting aspects of the orienting reflex are obviously of capital importance for the expedition of rehabilitation but, in one important respect, they are conflicting with a major current practice of speech therapy, namely, its emphasis upon the monotonous repetition of stereotyped learning exercises. This is just as true of education generally, for repetition is often described as the first law of learning.

Unlike signal-transmission in specific afferent paths, however, that in the nonspecific system, leading to the orienting reflex and facilitation of cortical input, attentuates rapidly and disappears upon stereotyped repetition of the evocative stimulus. Sharpless and Jasper,[358] Hernandez-Peón,[164] and others have shown that, with recurring presentation of the same signals which initially provoked orientation, the duration of arousal and related changes becomes progressively reduced and then stops altogether, and a stage called habituation ensues. This is not attributable to fatigue or other generalized impairment of the nonspecific system for, during habituation, whenever signals regain a novelty by some change in their parameters, full-blown orientation is again evoked. These findings indicate that the nonspecific neural system, which magnifies input signals and provokes orientation and attention to them, is built to respond only to novel signals. They imply, further, that the brain contains a converse mechanism, which responds to the stereotyped repetition of stimuli by actively blocking their transmission to the nonspecific system and so preventing orientation and attention to them.

The prepotent role of novelty in evoking the orienting reflex suggests that this reflex is not initiated directly by a stimulus, in the customary sense of the term, but rather by a change in its intensity, pattern, or other parameter. A comparison of present with previous stimulation seems of prime significance, with an orienting reflex being evoked at every point of disagreement. The concept of a cortical neuronal model has been proposed by Sokolov[365] to account for this induction of the orienting reflex by stimuli whose novelty is their characteristic feature. This model is conceived as a cortical cell assembly which preserves information about the modality, intensity, duration, and order of presentation of earlier stimuli, with which analogous aspects of novel stimulation may be compared. The orienting reflex is evoked whenever, upon such comparison, the parameters of the novel stimulus do not coincide with those of the model. This discordance, it is suggested, generates cortical discharge to the nonspecific core brain, triggering the orienting reflex. In the contrasting situation, when recurring stimuli are accordant with the cortical neuronal model, the cortex fails to excite the core system and the orienting reflex is not provoked. Moreover, upon repetition, such accordance of stimulus and model is proposed to generate feedback inhibition from the cortex, which blocks collateral afferent input to the core system and so promotes habituation.

These recent findings concerning the orienting reflex and habituation disclose a major conflict between a proposed primary law of learning and the way the brain actually works. They plainly imply that repetition is the first law, not of learning, but of habituation, whose influence upon learning is a negative, rather than a promoting one. Obviously, the promotion of novelty, rather than of repetition, should become a primary law of learning. Whenever afferent signals are repeatedly presented in a learning situation, each one should be made adequately distinctive, in some respect, from that preceding it, so as to provoke a recurring series of orienting reflexes and utilize their powerful amplification of cortical input signals as a resource in achieving learning. Should this prove impossible, recourse may be had, next, to a second law of learning—reinforcement.

Reference was similarly made earlier to the importance of utilizing reinforcement in the expedition of learning. A major field of current study is rapidly providing insights into the neurophysiological basis of reinforcement. Olds and Milner,[301] Delgado, Roberts, and Miller,[84] Lilly,[239] and others have identified reciprocal regions in the cephalic brain stem and the bordering area of its attachment to the hemisphere the direct experimental stimulation of which reproduces all the features of primary reward or punishment. With electrode placements in the positively reinforcing part of this limbic brain, and the animal trained to press a lever to stimulate the site of implantation, it repeatedly excites its own central nervous system, to the exclusion of all other activities, for long periods of time. Once an animal has stimulated the aversive part of this region, however, it will never do so again. Moreover, it will repeatedly press a lever to avoid recurring stimulation, by the experimenter, of this negatively reinforcing mechanism.

These limbic regions for positive and negative reinforcement are closely associated functionally with adjacent neural mechanisms for feeding, mating, and aggression or defense, serving the life- and race-preserving goals of innate behavior, the impelling nature of which is, in part, to be accounted for by the powerful degree to which its consummation is reinforced. The categories of innate behavior serving feeding or mating are conspicuously recurring: an appetitive phase leads to consummation and associated reinforcement, after which satiety brings the cycle to a transient end. Until consummation is achieved, however, the appetitive drives for feeding and mating are exceedingly potent

and resistant ones. Analogously, the categories of innate behavior serving aggression or defense, whose consummation consists of overcoming or avoiding aversive stimulation or punishment, are associated with drives to escape negative reinforcement. If anything, they are even more dominant and difficult to resist until consummation is attained. To whatever degree these reinforcement systems can be involved in a learning situation, their intrinsic potency and related immunity to habituation can provide a powerful resource in the acquisition and maintenance of learned behavior.

For a half century before the physiological basis of reinforcement was understood, it had been utilized effectively in the studies of conditional learning by Pavlov and his successors. Their experiments, undertaken with food-deprived dogs, consisted of the repeated pairing of an indifferent signal (bell) with the sight, taste, and ingestion of food, leading to unconditioned salivation, until the bell alone evoked a salivary response. In the avoidance conditioning of Bechterew, an indifferent signal (bell) was paired with a shock to the foot, causing the animal to withdraw its leg, until the bell alone evoked the flexor response. In the subsequent elaboration of operant conditioning, by Konorski and Skinner, a behavioral act (pushing a lever) was reinforced with a food reward, until the animal invariably pushed the lever, whenever it was hungry. The feature essential for the initiation and acquisition of these types of learned behavior was reinforcement: the positive reinforcement of a food reward in the case of approach learning, or the negative reinforcement of a noxious shock to the foot in the case of avoidance learning. Moreover, such reinforcement proved essential for the maintenance of learning, once acquired. When learned behavior had been established, subsequent withdrawal of reinforcement led to a kind of negative learning, or learning not to respond, called extinction, which tended to pass into the relaxation, drowsiness, and sleep of Pavlovian internal inhibition.

The powerful expedition of learning, either by positive or negative reinforcement, is attributable in considerable part to the marked facilitation and generalization of afferent signals, which such reward or punishment promotes. In recent experiments John and Killam,[189] Galambos,[120] and others have demonstrated a pronounced increase in the amplitude of afferent signals, and a generalization of their distribution in the brain, when either positive or negative reinforcement is introduced into a learning situation. In this respect, reinforcement resembles the orienting reflex, but the facilitation of input by reinforcement is far more persistent and, unlike that of the orienting reflex, does not attenuate or habituate upon repetition, short of that leading to consummation and ensuing satiety.

Indeed, when an afferent signal, initially facilitated by the orienting reflex, is monotonously repeated until habituation occurs, the introduction of reinforcement promptly overcomes habituation and augments the signal far beyond its original amplitude and central distribution. These striking capabilities for the amplification and generalization of afferent signals within the brain, as well as those for resisting and overcoming habituation, are testimony for the great influence which reinforcement can exert in the promotion of learning. Ideally learning should be initiated by orientation and then followed up to criterion and maintained by reinforcement, in the application of the renovated laws proposed.

Another major field of current study is exploring the interrelated involvement of these specific and nonspecific systems in the genesis of learning. The classical efforts of Pavlov to determine the physiological basis of learning were limited by the technical developments of his time. His concepts of the central neural events involved had necessarily to be derived largely from observations of external performance or behavior. By contrast, contemporary technical advances provide means of investigating the learning process more directly, by recording changes in electrical activity within regions of the brain where

events are actually proceeding. In much the same way that isotope-tagged chemicals are now introduced into and traced through metabolic processes in biochemical research, recent studies of learning employ repetitive flashes of light as tracer stimuli and monitor sequential changes in frequency-tagged responses during avoidance learning or conditioning to a paired tone. In these studies, the first photicly-labeled responses to be elicited by the tone alone are recorded from the nonspecific core of the brain stem. Only later do they appear in the cortex, initially with a widespread distribution that generally becomes restricted to the projection area of the unconditioned signal.[189,190,288,418]

Contrary to Pavlov's view that the cerebral cortex is the pre-eminent site of formation of novel temporary connections during learning, these findings imply that the nonspecific or polysensory nature of the subcortical core of the brain stem serves in establishing the first transmodal links, underlying stimulus equivalence which only secondarily become transferred to the cortex. Once the cortex is involved, however, the initially widespread and subsequently focal distribution of tagged responses confirm the succession of initial generalization and later differentiation identified by Pavlov in the establishment of all conditioned reflexes. Considered broadly, the sequence of events suggests a subcortical focus of and role in the initiation of conditioned learning, as well as its succeeding generalized transference to the cortex. The cortex is doubtless involved pre-eminently, however, in subsequent differentiation, probably by a gradual extinction, in the pattern of Sokolov's model of feedback inhibition, of all nonreinforced components. Ultimately, labeled responses persist only in the cortical projection area of the unconditioned signal, that is, in the analyzer with which reinforcement, immune to habituation, is or has become associated.

Other recent studies have revived and extended earlier interests in identifying pharmacological substances that promote the learning process. Recent studies of the facilitation of learning by such central neuronal stimulants as caffeine, strychnine, and picrotoxin have been reviewed by McGaugh.[268] In the further experiments of Bovet[44] the formation of a conditioned avoidance response in rats was both facilitated and accelerated by administration either of nicotine or thyroid hormone, the latter presumably by its general augmenting influence upon the metabolism of the brain. In continuation of this work, Bovet introduced a double procedure, whereby an animal was first conditioned to respond to a light stimulus and then trained not to respond when an acoustic signal was associated with the light. The action of drugs could then be tested upon both motor and inhibitory conditioning. Motor conditioning was facilitated by amphetamine and antagonized by the tranquilizer, chlorpromazine, while the inverse was true for inhibitory conditioning. The facilitatory effect of amphetamine was shown also to become progressively more marked during the deterioration of motor conditioning from continuous testing over several days. This latter effect is attributable in part to the well-known influence of amphetamine in promoting wakefulness and overcoming fatigue, but its direct excitation of the nonspecific core system, as in the case of the orienting reflex and reinforcement, doubtless contributes also to its facilitation of new learning. To the degree that neural links of the nonspecific core system utilize adrenergic transmitter substances, broken down by monamine oxidase, the monamine oxidase inhibitors and other "psychic energizers" might be tested for their possible promotion of learning in speech therapy and other rehabilitative efforts.

But what, in more general terms, I would like to propose is that, in view of the practical clinical problems involved and the mission orientation of this field, effort should be made to assemble, for testing and utilization in speech therapy, all of the clues provided by these various lines of study, with the goal of improving rehabilitation of the residual brain for communication, after the loss or impairment of a part of its substance and function by disease.

CHAIRMAN MILLIKAN: Are there comments?

DR. HIRSH: I cannot address myself to the general issue that Dr. Magoun raises concerning which lines of study are relevant, particularly as one orients toward the rehabilitation of disorders. It is very clear that there have been some reshapings within the speech pathology profession in recent years, not so much with respect to the nervous system, however, as to language and linguistics. However, this is an issue on which others can speak better than I.

I want to come back to a suggestion that Dr. Magoun raised, that came up in Dr. Teuber's early remarks. It has to do with this issue of transfer among modalities. As some of you may have gathered from earlier remarks, I believe that audition is rather special with respect to time, and I also believe that language is rather special with respect to audition.

I was very interested to hear Dr. Ettlinger and others present their information on transfer, or lack of it, in animals, and in some of the split brain preparations. I was also struck with the fact that, when you are dealing with the tactile and visual senses, you can talk about transfer because the objects in those two sense modalities have some common features, what John Locke called primary qualities, like shape and size, and you can compare the ability of a subject to discriminate forms with his hand, with that of discriminating forms with his eye. I do not know quite how to make the transfer between auditory-perceptual referents and other sensory modalities, the one exception being rhythmic patterning that you can test by ear, by touch, and by eye, as we did some years ago, to find that, initially, subjects are very poor in the nonauditory sense modalities but, if the training consists of what Dick Held would call mapping rhythmic perception in touch and vision on the original auditory one, then you can learn it.

With respect to defective operation, say, within the auditory-perceptual realm, just to take a specific example, if I were to take Professor Magoun's suggestion seriously about utilizing information sent in through several sensory modalities simultaneously, I would indeed, as he suggests, increase excitation. There would, as is suggested from physiological studies, be facilitation.

One of the difficulties with this language of ours is that we run out of words. A word like "facilitation" means one thing to a physiologist in his laboratory and means quite another thing in general conversation or even speculation. If I remember correctly, facilitation means either the lowering of a threshold or the increase of an amplitude. Surely, it must be true that you could find some cells or some groups of cells where excitation would be increased, that is, intersensory facilitation could be demonstrated from the physiological point of view. But from the perceptual point of view, I suspect we would find the inverse of facilitation, particularly when we are thinking, for example, of supplementing auditory input with visual input.

I think this may be the difficulty in the utilization of such schemes as visible speech to teach the deaf to talk; it may concern the interference effects where reading training is introduced too early in order to implement improved speaking, and I do not think that facilitation is represented in this kind of mixed-up input.

DR. CHASE: When we reflect on Dr. Hirsh's comments about augmenting the information going into a sensory system that is impaired, an important problem that comes to mind concerns investigation of the extent to which information that normally enters the nervous system through one sensory system might be reorganized for presentation to another sensory system. To my mind, the laboratory investigation of this issue would be more profitably guided by the results of behavioral experimentation than by what we know about the physiology of the major sensory systems.

When we reflect on the history of the use of "visible speech" to teach speech to the congenitally deaf child, it seems to me that two major problems reveal themselves. One problem concerns optimal periods for learning speech. Most of the children who have been used in visible speech experiments have been over ten years of age. This is probably an older age than would be ideal for such work.

The second problem concerns the manner in which a signal should be organized for presentation to the visual system, if it is to function as a correct template for learning speech motor gestures. It is possible that the auditory system operates selectively upon some critical subset of the acoustic representation of adult speech. If this is the case, we must determine the critical subset of information in adult speech in order to eliminate unnecessary information from the visual displays of speech signals.

Until there has been exhaustive exploration of these questions, I do not think that one can decide about the limitations of the visual system with respect to the processing of information about speech motor activity. Comparable issues are raised when we consider the problem of teaching the congenitally blind child models of three-dimensional space by mapping this information through the auditory system.

DR. SCHUELL: I do not know whether the principle of simultaneous visual and auditory stimulation works with children, but with adult aphasics it is an effective method for evoking responses that occur to neither stimulus mode alone. With a patient who can neither read nor repeat a word or a sentence, we are frequently able to evoke the desired response by presenting printed and spoken words together. Not only this, but after repeated paired presentations, the patient can respond appropriately to either stimulus presented alone.

Probably of all the neurophysiological principles we have tried to use experimentally, the principle of repetitive stimulation seems to produce the greatest facilitation of language in aphasia. It is not only effective for organizing responses the patient has not previously been able to produce but for obtaining recall from day to day and week to week.

There are other factors that are related to effecting verbal responses in aphasic patients. Meaningfulness of the stimulus is an important dimension. When we are dealing with language, it is very clear that familiarity, as opposed to novelty of stimulus, is an important factor. This principle includes the general frequency of usage of words and probably of structural units in the language, as well as the meaningfulness to the patient. It can easily be demonstrated that you can get verbal responses to stimuli that have occurred frequently in the patient's experience more readily than responses to items of lesser familiarity or lesser individual significance.

I remember one patient, for example, who was a judge, from whom I had been able to evoke only single-word responses. One day when I was presenting words simply to evoke responses, I said, "Homicide." He said excitedly, "Homicide—three degrees!" and proceeded to outline these degrees, one by one. He did not use complete sentences, but he combined words and produced more language than had previously been elicited, probably because a connection had been established to patterns previously well-organized in his brain.

The voluntary and involuntary aspects of behavior are extremely interesting in relation to aphasia. With adult aphasics you can get repetition from almost every patient, as soon as motor mechanisms are working well enough. It may take time, but this is almost always possible. When this is achieved, not only emotional responses and the other kinds of inferior utterances Hughlings Jackson described occur, but what Weisenburg and McBride called reactive responses, as well, with no particular emotional coloring.

For example, a hospital visitor once asked a patient with severe aphasia if he received his home town paper. The patient indicated that he did not. The visitor said, "Why not? Don't you have a subscription?" The patient replied, "Expired." This was a simple verbal association to the word "subscription."

Responses like this can be readily evoked in the clinic from any patient who can repeat. It is possible to get 100 different responses in a comparatively short period by providing verbal stimuli which have strong associational linkages. If you say *a cup of* -------, the patient says *coffee*; to *drive a*, he says *car*; to *bacon and* he says *eggs*; and so on. These are stimulus-bound responses, not voluntary speech. The patient who acquires some reactive speech tends to respond more normally outside the clinic, frequently producing responses appropriate to a situation. He remains unable to ask for a glass of water, to tell anyone where he lives, what kind of work he does, nor the names of his children. With severe aphasia we have not been able to move from reactive responses to voluntary speech. I wish someone could tell us how to cross this line. It is the point at which therapy most frequently fails, even with very intelligent and highly motivated patients.

DR. SILVERMAN: May I comment on Dr. Chase's comments. The history of educating deaf children is replete with attempts to accomplish what he has said should be accomplished. I agree we should continue to seek these.

For example, we have a number of competing criteria for an ideal phonetic symbol system. For example, we like to have a system that carries information about the phonemes, such as place and mode of articulation. The two Bells[22] developed such a system which was then called the system of visible speech, in which information was carried about what one does with the articulators. There were fundamental curves of palatal articulation, labial articulation, and so on, and even the size of the symbol conveyed information. The size one line high indicated a consonant; two lines high indicated a vowel.

A second criterion is that it be unambiguous. With the number of phonemes in the

English language and only 26 letters to work with, ambiguity is introduced. The third is that it be a perceptually easy one to take in.

The fourth is that we use the symbols of the culture, if we are to make the transfer into reading and some of the other kinds of linguistic skills that are necessary for the children. These are mutually exclusive criteria.

I welcome Dr. Chase's help and his comments. As I say, the continuing search for these systems, and I could outline a number of these, underline their need.

As for the suggestion of Dr. Magoun, maximizing conversion of excitability by using the different sensory systems, here we again run into the problem both of facilitation, perhaps, in the linguistic sense, and interference. My own view is that we need to study these developmentally. The time at which these are done I believe is important in a child's life, and also the way in which we manipulate, in a sense, the proportion in which we make stimuli available over the sensory systems, both visual and auditory. The kinds of reinforcement we give and associations which we create are also critical.

I believe here, from the rehabilitation point of view or, in our case, habilitation, lies one of our greatest challenges. I wish we had spent a little more time on Dr. Teuber's suggestions about shaping the input. Here, too, the shaping and the use of different sensory modalities may be one of our most fruitful areas of investigation in terms of application to the problems I deal with every day.

DR. GESCHWIND: I would like to second Dr. Hirsh's remarks. For the reasons which he pointed out it is difficult to conceive that cross-modal *transfer* is very important. Only a small number of stimuli can be mapped from one modality onto another. In fact, such mapping is possible only between vision and somesthesis and only for geometric features. Thus, it is difficult to see why a monkey should be built to recognize that a seen snake was of the same shape as a felt snake since he would clearly never have time to palpate a snake from end to end. It would be more

useful if he could learn to correlate the visual stimulus with the texture of the surface (including temperature, hardness, etc.) but in that case we would no longer be speaking of a geometrical mapping.

Obviously cross-modal *transfer* could never involve audition. I omit here deliberately the work on transfer of rhythms which I do not really believe to be relevant. Of general applicability and, I believe, of much greater importance is cross-modal association. What I mean here is the ability to link a stimulus in one modality to a stimulus in another modality, even when no geometrical mapping is possible.

Dr. Myers showed us that the visual, auditory, and somesthetic regions of cortex have no connections among themselves. On the other hand, the outflow from these regions probably converge eventually in certain locations. In particular, they probably converge in the limbic system. They also converge in the motor association cortex of the frontal lobe. Neither of these two systems of convergence is useful as language. Thus, there is an enormous number of visual stimuli but only perhaps 50 or 60 limbic responses. Hence, you could not create exclusive associations for all possible visual stimuli.

In man the situation changes. In the human it is possible to form associations between visual and auditory stimuli. I have pointed out elsewhere[130,132] reasons for believing that this is made possible by the development of the angular gyrus region in man. Since the number of auditory stimuli is for all practical purposes as great as that of visual stimuli, it is now possible to assign visual stimuli to auditory stimuli on a one-to-one basis. On this basis I believe the child learns the names of objects, that is, by learning to associate a seen or felt stimulus to its spoken name, that is, to an auditory stimulus.

DR. MORRELL: I am a little concerned about this discussion of multisensory facilitation and intermodal transfer. I would like to comment on one of the things I omitted from my presentation yesterday, and that is evidence that we have from evoked potential studies bearing upon the physiological character of the disturbances produced by particular central nervous system lesions which interfere with certain kinds of central activity. This really is essentially a plea against a global application of any principle, and for a very, very detailed examination of the actual deficit in every individual patient, so that any kind of rehabilitative measure or treatment is based entirely upon the particular deficit that that particular patient shows.

For example, we have studied some patients with what we have called auditory agnosia, or inability to comprehend verbal material, which is based upon the existence of discharging lesions in the left posterior temporal area. In studying these patients with evoked potential interactions, it has become clear that at least one of the characteristics of such lesions is that, when auditory responses of very high amplitude are obtained to auditory stimulation, it is impossible to use auditory stimuli as conditional stimuli in the kind of paradigm which Dr. Grey Walter outlined so well; that is, they do not provide the substrate that other sensory modalities do for transactional processes. In short, information gets into the auditory sphere, but it does not get out of it to form links with other areas. In this particular example, it would seem that increasing auditory input (even if simultaneously increasing visual or other kinds of input) in this situation disrupts behavior rather than allowing training or providing a basis for increased learning of material. Under such circumstances, it has been shown that learning is much easier through visual and tactile modalities than through the centrally injured acoustic modality.

This is different, then, from the deficit in deaf children or in peripheral injuries where, perhaps, it makes sense to step up the amplitude of the injured modality, of the auditory signal, and combine it with others and thus get mutual facilitation. In our case, that is, with central, irritative lesions having an effect on auditory perception, increasing the input

of auditory information has a disruptive effect. In such patients one should make very clear that the training procedures will be better based upon the utilization of non-involved sensory modalities. The general principle derived from this is that the deficit may be different in each patient, and it is the actual physiologic deficit in each particular patient which has to be looked at in order to plan a rational system of rehabilitation.

DR. PURPURA: I would like to comment on some remarks made by Dr. Hirsh. I am sure that Dr. Hirsh has sat in on many conversations and discussions with neurophysiologists, but I'm not quite sure he has come away from these meetings with a clear understanding of current concepts concerning mechanisms of "facilitation." One tends to talk about facilitation only in excitatory pathways when indeed one could obtain facilitation also of inhibitory elements. Such facilitation of inhibitory activity might be considered an important process for increasing contrast and sharpness as many others have proposed in mechanisms of "surround inhibition." Now the problem which is raised about gross potential actually reflect summated inhibitory activities, not excitatory events. For example, transcallosal activities may involve short latency excitation followed by long latency and prolonged inhibition. Such inhibitory processes are now well documented in all varieties of evoked responses.

The overt effects of brain stem reticular stimulation may appear to be generally excitatory, but intracellular recordings disclose that pyramidal neurons may be silenced during reticulo-cortical activation. Thus, many cells are turned off during arousal stimulation, whereas many are turned on. The latter may be inhibitory elements. Such an increase in inhibitory bombardment may be an effective mechanism for directing a new action. Loss of inhibition increases excitatory drives and causes these to exhibit positive feedback, oscillation, and probably nonpurposeful activity such as is seen in seizure states. It is likely that many of the functional interactions between cortex, basal ganglia, and thalamus are directed toward securing a greater inhibitory control of sensorimotor activities. Many of these events operate at the microtime level but also at the macrotime level.

The problem of inhibitory activities and inhibitory pathways seems to focus on the question of what one can interpret about anatomical connections alone. Given the demonstration of a connection from one site in cortex or one area of cortex to another, including interhemispheric connections, can it be inferred from these data whether the connection is excitatory or inhibitory? I am particularly unconcerned about the failures of Dr. Geschwind to find long anatomical connections between one cortical region and another. For me anatomy stops at the first synapse in a functional pathway. Relatively long latencies have been recorded in many cortico-cortical evoked responses. This strongly suggests multi-synaptic connections—and the more synapses the greater possibility for interaction, convergence, and integration. For this reason I think it is rather meaningless to insist on relationships based exclusively on direct connections between regions of brain.

Another point disturbs me in relation to some of Dr. Grey Walter's work. I am not sure that Dr. Grey Walter's Contingent Negative Variation (CNV) is indeed always an excitatory event. What is recorded is a large negative wave which may be positive in the depths of the cortex. It is of interest that negative waves in other types of responses are frequently associated with inhibitory postsynaptic potentials of cortical neurons. Perhaps, then, the CNV reflects an inhibitory "get-set" process for a correct response and not necessarily an excitatory event. It cannot be emphasized too strongly that what is so important for the elaboration of an integrated nervous system is the proper development and expression of inhibitory processes. Examination of inhibition and the synaptic pathways which produce inhibitory activities must be carried out with analytical tools that go far beyond the conventional anatomical

methods currently in use. Again, this is why I am not too disturbed by many of the negative findings obtained in conventional neuroanatomical studies aimed at defining relationships between different parts of the brain.

DR. ROSENBLITH: Professor Magoun's comments have had two facilitatory effects already: one, in removing a great deal of inhibition from the way in which the people around this table have perhaps not proclaimed their territories but at least their faith in the technics that they are using. I think such a reaffirmation of faith was the most important one. But, in a more profound way, he has focused upon the fact that many of those who deal with the organism as a whole do not have, at the present time, a philosophy, the knowledge, you might even say the myth, that tells them something about contemporary brain mechanisms instead of those that they have learned out of textbooks and discarded.

Second, he has also focused upon the necessity of a rationale for the way in which therapeutic and rehabilitative procedures are being carried on in the light of what has happened to recent study of brain mechanism. Both of these things I feel are very much needed.

Having said this, I must make a remark concerning the organization of this symposium that strikes me, perhaps at this stage of the symposium, as particularly peculiar. It is true that it was extremely important to hear Dr. Evarts talk about patterns of motor units and to have thereby shown what microphysiology, in this particular system, can do today. The fact that there was no presentation on what the auditory system is doing physiologically seems to me a lacuna upon which I have not yet heard any remarks.

Having said this, I will go a step further. I think I will agree with my friend Ira Hirsh when he says that time is the commodity that is of the essence in the auditory system. Indeed, if one studies the behavior of single units in the auditory system, what one is struck with is the fact of how enormously variable, flexible, and meaningfully coded the time patterns of unit activity are; how stimuli are being translated in a manner that makes later utilization of these time patterns extraordinarily useful and relevant. The time patterns not only are excitations, as Dr. Purpura indicated appropriately, but what are the long pauses that units of cortical and subcortical and other structures show when stimulated by a transient or a steady state? The fact that we have not heard this constitutes, to my way of thinking, a completely regrettable lacuna. I think it is probably one of those obvious things; it was too obvious to be thought of.

Let me go a little further in depth, however, and ask myself a couple more questions. We have talked here about single units. Dr. Teuber mentioned for us the multivalency of neurons, the fact that, in some sense, even in most afferent pathways, neurons turn out to be polyglots or, if not polyglots, at least people who listen to neighbors when they chatter in Polish.

It turns out, also, that anesthesia undoubtedly renders some of these units aphasic in several languages, whether in the classical order, or in the order of Polish first—I do not want to argue but it is very clear that, if you look at the behavior, and especially at the time pattern from single units that are in an unanesthetized preparation multisensorily interested, they very often will fall back upon a very much narrower way of dealing with external stimuli in the anesthetized animal.

Without detracting in any way from the extraordinarily beautiful work of Hubel and Wiesel, let me underline two important differences. As far as the auditory system is concerned, the units at the highest levels of the auditory system that have been studied are not beholden to a single stimulus. On the contrary, their specialization is a specialization in time patterns of response to a variety of stimuli. Therefore, the problems that do arise when one talks particularly about what might happen cross-modally is a very important problem, because it is not very clear to me—at least at this stage of what we know about the skin system, the visual system, and

the auditory system—that the neurons in these three systems, though many of them show influences of the other modalities, all behave the same way. As a matter of fact, my present belief is that they do not. Furthermore, it is very important to realize that, when one looks at a single unit and when one looks at an evoked response and when one talks about a hemisphere and when one talks about a given region, all these regions have an enormous population of neurons in a pattern of both specificity and something that one does not want to call randomness but that still carries with it the concept of populations. Therefore, the important thing is to understand what are the spatial temporal patterns of inhibition, activation, or whatever else you want to call it; and that if one talks about the way in which a particular region in the brain behaves, it is extraordinarily important that we have some kind of model in order to go from the behavior of single units to a behavior that represents something of a more integrated vote of a population, and how this vote reflects itself in other things.

The point that remains is that for the auditory system it might not be so terrible to think (from the point of view of the way in which it processes auditory information, including linguistic information)—to start out with the temporal patterns of activity as being at least something that is related to, shall we say, the surface structure of the way in which auditory stimuli are being coded; we should not immediately search, perhaps, for the universals that would tell us the way in which grammar might be encoded in there, but the mere fact of looking at the orderly structure of temporal patterns of information that come in essentially in a temporal way seems to me an absolutely necessary step in trying to understand how this system operates. Then we must also ask ourselves how activity from other senses, the general activation level of an organism, and orienting reflexes and contingent negative variation and similar type phenomena modulate these particular patterns. This is the type of task that I think can be carried on quite successfully, and it will get us a great step nearer the kind of problems of a basic nature that Professor Magoun has raised.

DR. GREY WALTER: I agree with everything that everybody has said.

The first point I would like to emphasize is one Dr. Teuber made: the importance of studies of development. In fact, a good deal of the material I described emerged from a laborious study of normal, disturbed, and autistic children, in which we gradually accumulated evidence that the Contingent Negative Variation is the most accurate measure of brain maturity we have. Children below three never show this effect. Children above about three can develop it with social support. At the age of 15 only half of our normal children showed consistent CNVs, and even students of about 20 often fail to show it, unless they are given powerful social support or competitive motivation. Disturbed children or autistic children rarely show the effect even in the mid-teens. In children with speech disorders one can sometimes identify the source of the difficulty by discovering the preferred sequence of stimulation for production of a Contingent Negative Variation. This is also reflected in adults with childish behavior, sometimes called psychopaths. They also respond in a childish fashion in this paradigm.

The next point is the question of neuropharmacology that Dr. Magoun raised. We must appreciate that the curves and patterns we throw on the screen are really reflections of chemical processes mediated by a vast complex of enzymatic processes, all of which are accessible to neuropharmacological intervention. I think this could be one of the most exciting fields in the future, to discover the compounds which will assist in the development of what we regard as desirable neuronal processes and prevent the undesirable ones. We have found, for example, that caffeine and the more sophisticated drugs, such as the amphetamines, will potentiate the Contingent Negative Variation even in people who don't

have it, for example, in a group of criminal psychopaths. For a while we can boost the Contingent Negative Variation to something like normal by exhibition of stimulant drugs. There is an enormous range of these drugs now, but this would need a special study which is beyond our capacity. One of the difficulties raised by Dr. Hirsh and Dr. Purpura is the total inadequacy in the present context of the excitation-inhibition dichotomy. We have to find new words or new meanings for these words.

Two years ago when I was addressing the Leningrad Physiological Society, there was heated argument in which they attempted to maintain the characteristic dialectic of excitatory and inhibitory processes. I pointed out, much as did Dr. Purpura, that people who do not have Contingent Negative Variation are not characterized by failure to respond but respond too soon; they jump the gun. Young children and psychopaths and other people in whom the Contingent Negative Variation is absent characteristically respond irregularly with anticipations as well as delays and the distribution of their responses is "normal" about the period when they are expected to respond. Normal people who do develop a CNV show something more like a Poisson distribution from the instant after the imperative stimulus. There is no doubt that this is a deferment of action, and a paradox arises. A simple illustration is when you have an alarm or phone call to wake you at a certain time. This is an excitatory stimulus, but it is also inhibitory because it stops you from waking too soon. The Contingent Negative Variation is an alarm in this sense. It defers action until an appropriate time and then promotes it. We do not get up from our chairs until a certain time has come; therefore, the Chairman is acting as an inhibitor. We are also stimulated to do things at the right time, when the Chairman tells us to do so.

In these complex systems it is quite inadequate to think in terms of excitatory and inhibitory processes or even of facilitation, occlusion, and so forth.

Next as to multimodal stimulation and its value in the operational problem of teaching children to hear or talk: it is true that a mere application of multimodal technic with flashback technic is futile. One of the most important features in the studies of Contingent Negative Variation is the great importance of stimulus interval; it is no good giving two visual stimuli together. This is a practical problem which we are faced with quite frequently in advising speech therapists and others treating children with hearing or speaking deficiencies: how to choose the sequence and interval of stimuli. Should they be auditory-visual or visual-auditory? What is the interval between the presentations to produce the optimum acquisition of information and skill? This seems to be a very important field for study in which we can use both physiological and behavioral estimates of performance.

Finally, a word about the general problem of integration of physiological studies. I think it is extremely important to combine information in these two categories simultaneously. The most valuable and helpful information we have obtained from experimental paradigms such as you saw is the simultaneous study of the electrophysiological (including autonomic) recordings with the psychological aspects of the presentations. Statistical comparison of performance of psychological results by hindsight with physiological changes is usually ambiguous, often confusing. If these observations are simultaneous, the amount of information is multiplied.

DR. EVARTS: I would like to expand on a point Dr. Teuber made about the types of insights one can get into the complex processes of the nervous system by starting on the output and working backward rather than starting at the input and working forward. In a way, I think perhaps the best person to have presented an integrated approach on output processing would have been someone like Dethier, who has worked with insect

sensory systems but in a context where he can relate the operation of a sensory system to the motor output of the insect. In fact, an understanding of the way in which the sensory systems are organized can often be best understood by looking at the output. This makes ontogenetic and phylogenetic sense in relation to the order in which the various parts of the nervous system develop: the nervous system has always developed in relation to the control of the motor output; this is what the nervous system is for.

DR. MYERS: Dr. Purpura's provocative comments invite a few observations. Dr. Purpura appears to suggest that the facts of anatomy may be ignored in favor of seemingly contradictory physiological findings. The rather specific and well-defined data of anatomy tell us on the one hand that there are highly organized, highly specific, and highly channelized pathways through which information may be transmitted between points within the nervous system. The degree of channelization and organization of these pathways does not allow for a broad diffusion of data between heterologous systems. By contrast and in apparent conflict with this there occur peculiar, so-called *multisensory* units widely disseminated within the nervous system. These *multisensory* units respond to stimuli originating from several sensory systems. Even with the use of gross electrodes evoked activity from the several sensory systems may be picked up in widespread cortical loci and even extensively within thalamus and brain stem in the cat.

It may be suggested that the term "multisensory" is a misnomer as applied to these neurons. The name itself implies a function for these units in sensation. However, contribution of such neurons to sensory functions has yet to be demonstrated. A less misleading designation for these units might be "multimodal." This designation lacks functional implications but still suggests that such units can be excited to activity by data or impulses derived from several different neural systems.

The multimodal neurons distributed widely in the brain and responding to stimuli applied to either body half seem not to serve higher order perceptual or memory functions. Animals with the cerebral commissures destroyed fail to give evidence for transfer of training within the tactile or visual spheres when patterned sensory stimuli are used. It follows that the multitude of multimodal units excited in the two hemispheres during training through one side of the body are later incapable of contributing to correct performance on transfer testing through the other side of the body. The reported training transfer in commissure-sectioned animals when using stimuli such as brightness or flicker frequency suggests, however, that multimodal units may contribute to perceptual processes at a more primitive level.

Other functional possibilities might be suggested for multimodal neurons. Sensory systems, whether auditory, visual, or tactual, ultimately must have access to the motor reaction mechanism to guide or affect motor response. Certain of the neurons within the motor mechanism may thus be responsive in a more or less direct fashion to stimuli originating in several or all of the sensory systems. Such neurons, though fired by sensory stimuli, still must be considered motor in function. Multimodal units alternatively might serve an alerting or attention function. The degree of dissemination and the intensity of response of multimodal units has been shown to relate to the significance or degree of unexpectedness of a sensory signal rather than to its energy. Startling or significant signals produce generalized effects throughout the cerebrum.

It is not clearly known through what anatomical pathways the multimodal neurons may be excited. Data presented in the present symposium suggest that cerebral associational pathways do not likely account for these heterologous excitations. Rather more likely is an excitation from below through corticopetal diffuse pathways by means of thalamus.

While multimodal neurons may not contribute directly to memory or perceptual processes, there is evidence that the anatomic mechanism identified with the multi-modal system has profound contributions to make to the proper functioning of cortical sensory systems. Lesions in brain-stem tegmentum impinging upon this system produce profound and lasting deficits in visual perceptual processes in the cat. Similar lesions disrupt function as well in other sensory systems. Thus, diffuse system centers in the brainstem seem to have a profound generalized impact on cortical physiology. The activities of multimodal units may represent ripples or reflections of the functioning of this diffuse system perhaps in relation to levels of excitation. These brain-stem systems are poorly known both anatomically and physiologically but seem to be of greater importance to less evolved forms than to the primate.

In summary, the functional implications of multimodal units are not known. Several logically possible roles for such units are suggested, none of which would rule out the occurrence or diminish the importance of highly organized and channelized pathways within the nervous system. Rather, these two types of mechanisms may occur anatomically intermingled and serve quite different roles in the total functioning of the organism. Multisensory mixing in relation to these units likely occurs in brainstem or thalamus.

CHAIRMAN MILLIKAN: Dr. Masland, will you continue?

Lacunae and Research Approaches to Them. III.

RICHARD L. MASLAND

National Institute of Neurological
Diseases and Blindness
Bethesda, Maryland

POSSIBLY FROM A somewhat more simple-minded approach there may still be a few other rays of light cast on some of the difficult problems which we have been discussing.

First I would like to consider the problem of the input. I was tremendously impressed by Dr. Hirsh's description of the varied parameters of speech and language and with the great diversity of input signal with which the nervous system has to deal. We speak of spectral pattern, serial order, stress, rhythm, and probably many other parameters with which I am personally completely unacquainted. It impressed me that there must be a great deal of redundancy within this system, and I wonder whether every individual relies on the same items of information for the major recognition of language.

Hirsh pointed out that he has been concerned with a search for systematic confusions as an indication of the use of cues and of the method of interpretation used. If, in fact, this thesis of redundancy is correct, and particularly if there are individual differences in the utilization of various cues, then the search for systematic confusions becomes very much more difficult, indeed.

I come back to the thesis which has previously been presented that one of the most fruitful sources of information on this point, and many others like it, is through the careful study of language development in children, using data derived from large numbers of carefully studied individuals. Certainly a more precise knowledge of the nature of the task involved in communication and of the mechanisms which are used will give us important data regarding the characteristics of the nervous system which will be required to handle this task. Through the course of time the technic of communication has been fashioned to suit the accomplishments and capabilities of the nervous system. Possibly this was one of the important contributions of Dr. Chomsky in pointing out the capability of the child automatically to learn a great portion of our grammar which does not appear in the textbook. I am not myself convinced that the fact that this does not appear in the textbook necessarily means that it is not learned behavior.

Another major focus of this Conference has been the nature of cerebral dominance—an almost unique feature of the human nervous system which is of paramount importance. In this connection a very interesting point was emphasized by Mishkin[286] at the conference on Interhemispheric Relations and Cerebral Dominance. He showed that intermodal association is more readily accomplished within a single hemisphere than it is accomplished when the utilization of both hemispheres is required.

The experiment presented was quite a simple one. As shown in Figure 52, first produce in monkeys a lesion in the occiput and a lesion in the appropriate area of the temporal lobe concerned with interpretation of complex visual symptoms. If both lesions are in a single hemisphere, you find little, if any, deficit except in homonymous hemianopsia, which corresponds to this occipital lesion.

If, on the other hand, the temporal-lobe lesion is made in the other hemisphere from the occipital, then you find that there is a deficit of performance. In other words, the ability of the remaining occipital lobe to interact with the temporal lobe of the contralateral hemisphere is less than is its ability to interact with one on the same side. As long as you have an intact occipital and temporal area on one side, the animal can perform reasonably well. When an interhemispheric reaction is required, there is a deficit of performance. Of course, if one sections the corpus callosum, then this becomes a profound deficit. I think this may give us a clue, from the teleological point of view, as to the importance of hemisphere dominance. When the nervous system is concerned with activities which require complex intermodality associations, it becomes a matter of efficiency for these to be accomplished within a single hemisphere.

There have been alluded to in this meeting several possible bases or characteristics of cerebral dominance. The first is that which Dr. Milner has presented here and elsewhere, that the outstanding characteristic of the dominant hemisphere is its ability to handle symbols; that activities requiring the use of symbols require the integrity of the left hemisphere but that certain nonsymbolic acts or interpretation or recognition of objects having no symbolic meaning involve the right hemisphere. If one accepts the thesis, which apparently is still at issue, that language requires intermodality associations, then it would seem appropriate that the symbol formation would be more readily accomplished within a single hemisphere.

We have even gone so far in this Conference as to suggest the thesis that, according to the concept which has been rather popular in the Soviet Union,[250,251] language is used as a means of controlling other behavior. If this is true, then the fact that language becomes centered in the left hemisphere might mean that this is the basis upon which that hemisphere has become dominant in other respects. This, I think, has been suggested in the course of this Conference. I find it doubtful to accept this

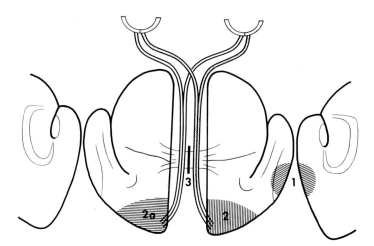

Fig. 52. Results of lesions in occiput and temporal lobes and sections of corpus callosum. 1: Lesion of lateral temporal lobe. 2: Lesion of ipsilateral occiput. 2a: Lesion of contralateral occiput. 3: Section of corpus callosum. 1 plus 2 produces no deficit. 2 plus 2a produces moderate deficit. 1 plus 2a and 3 produced severe deficit (after Mishkin[286]).

234

BRAIN MECHANISMS UNDERLYING SPEECH AND LANGUAGE

thesis since even deaf illiterate people are right-handed. It would appear that handedness is something that appears aside from language, that cerebral dominance is something that appears aside from spoken language, at least, and probably precedes it. I would personally suspect that language is in the left hemisphere because that hemisphere is dominant rather than that the reverse is the case.

A second possible characteristic of cerebral dominance has also been alluded to, and I think Dr. Hirsh, again, has been most helpful in emphasizing the fact that language and hearing differ so strikingly from the other senses in their preoccupation with time. I have been intrigued with the possibility that maybe it is the integration of time-bound activities which centers in the left hemisphere and that it is preoccupation with space-bound activities which might center in the right hemisphere. This is a nice, tidy concept. It seemed to me for a while that this was being supported by such interesting observations as those presented by Dr. Benton regarding the spatial preoccupation of the right temporoparietal region. I find myself a little shaken, however, by the reports of Dr. Geschwind, Dr. Gazzaniga, and Dr. Sperry of the split-brain preparations, which throw into question the evidence that spatial perception is integrated in the right hemisphere.

In this respect, the observation has been made that, when one has a lesion in the right temporoparietal region, the individual develops a lack of concern for or recognition of events occurring on the left side of his body or, in fact, a loss of appreciation of the existence of the left side of his body. This has been taken to indicate that this area is concerned with spatial representation and body image. But it occurs to me that this information which comes to the right parietal region, under normal circumstances, is carried across the corpus callosum to the temporoparietal region of the left hemisphere, which is so clearly crucial in overall intel-

ligence and certain other integrated functions.

What is going to be the reaction of this left hemisphere if, in fact, it is deprived of information coming from the right side of the brain? It seems to me that this hemisphere is going to say, "The left side of my body doesn't exist." And, far from indicating that it is the right side which is concerned with body image, it seems to me that these data support the thesis that it is the left hemisphere which integrates the total picture and that, when the left hemisphere is deprived of the information from the right, it simply behaves as though it were not present.

Let us also remember that in many of these experiments these individuals are being asked to give spoken responses as to what they are observing and to write with their right hand. If we consider these patients to be the equivalent of a split-brain preparation, then we know that the individual with this split cannot speak about what goes on in the contralateral hemisphere. He cannot describe it unless he describes it with his left hand.

These considerations have shaken me rather seriously and caused me to feel that many of our observations and much of our psychological testing is going to have to be re-evaluated in terms of the output channels which we have utilized for reporting the subjective experiences of our subjects.

A third possibility of cerebral dominance is the thesis that really the left hemisphere has to serve as the trigger mechanism or as the primary initiator of activity. Let us consider the instance of a split-brain preparation. I gather that these individuals talk naturally, that they walk down the street in a reasonable fashion, that they are able to dress themselves. How are those coordinated functions carried out if the two hemispheres are, in fact, as independent as this operation would lead you to believe they are? I am sorry that Dr. Lansdell did not report for Dr. Maitland Baldwin on their split-brain activities. I believe Dr. Baldwin has split even further down in his chimpanzees, and they still behave in a remarkably intact fashion. How is it that this takes place? I am assuming that there is a much greater feedback from the proprioceptive and even spinal areas of these individuals than might be recognized, that, in fact, if the individual starts to talk, this triggers a proprioceptive input into the nondominant hemisphere, which then locks into a long remembered pattern, and that, in fact, the speech mechanism of the right hemisphere and of the left hemisphere are locked through this feedback mechanism into a relatively normal procedure.

Let us recognize that either hemisphere has considerable control over both sides of the body and that if one hemisphere, in fact, triggers something off, both sides may then be interacting. In this connection, this may be some explanation, also, for the very interesting phenomenon described by Dr. Falconer in his patient with epilepsy. Maybe there is something also to the thesis that the right hemisphere is more involved in emotional activities. Possibly it is that under emotional circumstances an act can be initiated in the nondominant hemisphere which ordinarily is triggered off only by the activation of the dominant hemisphere. In this connection, from a practical point of view, I wonder how much we can accomplish in the nondominant hemisphere of the aphasic. I gather from Dr. Sperry's report that the individuals with the split brain were able to appreciate written words in the field of vision on their nondominant side and to respond to that. It would be very interesting to know whether, in fact, the aphasic individual, or the individual with a lesion, can perform in this fashion with his nondominant hemisphere. I see no reason why he should be any worse. Is it possible that this might ultimately be a useful device to assist in the retraining of the aphasic, particularly since it is evident that in the split-brain

individual there is a carry-over from one hemisphere to the other through some of these mechanisms which I have been discussing.

It is important to note from what Dr. Schuell has said in regard to severe aphasics that even the most severe aphasic has not lost speech; the patterns for speech are still there. Maybe the patterns for language are lost but the motor mechanism of speech exists. The problem is how to key into it, how to set this mechanism in motion. This appears to be what is lacking in the aphasic.

This conference has given me a greater respect, I think, for the work of Dr. Samuel T. Orton[302] who, observing a group of children with language disabilities, developed the concept that, in certain instances, these disturbances related to an improper coordination or interaction between the two hemispheres. Dr. H. G. Birch has recently studied a group of these children and finds that he does not confirm any relationship with handedness, but he does find that, in the children with specific dyslexia, there is a confusion of body image and of right-left orientation. It would be interesting to know whether in a group of such children one would find the differences in laterality of perception such as Dr. Milner has demonstrated in a group of other individuals. Do these individuals with specific dyslexia show an equivalence of sensitivity to visual and auditory stimuli in the two hemispheres? If so, it gives a little more support to the procedures which have at times been recommended of concentrating on sensory, auditory, and visual input and utilization of one side of the body in this group of individuals. I do not know whether anyone has attempted, for example, flashing word pictures into one or another field of vision of a group of dyslexic children to see whether they then show the strephosymbolia which is so characteristic of this disorder.

CHAIRMAN MILLIKAN: Are there comments? Dr. Darley, will you proceed?

Lacunae and Research Approaches to Them. IV.

FREDERIC L. DARLEY

Mayo Clinic
Rochester, Minnesota

ASKED TO REFLECT as a speech pathologist on the impact of this Conference, I would like to respond with comments in three areas. First, I believe we need to solve some evident problems concerned with the identification of language phenomena and with terminology. It seems to me there are some problems here in several areas we have been talking about. For example, let us talk about aphasia.

Not everything called aphasia by someone is, indeed, aphasia. The question has arisen: Is aphasia caused by a lesion of subcortical structures? We have heard Dr. Myers point out that lesions or stimulation of the thalamus lead to confusion or dementia. This might overwhelm or obscure any language deficit, if it were present; or this confusion itself may simply be mistaken for aphasia. Language performance in diffuse degenerative disease bears certain resemblances to and displays certain differences from aphasia. As we previously learned, ictal speech automatisms differ from ictal aphasia. So these constitute one set of distinctions that we obviously have to make.

Another relates to behaviors which have traditionally gone by the name of aphasia but which are distinguishable from it. When we review the behavior that Broca described, which has since gone by the name of motor aphasia, many of us believe it should be called by a name other than aphasia because it is in a different, a nonlinguistic, dimension. One of the latest to point this out is Wep-man[405] in 1955 and again in a revised statement in 1960.[404] The gropings of the motor aphasic patient for correct positioning of his articulators, his clumsiness in finding the correct pattern of movement to produce a polysyllabic word, his near misses phonemically, and his retrials are predominant. And in the kind of patient I am talking about, they are coupled, as Broca pointed out, with no reduction in auditory comprehension and no disability in expressing himself fluently in writing. In other words, his performance represents no cross-modality impairment in the use of language symbols but a specific modality-bound deficit, better labeled an apraxia, to be exact, an oral verbal apraxia.

Now, Bay does not call this apraxia; he calls it cortical dysarthria,[21] emphasizing that it is more in the sphere of motor impairment than in the sphere of linguistic impairment. But he insists that we must not consider it aphasia. This is no idle semantic exercise, some of us feel, because the treatment of these patients is certainly different from the treatment of those whom we call aphasic. What I have to do with this apraxic patient only puzzles and does not help the aphasic patient, and if I were to do with the apraxic patient what I do with the aphasic patient, he would be only offended; he does not need general language stimulation.

Another set of distinctions pertains to dysarthria. In contrast to the patient with an oral verbal apraxia is the person who presents a motor speech problem due to paralysis, weakness, or incoordination. But dysarthria[1] is not dysarthria.[2] What shall we let the term "dysarthria" encompass? Originally, it simply referred to an affection of articulation, but nowadays we extend it to include neurogenic problems in all the basic aspects of execution of the speech act: respiration, phonation, articulation, resonance, and prosody. And these are differentially disturbed in lower motor neuron lesions, bilateral upper motor neuron lesions, extrapyramidal lesions characterized by hyperkinesia, those characterized by hypokinesia, and cerebellar lesions. The term "dysarthria," then, covers multiple variables. We need some modifiers to identify the systems involved and the phenomena that typify each system involved.

These are some of the areas in which I think our terminology needs disciplining. It is evident that all our studies to date are not of equal importance or validity in terms of this requirement of exact differential identification and designation. I think we have seen in this Conference a wide range represented, from the description of the exquisitely detailed analysis of the speech and motor behavior under multiple conditions of Dr. Sperry and Dr. Gazzaniga's three patients, to a broad statement about the fact that in one study half the patients had a receptive problem and half had an expressive one. Throughout the literature labels are used without due care, and that is one reason why Dr. Sperry could allude without contradiction to "the almost paralyzing complexity and contradictoriness of the literature."

Perhaps the time has come, before we rush on to gather more data, to review critically what we can stand on in terms of adequency of identification and designation. What data should we ignore since the terminology was fuzzy and the observations of behavior were too restricted or too uncontrolled? What studies warrant replication to reveal whether what seemed to emerge as a germ of truth was, in fact, believable? What re-examina-

tions of concepts are required because they were framed in terms or thrust into classifications which were armchair and *a priori?* Perhaps we need a kind of International Standards Organization for aphasia terminology and classification!

To do this kind of critical review surely requires unusual courage and scintillating scholarship, and who is good enough and brave enough to do it? But if it is not done, at a Conference like this ten or 25 years hence won't we be talking in the same vague way about the meaning of some of the things we have been trying to stand on?

The second thing I want to talk about is really closely related to this. What I guess we are engaged in here is a confrontation that invites a kind of matching up—an interlocking—of batches of phenomonology. We are trying to hook up some language phenomenology the clinician tries to understand and cope with every day with some neurophysiological phenomenology revealed in the laboratory. I have been impressed with the beauty of some of the neurophysiological work detailing ever so explicitly the phenomenology. I am less enchanted with the methodology and the detail of the language phenomenology. I think when it comes to saying something about language that we, as speech pathologists, clinical psychologists, and others have been too blithe in applying labels, as I have already said, and then letting the words we use do our thinking for us.

Remember Dr. Sperry's words: "Perhaps patients are deliberate nonconformists." Surely their likenesses are exceeded by their differences. We must see and never forget that the patients we ultimately push into one category or another do not, because they are there, represent a unitary population. As Dr. Geschwind pointed out, patients with trouble in comprehending are not all alike. Some of them can repeat but not understand words. Some can neither repeat nor understand. Some can read words and not numbers. Some can follow written but not oral commands.

What do we need, then, if we are going

to elaborate the language phenomenology? I think we have to fragment the patient's behavior and specify in greater detail what he can and can not do under what circumstances in what time frame? We have to do standardized, detailed testing. It is not enough to sort through our pockets and present miscellaneous objects to the patient to respond to, nor is it enough to trust to a brief screening test, though such a test may be useful for other purposes. I think the coverage of many combinations of stimulus and response modes, each in adequate depth, requires a pattern of detailed appraisal such as Dr. Schuell's Minnesota Test of Differential Diagnosis of Aphasia.[345]

Hopefully, too, the test vehicle should permit quantification and easy comparison of serial performances, as Porch's Index of Communicative Ability[320] promises to do. And I think the testing should make allowance for flexibility in expansion of parts of the test where warranted so that one's clinical ingenuity will not be inhibited. I think speech pathologists and clinical psychologists should not be content with anything less than systematic, comprehensive, deep testing as they play a crucial role in language appraisal in this cooperative venture of understanding and helping the language-impaired individual.

Third, in order to present some of the gaps in our knowledge, I would like to suggest a whole different way the Conference might have been organized—and no criticism is implied, Dr. Millikan. But what if this had been called "Language Development and Change from the Cradle to the Grave?" These are some of the questions that I and my colleagues in speech pathology and audiology, in education of the deaf, and in special education would inject into the discussion.

What is the nature of the process by which we acquire language? How do we learn a language symbol system? Do we learn it the same way we learn nonverbal symbol systems —mathematical, artistic, spatial, etc.? How are our uses of various symbol systems related?

Then, what goes awry? What are the up-to-now undefined developmental aplasias, to use Dr. Hardy's term, that account for the nonacquisition of language by youngsters who are clearly neither hard of hearing nor mentally retarded? Can we, by a variety of appraisal methods, develop a profile showing how the relevant variables (input, cognition, output) are patterned in these children? The Illinois Test of Psycholinguistic Abilities[264] is an effort to profile some of these variables. There are other variables—psychosocial ones —that need to be profiled, too.

Some information about physical variables must await autopsy, apparently, but how badly we need this kind of information, there being, to my knowledge, only one report in the literature on the postmortem of an individual judged to be congenitally aphasic, a report by Landau, Goldstein, and Kleffner.[214]

Back to the live children: can we discern how alerting and attention mechanisms function in normal language learning and, again, in the disordered learning of children who are dyslexic, or who are aphasic, the uninhibited, overactive and destructive children, children with multiple physical intellectual and emotional problems?

Moving to the question Dr. Bosma raised, how do disorders of the sensory apparatus of the oral mechanism relate to speech disorders? Taking one example, our athetoid children: how much of their communication problem is due to sensory deprivation or sensory distortion?

Further, if there is an instinctive basis for language learning, if we must hypothesize deep structures whose existence is a prerequisite to language learning, what are the prerequisites to the utilization of these instinctive mechanisms? How much speech, of what kind, must the child be stimulated with before he will learn, and what are the time limits within which realization of this language potential must occur? If the child is to master language, must the prerequisite be met by age three, five, eight, or twelve?

Skipping over all the intervening years,

with the coming of the stroke, the trauma, the neoplasm, or the infection, we have a whole new set of questions. In the aphasic patient, what is the nature of the task involved in relearning? How is it different, if it is different, from original learning? What is the speech pathologist doing in his remedial program? Is he educating? We do not think so. Is he stimulating, fostering recall of language patterns? How does this take place? Can we help the aphasic patient most in unimodality stimulation or multimodality stimulation? How do we program the presentation of the stimuli? We may ask if what we are trying to get our patients to do in aphasic therapy is linguistically and neurologically unsound. Perhaps we are trying to get our patients to talk the way we write. The sentences we encourage them to produce may resemble the sentences the linguist writes on the board which are a far cry from the sentences that same linguist feeds into this microphone. Are we trying to teach patterns they almost never hear?

As Dr. Schuell asked earlier, can we somehow exploit the patient's ability to produce automatic-reactive speech and get him to produce more volitional-propositional speech, or must these remain separate if, indeed, they are separate?

How can we explain the patient's blocks on one hand and his uninhibited reflections of an irrelevant stimulus on the other hand? What are the gating mechanisms? How do they go awry? In the case of the patient not aphasic but dysarthric, what are the mechanisms that account for distinctive patterns of dysarthria? Do cortical and subcortical lesions result in different kinds of dysarthria, as suggested yesterday? This is not to be answered by a casual listening and saying, "I think so" or "I don't think so," but by careful fractionation into the dimensions of motor speech performance, critical listening, and instrumental analysis.

Ladies and gentlemen, hopefully we in speech pathology and in audiology, in clinical and experimental psychology, in clinical neurology and psychiatry, in neuroanatomy, neurophysiology, and neurochemistry can develop more and more low-order laws concerning human and perhaps subhuman language behavior. These laws ultimately will be encompassed and integrated by a unifying theory, whether one developed by the linguists or another. But we need old data critically re-examined and new data vigorously collected, analyzed, and interpreted, and generously shared in our journals and our books, and in experiments in cross-professional fertilization like this one, for which we are most sincerely grateful.

CHAIRMAN MILLIKAN: Any comments?

DR. JAMES F. BOSMA: May I briefly mention oral stereognosis, as a form of cross-modal perception which is currently under study in normal and in neurologically impaired subjects in a collaborative project of the National Institute of Dental Research.[42]

The development of oral stereognosis abilities in children has been observed by McDonald and Aungst[266] and by Shelton, Hetherington, and Arndt.[359] In the testing routine the children are first visually oriented to the forms and practice visual matching. Unknown forms are then placed in the mouth and the subject attempts to select a duplicate from an array of 20 or 25 forms before him. During the grade school years discrimination progresses from an average of eight (at five years) to 20 (at 16 years) or 25 standard shapes developed at NIDR and at the Pennsylvania State University.

CHAIRMAN MILLIKAN: Other comments?

DR. ARTHUR L. BENTON: I could not agree more with Dr. Darley about the sad state of terminology and classification in the field of aphasia. I doubt there would be any disagreement among us.

However, I shudder at the thought that these questions will be decided by an international commission, either by an elite or by a democratic process; really we would be carrying democracy too far. Obviously there are good reasons for this confusion. We don't know the facts. The obvious prescription, I think, is investigative work to determine the most useful definitions, the most useful classifications, for different purposes. Thus we might have different classifications for pathology, for purposes of re-education, and so on. We need this investigative work. It is also evident why we don't have this empirical underpinning at the present time. This calls for tedious, time-consuming longitudinal work, for example, comparing symptomatology with response to treatment. We might want to do this but we really cannot, because our treatments vary from case to case. This is the sad state of the art but it cannot be corrected by fiat.

DR. BRUCE KONIGSMARK: I would like to make one comment in conjunction with the point brought up by Dr. Carhart. The experiments of nature can well be utilized, I think, in shedding more light on aphasia in children. Much work has been done on the pathology of aphasia in adults, but very little, as Dr. Darley has mentioned, has been completed in the pathology of childhood aphasia. This lack should and can be remedied, I think, if everyone who works in the field is conscious of it and gains permission for autopsy, seeing to it that these cases are examined as completely as possible so that correlation can be made between the clinical status and the deficits in the nervous system that can be found out by adequate study.

CHAIRMAN MILLIKAN: Other comments?

DR. RAYMOND CARHART: During this Conference we have heard a tremendous number of stimulating things about language, speech, and the brain mechanisms underlying them. Now it might be well to reiterate something we probably should remember as we leave this Conference, namely, there are really two distinct behaviors involving verbal language, at least insofar as the child or adult who has mastered language is concerned. Specifically, the reception of speech as it goes on within all of us is a very different process, in a multitude of ways, from the process of producing speech. When we receive speech, we are awaiting the temporal sequences Dr. Hirsh described for us so well. Here we must await the sequences to complete a meaning someone else is transmitting to us. When we produce speech, we are searching from moment to moment for the symbols with which to phrase a concept that we wish to express. In this second instance we must keep selecting the verbal elements required for that expression and we must then produce the necessary speech sequences. Inevitably the brain mechanisms underlying receptive and expressive language functions are distinctive in many important ways.

Concluding Remarks

DR. BROSIN: We are at the end. May I, on behalf of the assembly, move thanks to NINDB and to our Chairman and his colleagues for this excellent Conference.

DR. BENTON: I second it. (Applause)

MR. RICHARD C. BAIN: I want to say that, for me this was a marvelous thing. Why I should be here is a good question, because I don't have your special knowledge or use the language you use—except that, in one sense, I perhaps am a special kind of physician who has just one client, and that is me. I have gone through many of the problems which you have talked about, and I am trying to recover so far as I can myself. I think I was, as some people have said, a global aphasia. I could hear the words but I couldn't understand the words and could not say them. I could not read, and I could not do anything, so to speak. Physically, I had trouble but fortunately I corrected that.

The thing I want to say is this, that when we come out of the darkness and we begin to be conscious, it is a pretty difficult thing for us to know where our problems are. Had I lost a leg or an arm, I would have known immediately, as soon as I came to, that I would have to find other ways of doing things because I knew where the trouble was. But I did not know, and do not really know yet, and neither do you, where the real problems are.

But the important thing that came finally to help me was to realize and to believe that I must accept what I cannot do the same way I did before, but to try and search for other ways of doing it—and also that I had to learn to hang onto patience. Thank you all.

CHAIRMAN MILLIKAN: A few concluding remarks. During the first 24 hours of this Conference, I was asked by 21 people, "What is the purpose of this Conference?" You have had displayed before you, following by discussion, information concerning a spectrum, at one end of which was the individual cell or two or three cells and at the opposite end of which was the sentence "What disturbed John was being misunderstood by everyone." If those 21 individuals who asked the question "What is the purpose of this Conference?" have found no answer, then I, at this particular time of year, would suggest that Dr. Chomsky's sentence be extended one line upwards and that those individuals ask themselves, after they return home, a question so frequently put by the six or seven year old child, "Is there a Santa Claus?" And, if they are unable to answer *that* question, they should go on to the "Letters to the Editor" in the *New York Herald-Tribune* of half a century ago, where the question is answered! If the interrogators, after reading that answer still find no answer to their question, they should stop asking it!

The program committee consisted of Dr. H. W. Magoun, Dr. Raymond Adams, and myself. We wish to thank the following consultants who met with us: Drs. Hirsh, Geschwind, Chomsky, and Teuber. To NINDB, which furnished many kinds of support, and particularly to Dr. Richard Masland, who consulted with all of us concerning many problems relating to this Conference, I wish to extend the program committee's thanks. Thank you all for coming.

References

1. Adey, W. R.: Hippocampal mechanisms in process of memory. In M. A. B. Brazier (Ed.): *Brain Function Vol. II. RNA and Brain Function; Memory and Learning.* Los Angeles: University of California Press, 1964, pp. 233-276.

2. ——: Neurophysiological correlates of information and transaction and storage in brain tissue. In E. Stellar and J. W. Sprague (Eds.): *Progress in Physiological Psychology,* Vol. I. In press.

3. ——: Dunlop, C. W., and Hendrix, C. E.: Hippocampal slow waves. *Arch. Neurol.* 3:74-90, 1960.

4. Akelaitis, A. J.: A study of gnosis, praxis, and language following section of the corpus callosum and anterior commissure. *J. Neurosurg.* 1: 94-102, 1944.

5. ——: Studies on the corpus callosum: II. The higher visual functions in each homonymous field following complete section of the corpus callosum. *Arch. Neurol. Psychiat.* 45:788-796, 1941.

6. ——: Studies on the corpus callosum. VI. Orientation (temporal-spatial gnosis) following section of the corpus callosum. *Arch. Neurol. Psychiat.* 48:914-937, 1942.

7. ——: Studies on the corpus callosum. VII. Study of language functions (tactile and visual lexia and graphia) unilaterally following section of the corpus callosum. *J. Neuropath. Exper. Neurol.* 2: 226-262, 1943.

8. Alajouanine, T., Castaigne, P., Sabouraud, O., and Contamin, F.: Palilalie paroxystique et vocalisations itératives au cours de crises épileptiques par lésion interessant l'aire motrice supplémentaire. *Rev. Neurol.* 101: 685-697, 1959.

9. Alema, G., and Donini, G.: Sulle modificazioni cliniche ed elettroencefalografiche da introduzione intracarotidea di iso-amil-etil-barbiturate di sodio nell'uomo. *Boll. Soc. Ital. Biol. Sper.* 36:900-904, 1960.

10. ——: Perria, L., Rosadini, G., Rossi, G. F., and Zattoni, J.: Functional deactivation of the brain stem and level of consciousness in man. *J. Neurosurg.* In press.

11. ——, and Rosadini, G.: Données cliniques et E.E.G. de l'introduction d'Amytal sodium dans la circulation encéphalique concernant l'état de conscience. *Acta Neurochir.* 12: 240-257, 1964.

12. ——, ——, and Rossi, G. F.: Psychic reactions associated with intracarotid amytal injection and relation to brain damage. *Excerpta Med. Internat. Congress Ser.* No. 97, p. 137, 1961.

13. ——, ——, and ——: Sugli effetti psichici dell' introduzione intracarotidea di Amytal. *Riv. Sper. Freniat.* 85: 166-169, 1961.

14. Arrigoni, G., and De Renzi, E.: Constructional apraxia and hemispheric locus of lesion. *Cortex* 1:170-197, 1964.

15. Barlow, J. S.: Rhythmic activity induced by photic stimulation in relation to intrinsic alpha activity of the brain in man. *Electroenceph. Clin. Neurophysiol.* 12:317-326, 1960.

16. ——: Rovit, R. L., and Gloor, P.: Correlation analysis of EEG changes induced by unilateral intracarotid injection of amobarbital. *Electroenceph. Clin. Neurophysiol.* 16:213-220, 1964.

17. Bastian, J., Eimas, P., and Liberman, A. M.: Identification and discrimination of a phonemic contrast induced by silent interval. *J. Acoust. Soc. Amer.* 33:842, 1961.

18. Bates, J. A. V., and Ettlinger, G.: Posterior biparietal ablations in the monkey. *Arch. Neurol.* 3:177-192, 1960.

19. Battersby, N. W., Bender, M. B., Pollack, M., and Kahn, R. L.: Unilateral "spatial agnosia" (inattention). *Brain* 79:68-93, 1956.

20. Bay, E.: Der Gegenwartige stand der Aphasie-Forschung. *Folia Phoniat.* 4:9-30, 1952.

21. ——: Principles of classification and their influence on our concepts of aphasia. In A. V. S. DeRueck and Maeve O'Connor (Eds.): *Disorders of Language.* Boston: Little, Brown and Co., 1964, pp. 122-139.

22. Bell, A. G.: *The Mechanism of Speech.* New York: Funk and Wagnalls, 1916.

23. Bennet, F. E.: Intracarotid and intravertebral metrazol in petit mal epilepsy. *Neurology* 3:668-673, 1953.

24. Benton, A. L.: *Right-left Discrimination and Finger Localization: Development and Pathology.* New York: Hoeber, 1959.

25. ——: The visual retention test as a constructional praxis task. *Confin. Neurol.* 22: 141-155, 1962.

26. ——, and Fogel, M. L.: Three-dimensional constructional praxis: A clinical test. *Arch. Neurol.* 7:347-354, 1962.

27. Berlin, C. I., Chase, R. A., Dill, A., and Hagepanos, T.: Auditory findings in temporal lobectomized patients (abstract). *Asha* 7: 386, 1965.

28. Bever, T. G., Fodor, J. A., and Weksel, W.: On the acquisition of syntax: A critique of contextual generalization. *Psychol. Rev.* 72: 467-482, 1965.

29. Bingley, T., Mental symptoms in temporal lobe epilepsy and temporal lobe gliomas. *Acta Psychiat. Neurol. Scand.* 33: Suppl. 120, 1958.

30. Birch, H. G., and Lefford, A.: Intersensory development in children. *Monographs Soc. Child Develop.* 28: 1-47, 1963.

31. Black, P., and Myers, R. E.: A neurological investigation of eye-hand control in the chimpanzee. In G. Ettlinger (Ed.): *Functions of the Corpus Callosum.* London: Churchill, 1965, pp. 47-59.

32. ——, and ——: Visual function of the forebrain commissures in the chimpanzee. *Science* 146: 799-800, 1964.

33. Blank, M., and Bridger, W. H.: Cross-modal transfer in nursery-school children. *J. Comp. Physiol. Psychol.* 58:277-282, 1964.

34. Bocca, E., and Calearo, C.: Central hearing processes, Chapt. 9. In J. Jerger (Ed.): *Modern Developments in Audiology.* New York: Academic Press, 1963.

35. Bogen, J. E., Fisher, E. D., and Vogel, P. J.: Cerebral commissurotomy; a second case report. *J.A.M.A.* 194:1328-1329, 1965.

36. ——, and Vogel, P. J.: Cerebral commissurotomy in man; preliminary report. *Bull. Los Angeles Neurol. Soc.* 27: 169-172, 1962.

37. ——, and ——: Treatment of generalized seizures by cerebral commissurotomy. *Surg. Forum* 14:431-433, 1963.

38. Bonhoeffer, K.: Klinischer und anatomischer Befund zur Lehre von der Apraxie und der "motorischen Sprachbahn." *Mschr. Psychiat. Neurol.* 35:113-128, 1914.

39. Bonin, G., von: Anatomical asymmetries of the cerebral hemispheres. In V. B. Mountcastle (Ed.): *Interhemispheric Relations and Cerebral Dominance.* Baltimore: Johns Hopkins Press, 1962, pp. 1-6.

40. ——, and Bailey, P.: *The Neocortex of Macaca Mulatta.* Urbana: University of Illinois Press, 1947.

41. Boring, E. G.: *A History of Experimental Psychology*, 2nd ed. New York: Appleton-Century-Crofts, 1950.

42. Bosma, J. F. (Ed.): *Symposium on Oral Sensation and Perception.* Springfield, Ill.: Charles C Thomas, in press.

43. Bouillaud, J.: Cited by H. Head in *Aphasia and Kindred Disorders of Speech*, Vol. 1. Cambridge: Cambridge University Press, 1926, p. 16.

44. Bovet, D., and Gatti, G. L.: Pharmacology of instrumental avoidance conditioning. In: *Pharmacology of Conditioning, Learning and Retention.* New York: Pergamon Press, 1965, pp. 75-89.

45. Bowlby, J.: *Maternal Care and Mental Health.* Geneva: World Health Organization, 1952.

46. Brain, R.: *Speech Disorders.* London: Butterworth, 1961.

47. Branch, C., Milner, B., and Rasmussen, T.: Intracarotid sodium amytal for the lateralization of cerebral speech dominance. *J. Neurosurg.* 21: 399-405, 1964.

48. Brazier, M. A. B.: Long persisting electrical traces in the brain of man and their possible relationship to higher nervous activity. *Electroenceph. Clin. Neurophysiol. Suppl.* 13:347-358, 1960.

49. Bremer, F.: Un aspect de la physiologie du corps calleux. *Arch. Int. Physiol.* 61: 110-113, 1953.

50. ——, and Stoupel, N.: Facilitation et inhibition des potentiels évoqués corticaux dans l'éveil cérébral. *Arch. Int. Physiol. Biochim.* 67: 240-275, 1959.

51. Bremond, J. C.: Sur quelques propriétés réactogènes du motif du signal acoustique de défense territoriale du Rouge-gorge (Erithacus rubecula L.). *C. R. Acad. Sci.* (Paris) 259:3365-3366, 1964.

52. Bremond, J. C., Valeur reactogene des frequences acoustiques dans le signal de défense territoriale du Rouge-gorge (Erithacus rubecula L.). *C. R. Acad Sci.* (Paris) 260: 2910-2913, 1965.

53. Broadbent, D. E.: *Perception and Communication.* New York: Pergamon Press, 1958.

54. ——: The role of auditory localization in attention and memory span. *J. Exper. Psych.* 47:191-196, 1954.

55. ——, and Gregory, M. Accuracy of recognition for speech presented to the right and left ears. *Quart. J. Exper. Psychol.* 16: 359-360, 1964.

56. Broca, P.: Sur la faculté du langage articulé. *Bull. Soc. Anthropol.* 4:493-494, 1865.

57. Burton, D., and Ettlinger, G.: Cross modal transfer of training in monkeys. *Nature* 186: 1071-1072, 1960.

58. Busnel, R. G., and Bremond, J. C.: Recherche

du support de l'information dans le signal acoustique de défense territoriale du Rouge-gorge (Erithacus rubecula L.). *C. R. Acad. Sci.* (Paris) 254: 2236-2238, 1962.

59. Chang, H.-T., Ruch, T. C., and Ward, A. A., Jr.: Topographical representation of muscles in motor cortex of monkeys. *J. Neurophysiol.* 10: 39-56, 1947.

60. Charlton, M.: Presentation at Academy of Aphasia, Niagara Falls, Ontario, 1964.

61. Charney, E. J.: Postural configurations in a psychotherapy film. *Psychosom. Med.* In press.

62. Chase, R. A.: Abnormalities in motor control secondary to congenital sensory deficits; a case study, Chapt. 16. In J. F. Bosma (Ed.): *Symposium on Oral Sensation and Perception.* Springfield, Ill.: Charles C Thomas, in press.

62a. ——: An information-flow model of the organization of motor activity. I. Transduction, transmission and central control of sensory information. *J. Nerv. Ment. Dis.* 140:239-251, 1965.

63. ——: An information-flow model of the organization of motor activity. II: Sampling, central processing and utilization of sensory information. *J. Nerv. Ment. Dis.* 140: 334-350, 1965.

64. ——: Developmental study of changes in behavior under delayed auditory feedback. *J. Genet. Psychol.* 99:101-112, 1961.

65. Cherry, E. C.: Some experiments on the recognition of speech with one and with two ears. *J. Acoust. Soc. Amer.* 25:975-979, 1953.

66. Chomsky, N.: A review of B. F. Skinner's "Verbal Behavior." *Language* 35:26-58, 1959; reprinted in J. A. Fodor and J. J. Katz (Eds.): *The Structure of Language.* Englewood Cliffs, N.J.: Prentice-Hall, 1964.

67. ——: *Aspects of a Theory of Syntax.* Cambridge, Mass.: MIT Press, 1965.

68. ——: *Syntactic Structures.* The Hague: Mouton and Cie, 1957.

69. Chow, K. L.: Effects of partial extirpation of the posterior association cortex on visually mediated behavior in monkeys. *Comp. Psychol. Monogr.* 20:187-217, 1951.

70. Cole, M., Chorover, S. L., and Ettlinger, G.: Cross-modal transfer in man. *Nature* 191: 1225-1226, 1961.

71. Conel, J. L.: *The Postnatal Development of the Human Cerebral Cortex, Vol. VII. The Cortex of the Four-Year Child.* Cambridge, Massachusetts: Harvard University Press, 1963.

72. Connolly, C. J.: *External Morphology of the Primate Brain.* Springfield, Ill.: Charles C Thomas, 1950.

73. Conrad, K.: Das Korperscheima; Eine Kritische Studie und der Versuch einer Revision. *Z. Ges. Neurol. Psychiat.* 147:346-369, 1933.

74. ——: Strukturanalysen hirnpathologischer Fälle. IV. Zum. Problem der Leitungsaphasie. *Deutsch. Z. Nervenheilk.* 159: 188-228, 1948.

75. Corkin, S.: Tactually-guided maze learning in man: Effects of unilateral cortical excisions and bilateral hippocampal lesions. *Neuropsychologia* 3:339-351, 1965.

76. Costa, L. D., and Vaughan, H. G.: Performance of patients with lateralized cerebral lesions. I. Verbal and perceptual tests. *J. Nerv. Ment. Dis.* 134:162-168, 1962.

77. Critchley, M.: Dax's law. *Int. J. Neurol.* 4: 199-206, 1964.

78. ——: The drift and dissolution of language. *Proc. Roy. Soc. Med.* 57: 1189-1198, 1964.

79. DaPian, R., Bricolo, A., Dalle Ore, G., and Perbellini, D.: Amytal sodico intracarotideo. *G. Psichiat. Neuropat.* 89:885-912, 1961.

80. Darwin, C. R.: *The Expression of Emotions in Man and Animals.* New York: Philosophical Library, 1955.

81. Dejerine, J.: Contribution à l'étude anatomo-pathologique et clinique des différentes variétés de cécité verbale. *Mém. Soc. Biol.* 4:61-90, 1892.

82. ——: *Semeiologie des Affections du Système Nerveux.* Paris: Masson et Cie, 1914.

83. ——: Sur un cas de cécité verbale avec aphasie suivi d'autopsie. *Bull. Soc. Anat.* p. 481, 1880.

84. Delgado, J. M. R., Roberts, W. W., and Miller, N. E.: Learning motivated by electrical stimulation of the brain. *Amer. J. Physiol.* 179:587-593, 1954.

85. Denny-Brown, D., and Chambers, R. A.: The parietal lobe and behaviour. *Res. Publ. Ass. Res. Nerv. Ment. Dis.* 36:36-117, 1958.

86. deSaussure, F.: *Cours de Linguistique Générale,* 3rd ed. Paris: Payot, 1931.

87. Diamond, I. T., and Neff, W. D.: Ablation of temporal cortex and discrimination of auditory patterns. *J. Neurophysiol.* 20:300-315, 1957.

88. DiChiro, G.: Angiographic patterns of cerebral convexity veins and superficial dural sinuses. *Amer. J. Roentgenol.* 87:308-321, 1962.

89. Dirks, D.: Perception of dichotic and monaural verbal material and cerebral dominance for speech. *Acta Otolaryng.* 58:73-80, 1964.

90. Downer, L. J. de C.: Changes in visually guided

behavior following mid-sagittal section of optic chiasm and corpus callosum in monkey (Macaca mulatta). *Brain* 82:251-259, 1959.

91. Driver, M., Falconer, M. A., and Serafetinides, E. A.: Ictal speech automatism reproduced by activation procedures. *Neurology* 14: 455-463, 1964.

92. Dubois, J., Hécaen, H., Angelergues, R., Maufras, du Chatelier, A., and Marcie, P.: Étude neurolinguistique de l'aphasie de conduction. *Neuropsychologia* 2:9-44, 1964.

93. Duensing, F.: Raumagnotische und ideatorisch-apraktische Störung des Gestaltenden Handelns. *Deutsch. Z. Nervenheilk.* 170:72-94, 1953.

94. Dukoff, V. (translator): *Comparative Anatomy of the Cerebral Cortex of Mammalians.* U. S. Department of Commerce technical translation #65-30769, April 19, 1965, Washington, D. C.: Joint Publication Research Service, 1965.

95. Dumont, S., and Dell, P.: Facilitation réticulaire des mécanismes visuels corticaux. *Electroenceph. Clin. Neurophysiol.* 12: 769-796, 1960.

96. Eccles, J.: *The Brain and the Unity of Conscious Experience.* Cambridge, England: University Printing House, 1965.

97. Economo, C. von, and Horn, L.: Über Windungsrelief, Masse und Rindenarchitektonik der Supratemporalfläche, ihre individuellen und ihre Seitenunterschiede. *Z. Ges. Neurol. Psychiat.* 130: 678-757, 1930.

98. Edwards, A. E., and Auger, R.: The effect of aphasia on the perception of precedence. *Proceedings of the 73rd Annual Convention of the American Psychological Association,* 1965, pp. 207-208.

99. Efron, R.: An extension of the pulfrich stereoscopic effect. *Brain* 86:295-300, 1963.

100. ——: Temporal perception, aphasia, and déjà vu. *Brain* 86:403-424, 1963.

101. ——: The effect of handedness on the perception of simultaneity and temporal order. *Brain* 86: 261-284, 1963.

102. ——: The effect of stimulus intensity on the perception of simultaneity in right and left-handed cases. *Brain* 86:285-294, 1963.

103. Ehrenwald, H.: Storung der Zeitauffassung der raumlichen Orientierung des Zeichnens und des Rechnens bei einem Hirnverletzten. *Z. Ges. Neurol. Psychiat.* 132:518-569, 1931.

104. Eisenson, J.: Language and intellectual findings associated with right cerebral damage. *Lang. Speech* 5:49-53, 1962.

105. Erickson, T. C.: Spread of the epileptic discharge. *Arch. Neurol. Psychiat.* 43: 429-452, 1940.

106. Ettlinger, G.: Cross-modal transfer of training in monkeys. *Behaviour* 16:56-65, 1960.

107. ——: Defective identification of fingers. *Neuropsychologia* 1:39-46, 1963.

108. ——, and Blakemore, C. B.: Cross-modal transfer of conditional discrimination training in monkeys. *Nature* 210:117-118, 1966.

109. Evarts, E. V.: Pyramidal tract activity associated with a conditioned hand movement in the monkey. *J. Neurophysiol.* 29:1011-1027, 1966.

110. ——: Relation of discharge frequency to conduction velocity in pyramidal tract neurons. *J. Neurophysiol.* 28:216-228, 1965.

111. ——: Temporal patterns of discharge of pyramidal tract neurons during sleep and waking in the monkey. *J. Neurophysiol.* 27:152-171, 1964.

112. Fairbanks, G.: Test of phonemic differentiation: The rhyme test. *J. Acous. Soc. Amer.* 30:596-600, 1958.

113. Falconer, M. A., and Serafetinides, E. A.: A follow-up study of surgery in temporal lobe epilepsy. *J. Neurol. Neurosurg. Psychiat.* 26:154-165, 1963.

114. ——, ——, and Corsellis, J. A. N.: Etiology and pathogenesis of temporal lobe epilepsy. *Arch. Neurol.* 10:233-248, 1964.

115. Fantz, R. L., Ordy, J. M., and Udelf, M. S.: Maturation of pattern vision in infants during the first six months. *J. Comp. Physiol. Psychol.* 55:907-916, 1962.

116. Feindel, W., and Penfield, W.: Localization of discharge in temporal lobe automatism. *Arch. Neurol. Psychiat.* 72: 605-630, 1954.

117. Fodor, J. A.: Could meaning be an r_m? *J. Verbal Learn. Verbal Beh.* 4: 73-82, 1965.

118. ——, and Bever, T. G.: The psychological reality of linguistic segments. *J. Verbal Learn. Verbal Beh.* 4:414-420, 1965.

119. Foix, C.: Aphasies. In G. E. H. Roger, F. Widal, and P.-J. Teissier (Eds.): *Nouveau Traité de Médecine et de Thérapeutique.* Paris: Masson et Cie, 1928, pp. 135-213.

120. Galambos, R.: Neurophysiological studies on learning and motivation. *Fed. Proc.* 20: 603-608, 1961.

121. Garrett, M., Bever, T. G., and Fodor, J. A.: The active use of grammar in speech perception. *J. Percep. Psychophysiol.* 1:30-32, 1966.

122. Gazzaniga, M. S.: Psychological properties of

the disconnected hemispheres in man. *Science* 150:372, 1965.

123. ——, Bogen, J. E., and Sperry, R. W.: Observations on visual perception after disconnection of the cerebral hemispheres in in man. *Brain* 88: Part II, 221-236, 1965.

124. ——, ——, and ——: Some functional effects of sectioning the cerebral commissures in man. *Proc. Nat. Acad. Sci. U. S. A.* 48: Part 2, 1765-1769, 1962.

125. ——, and Sperry, R. W.: Language in human patients after brain bisection. *Fed. Proc.* 24:522 (abstract), 1965.

126. ——, and ——: Simultaneous double performance ability following brain bisection in man. *Psychon. Sci.* In press.

127. ——, and ——: Some comparative effects of disconnecting the cerebral hemispheres. *Fed. Proc.* 23:359 (abstract), 1964.

128. ——, and ——: Visuomotor control in monkey following brain lesions. *Fed. Proc.* 25: 393 (abstract), 1966.

129. Geschwind, N.: Alexia and colour-naming disturbance. In G. Ettlinger (Ed.): *Functions of the Corpus Callosum*. London: Churchill, 1965.

130. ——: Disconnexion syndromes in animals and man. *Brain* 88:237-294, 1965.

131. ——: The anatomy of acquired disorders of reading. In J. Money (Ed.): *Reading Disability*. Baltimore: Johns Hopkins Press, 1962, pp. 115-129.

132. ——, and Fusillo, M.: Color-naming defects in association with alexia. *Tr. Amer. Neurol. Ass.* 89:172-176, 1964.

133. ——, and Kaplan, E.: A human cerebral deconnection syndrome. *Neurology* 12:675-685, 1962.

134. Ghent, L.: Developmental changes in tactual thresholds on dominant and nondominant sides. *J. Comp. Physiol. Psychol.* 54:670-673, 1961.

135. Gibbs, E. L., Gibbs, F. A., and Fuster, B.: Psychomotor epilepsy. *Arch. Neurol. Psychiat.* 60:331-339, 1948.

136. Gibson, E. J.: Perceptual development. *In* H. W. Stevenson (Ed.): *Child Psychology* (62d Yearbook, NSSE). Chicago: University of Chicago Press, 1963, pp. 144-195.

137. ——, Gibson, J. J., Pick, A. D., and Osser, H.: A developmental study of the discrimination of letter-like forms. *J. Comp. Physiol. Psychol.* 55:897-906, 1962.

138. Gilden, L., Vaughan, H. G., Jr., and Costa, L. D.: Summated EEG potentials with voluntary movement. *Electroenceph. Clin. Neurophysiol.* 20: 433-438, 1966.

139. Gilman, S., MacFayden, D. J., and Denny-Brown, D.: Decerebrate phenomena after carotid amobarbital injection. *Arch. Neurol.* 8:662-675, 1963.

140. Glanzer, M.: Psycholinguistics and verbal learning. Paper read at Verbal Behavior Conference, New York, September, 1965. To appear in a volume edited by K. Salzinger and published by McGraw-Hill, New York.

141. Glickstein, M., Arora, H. A., and Sperry, R. W.: Delayed-response performance following optic tract section, unilateral frontal lesion, and commissurotomy. *J. Comp. Physiol. Psychol.* 56:11-18, 1963.

142. Goldiamond, I.: Stuttering and fluency as manipulatable operant response classes. In L. Krasner and L. P. Ullman (Eds.): *Research in Behavior Modification*. New York: Holt, Rinehart and Winston, 1965, pp. 106-156.

143. Goldstein, K.: Die amnestische und die zentrale Aphasie (Leitungsaphasie). *Arch. Psychiat. Nervenkr.* 48:314-343, 1911.

144. Goldstein, K.: Zur Lehre von der motorischen Apraxie. *J. Psychol. Neurol.* 11:169-187, 270-283, 1908.

145. Greenberg, J. H. (Ed.): *Universals of Language*, 2nd ed. Cambridge, Mass.: MIT Press, 1966.

146. Gwinner, E., and Kneutgen, J.: Über die biologisch Bedeutung der "Zweckdienlichen" Anwendung erlernter Laute bei Vogeln. *Z. Tierpsychol.* 19:692-696, 1962.

147. Harlow, H. F.: The heterosexual affectional system in monkeys. *Amer. Psychol.* 17:1-9, 1962.

148. Head, H.: *Aphasia and Kindred Disorders of Speech*. Cambridge, England: Cambridge University Press, 1926 (2 vols.).

149. Hebb, D. O.: Intelligence in man after large removals of cerebral tissue: Defects following right temporal lobectomy. *J. Genet. Psychol.* 21:437-446, 1939.

150. Hécaen, H.: Clinical symptomatology in right and left hemispheric lesions. In V. B. Mountcastle (Ed.): *Interhemispheric Relations and Cerebral Dominance*. Baltimore: Johns Hopkins Press, 1962, pp. 215-243.

151. ——, and de Ajuriaguerra, J.: L'apraxie de l'habillage; Ses rapports avec la planotopokinésie et les troubles de la somatognosie. *Encéphale* 8-9-10:113-144, 1945.

152. ——, and ——: Les Gauchers. *Prévalence Manuelle et Dominance Cérébrale* Paris: Press Universitaires de France, 1963.

153. ——, ——, and Massonet, J.: Les troubles visuoconstructifs par lésion pariéto-occipitale droite. Rôle des perturbations vestibulaires. *Encéphale* 40:122-179, 1951.

154. ——, and Angelergues, R.: Epilepsie et troubles du language. *Encéphale* 49:138-169, 1960.

155. ——, and ——: Etude anatomo-clinique de 280 cas de lésions rétrorolandiques unilatérales des hémispheres cérébraux. *Encéphale* 50:533-562, 1961.

156. ——, and ——: La Cécité Psychique. Paris: Masson et Cie, 1963.

157. ——, and ——: Localization of symptoms in aphasia. In A. V. S. de Rueck and Maeve O'Connor (Eds.): *Disorders of Language.* Boston: Little, Brown and Co., 1964, pp. 222-256.

158. ——, ——, and Douzenis, J.: Les agraphies. *Neuropsychologia* 1:179-208, 1963.

159. ——, Penfield, W., Bertrand, C., and Malmo, R.: The syndromes of apractognosia due to lesions of the minor cerebral hemisphere. *Arch. Neurol. Psychiat.* 75:400-434, 1956.

160. Held, R.: Exposure history as a factor in maintaining stability of perception and coordination. *J. Nerv. Ment. Dis.* 132:26-32, 1961.

161. ——, and Hein, A.: Movement-produced stimulation in the development of visually guided behavior. *J. Comp. Physiol Psychol.* 56:872-876, 1963.

162. Henschel, G.: Bullfinch and canary. *Nature* 67:609-610, 1903.

163. Hermelin, B. T., and O'Connor, N.: Recognition of shapes by normal and subnormal children. *Brit. J. Psychol.* 52:281-284, 1961.

164. Hernandez-Peón, R.: Reticular mechanisms of sensory control. In W. A. Rosenblith (Ed.): *Sensory Communication.* New York: John Wiley and Sons, 1961, pp. 497-520.

165. Hershenson, M.: Visual discrimination in the human newborn. *J. Comp. Physiol. Psychol.* 58:270-276, 1964.

166. Hilpert, P.: Die Bendeutung des linken Parietallappens fur das Sprechen. Ein Breitrag zur Lokalisation der Leitungsaphasie. *J. Psychol. Neurol.* 40:225-255, 1930.

167. Hirsh, I. J.: Auditory perception of temporal order. *J. Acoust. Soc. Amer.* 31:759-767, 1959.

168. ——: Perception of Speech. In *Symposium on Sensorineural Hearing Processes and Disorders.* Boston: Little, Brown and Company, in press.

169. ——, Bilger, R. C., and Deatherage, B. H.: The effects of auditory and visual background on apparent duration. *Amer. J. Psychol.* 69:561-574, 1956.

170. ——, and Sherrick, C. E.: Perceived order in different sense modalities. *J. Exper. Psychol.* 62:423-432, 1961.

171. Hoeft, H. J.: Klinisch-anatomischer Breitrag zur Kenntnis der Nachsprechaphasie (Leitungsaphasie). *Deutsch. Z. Nervenheilk.* 175: 560-594, 1957.

172. Hoff, H.: Die Lokalisation der Aphasie. Proceedings of the VIIth International Congress of Neurology, (Rome), 1961, pp. 555-568.

173. Holmes, H. L.: Disordered perception of auditory sequences in aphasia. Unpublished Ph.D. Thesis, Harvard University, 1965.

174. House, A. S., Williams, C. E., Hecker, M. L., and Kryter, K. D.: Articulation testing methods: Consonantal differentiation with a closed response set. *J. Acoust. Soc. Amer.* 37:158-166, 1965.

175. Howes, D., and Geschwind, N.: Quantitative studies of aphasic language. In D. McK. Rioch and E. A. Weinstein (Eds.): *Disorders of Communication* (Proceedings of the Association for Research in Nervous and Mental Disease), Baltimore: Williams and Wilkins, 1964, pp. 229-244.

176. Hubel, D. H.: Single unit activity in striate cortex of unrestrained cats. *J. Physiol.* 147:226-238, 1959.

177. ——, and Wiesel, T.: Receptive fields and functional architecture in two non-striate visual areas (18 and 19) of the cat. *J. Neurophysiol.* 28:229-289, 1965.

178. ——, and ——: Receptive fields of cells in striate cortex of very young, visually inexperienced kittens. *J. Neurophysiol.* 26:994-1002, 1963.

179. Hughes, G. W., and Halle, M.: Spectral properties of fricative consonants. *J. Acoust. Soc. Amer.* 28:302, 1956.

180. Hydén H.: RNA—a functional characteristic of the neuron and its glia. In M. A. B. Brazier (Ed.): *Brain Function, Vol. II. RNA and Brain Function; Memory and Learning.* Los Angeles: University of California Press, 1964, pp. 29-68.

181. Iannone, M., and Morrell, F.: Experience with intracarotid amytal in man. *Electroenceph. Clin. Neurophysiol.* 13:305, 1961.

182. Ingle, D. J.: The use of the fish in neuropsychology. *Perspect. Biol. Med.* 8:241-260, 1965.

183. Jackson, J.H.: Cited by H. Head in *Aphasia*

and Kindred Disorders of Speech, Vol. 1. Cambridge: Cambridge University Press, 1926, pp. 30-53.

184. ———: On the nature of the duality of the brain. In J. Taylor (Ed.): *Selected Writings of John Hughlings Jackson*. London: Hodder and Stoughton, 1932.

185. Jakobson, R., and Halle, M.: *Fundamentals of Language*. 's-Gravenhage: Mouton and Co., 1956.

186. Janota, O.: Sur l'apraxie constructive et sur les troubles apparents de l'aperception et de l'expression des rapports spatiaux, *Encéphale* 2:173-211, 1938.

187. Jerger, J., Audiological manifestations of lesions in the auditory nervous system. *Laryngoscope* 70:417-425, 1960.

188. ———: Auditory tests for disorders of the central auditory mechanism, Chapt. 5. In W. S. Fields and R. R. Alford (Eds.): *Neurological Aspects of Auditory and Vestibular Disorders*. Springfield, Ill.: Charles C Thomas, 1964.

189. John, E. R., and Killam, K. F.: Electrophysiological correlates of avoidance conditioning in the cat. *J. Pharmaco. Exper. Therap.* 125:252-274, 1959.

190. ———, Ruchkin, D. S., and Villegas, J.: Signal analysis and behavioral correlates of evoked potential configurations in cats. *Ann. New York Acad. Sci.* 112:362-420, 1964.

191. Jung, R., Kornhuber, H. H., and Da Fonseca, J. S.: Multisensory convergence on cortical neurons: Neuronal effects of visual, acoustic and vestibular stimuli in the superior convolutions of the cat's cortex. In G. Moruzzi, A. Fessard, and H. H. Jasper (Eds.): *Progress in Brain Research*, Vol. 1. Amsterdam: Elsevier, 1963, pp. 207-240.

192. Kalischer, O: Das Grosshirn der Papageien in anatomischer und physiologischer Beziehung. Abh. Preuss. Akas. Wiss. No. IV, 1905.

193. Katz, J.: The use of staggered spondaic words for assessing the integrity of the central auditory nervous system. *J. Audit. Res.* 2:327-337, 1962.

194. Katz, J. J., and Postal, P. M.: *An Integrated Theory of Linguistic Descriptions*. (MIT Research Monograph Number 26). Cambridge, Mass.: MIT Press, 1964.

195. Kelemen, G.: Structure and performance in animal language. *Arch. Otolaryng.* 50:740-744, 1949.

196. Kelvin, R. P., and Mulik, A.: Discrimination of length by sight and touch. *Quart. J. Exper. Psychol.* 10:187-192, 1958.

197. Kennard, M. A.: Alterations in response to visual stimuli following lesions of frontal lobe in monkeys. *Arch. Neurol. Psychiat.* 41:1153-1165, 1939.

198. Kimura, D.: A note on cerebral dominance in hearing. *Acta Otolaryng.* 56:617-618, 1963.

199. ———: Cerebral dominance and the perception of verbal stimuli. *Canad. J. Psychol.* 15:166-171, 1961.

200. ———: Left-right differences in the perception of melodies. *Quart. J. Exper. Psychol.* 16:355-358, 1964.

201. ———: Right temporal-lobe damage. *Arch. Neurol.* 8:264-271, 1963.

202. ———: Some effects of temporal-lobe damage on auditory perception. *Canad. J. Psychol.* 15:156-165, 1961.

203. Kinsbourne, M., and Warrington, E.: A study of finger agnosia. *Brain* 85:47-66, 1962.

204. Klein, R.: Ueber die empfindung der Korperlichkeit. *Z. Ges. Neurol.* 126:453-472, 1930.

205. Kleist, K.: *Gehirnpathologie*. Leipzig: Barth, 1934.

206. ———: Ueber Leitungsaphasie und grammatische storungen. *Mschr. Psychiat. Neurol.* 40:118-199, 1916.

207. Konorski, J.: Analiza patofizjologiczna Róznych Rudzajów Zaburzén Mowy I Próba ich Klasyfikacji. *Rozpr. Wydz. Nauk Med.* 2:11-32. 1963.

208. Kornhuber, H. H., and Deecke, L.: Hirnpotentialänderungen beim Menschen vor und nach Willkurbewegungen dargestellt mit Magnetbandspeicherung und Ruckwartsanalyse. *Arch. Ges. Physiol.* 218:52, 1964.

209. Kornhuber, H. H., and Deecke, L.: Hirnpotentialänderungen bei Willkürbewegungen und passiven Bewegungen des Menschen: Bereitschaftspotential und reafferente Potentiale. *Arch. Ges. Physiol.* 284:1-17, 1965.

210. Krasner, L.: Verbal conditioning and psychotherapy. In L. Krasner and L. P. Ullmann (Eds.): *Research in Behavior Modification*. New York: Holt, Rinehart and Winston, 1965, pp. 211-228.

211. Lade, B. I., and Thorpe, W. H.: Dove songs as innately coded patterns of specific behaviour. *Nature* 202:366-368, 1964.

212. Ladefoged, P., and Broadbent, D. E.: Perception of sequences in auditory events. *Quart. J. Exper. Psychol.* 13:162-170, 1960.

213. Lambert, W.: In C. Osgood and M. Miron (Eds.): *Approaches to the Study of Aphasia*. Urbana: University of Illinois Press, 1963.

214. Landau, W., Goldstein R., and Kleffner, F.: Congential aphasia: a clinicopathologic study. *Neurology* 10:915-21, 1960.

215. Lane, H., and Shepphard, W.: Development of the prosodic features of infants' vocalizing. Paper read at Language Development Conference, sponsored by National Institute of Child Health and Human Development, Ann Arbor, Michigan, October, 1965. To appear in volume edited by E. Martin, Academic Press.

216. Lange, J.: Agnosien und Apraxien, Vol. 6. In O. Bunke and O. Foerster (Eds.): *Handbuch der Neurologie*. Berlin: Springer, 1937, pp. 807-960.

217. Lansdell, H.: Sex differences in hemispheric asymmetries of the human brain. *Nature* 203:550, 1964.

218. ——: The effect of neurosurgery on a test of proverbs. *Amer. Psychol.* 16:448 (abstract), 1961.

219. Lansdell, H. C., Two selective deficits found to be lateralized in temporal neurosurgery patients. Paper read at 32nd Annual Meeting of Eastern Psychological Association, Philadelphia, 1961.

220. Lansdell, H., Purnell, J. K., and Laskowski, E. J.: The relation of induced dysnomia to phoneme frequency. *Lang. Speech* 6:88-93, 1963.

221. ——, and Urbach, N.: Sex differences in personality measures related to size and side of temporal lobe ablations. *Proceedings of the 73rd Annual Convention of the American Psychological Association*, 1965, pp. 113-114.

222. Lansdell, J. P.: Verbal factors involved in the identification of photographed objects presented at an accelerated rate. Unpublished M.A. thesis, University of Maryland, 1965.

223. Lashley, K. S.: The problem of serial order in behaviour. In L. A. Jeffress (Ed.): *Cerebral Mechanisms in Behaviour*. New York: John Wiley and Sons, 1951, pp. 112-136.

224. Lenneberg, E.: The capacity for language acquisition. In J. A. Fodor and J. J. Katz (Eds.): *The Structure of Language*. Englewood Cliffs, N.J.: Prentice-Hall, 1964.

225. Lennox, W. G.: Phenomena and correlates of the psychomotor triad. *Neurology* 1:357-371, 1951.

226. Lettvin, J., Maturana, H. R., McCulloch, W. S., and Pitts, W. H.: What the frog's eye tells the frog's brain. *Proc. IRE* 4:1940-1951, 1959.

227. Liberman, A. M.: Some results of research on speech perception. *J. Acoust. Soc. Amer.* 29:117, 1957.

228. Liberman, A. M., Cooper, F. S., Harris, K. S., and MacNeilage P. F.: *A Motor Theory of Speech Perception*. (Proceedings of Speech Communication Seminar.) Stockholm: Royal Institute of Technology, 1963.

229. Liberman, A. M. et al.: An effect of learning on speech perception: The discrimination of durations of silence with and without phonemic significance. *Lang. Speech* 4:175, 1961.

230. Liberman, A. M., Harris, K., Hoffman, H. S., and Griffith, B. C.: The discrimination of speech sounds within and across phoneme boundaries. *J. Exper. Psych.* 54:358-368, 1957.

231. Liepmann, H.: Das Krankheitsbild der Apraxie "motorischen Asymbolie". *Mschr, Psychiat. Neurol.* 8:15-44, 102-132, 182-197, 1900.

232. ——: Die linke Hemisphäre und das Handeln. In *Drei Aufsätze aus dem Apraxiegebeit*. Berlin: Karger, 1905, pp. 17-50.

233. ——, and Maas, O.: Fall von linksseitiger Agraphie und Apraxie bei rechtsseitiger Lähmung. *J. Psychol. Neurol.* 10:214-227, 1907.

234. Lilly, J. C.: Airborne sonic emissions of Tursiops truncatus (M). *J. Acoust. Soc. Amer.* 36:1007 (abstract), 1964.

235. ——: Animals in aquatic environment: Adaptation of the mammals to the ocean. In *Handbook of Physiology: Environment*. Washington, D.C.: American Physiological Society, 1964, pp. 741-757.

236. ——: Correlations between neurophysiological activity in the cortex and short-term behavior in the monkey. In H. F. Harlow and C. N. Woolsey (Eds.): *Biological and Biochemical Bases of Behavior*. Madison: University of Wisconsin Press, 1958, pp. 83-100.

237. ——: Critical brain size and language. *Perspect. Biol. Med.* 6:246-255, 1963.

238. ——: Distress call of the bottlenose dolphin: stimuli and evoked behavioral responses. *Science* 139:116-118, 1963.

239. ——: Learning motivated by subcortical stimulation: The start and stop patterns of behavior. In H. H. Jasper (Ed.): *Reticular Formation of the Brain*. Boston: Little, Brown and Company, 1958.

240. ——: *Man and Dolphin*. Garden City, N.Y.: Doubleday and Company, 1961.

241. ——: Modern whales, dolphins and porpoises, as challenges to our intelligence. In A. Montagu and J. C. Lilly (Eds.): *The Dolphin in History*. (Symposium given at Clark Memorial Library, 1962.) Los Angeles: University of California Press, 1963, pp. 31-54.

242. ——: Vocal behavior of the bottlenose dolphin. *Proc. Amer. Philos. Soc.* 106:520-529, 1962.

243. ——: Vocal mimicry in Tursiops: Ability to match numbers and durations of human vocal bursts. *Science* 147:300-301, 1965.

244. ——, and Miller, A. M.: Operant conditioning of the bottlenose dolphin with electrical stimulation of the brain. *J. Comp. Physiol. Psychol.* 55:73-79, 1962.

245. ——, and ——: Sounds emitted by the bottlenose dolphin. *Science* 133:1689-1698, 1961.

246. ——, and ——: Vocal exchanges between dolphins. *Science* 134:1873-1876, 1961.

247. Lindauer, M.: *Communication among Social Bees.* Cambridge, Mass.: Harvard University Press, 1961.

248. Lowe, A. D., and Campbell, R. A.: Temporal discrimination in aphasoid and normal children. *J. Speech Hear. Res.* 8:313-314, 1965.

249. Luria, A. R.: Factors and forms of aphasia. In A. V. S. de Reuck, and Maeve O'Connor (Eds.): *Disorders of Language.* Boston, Little, Brown and Co., 1964, pp. 143-167.

250. ——: *Higher Cortical Functions in Man.* New York: Basic Books, 1964.

251. ——: *The Regulation of Speech in Normal and Abnormal Behavior.* New York: Pergamon Press, 1960.

252. Maas, O.: Ein Fall von linksseitiger Apraxie und Agraphie. *Neurol. Zbl.* 26:789-792, 1907.

253. Magoun, H. W.: *The Waking Brain,* 2nd ed. Springfield, Ill.: Charles C Thomas, 1965.

254. ——, Darling L., and Prost, J.: The evolution of man's brain. In M. A. B. Brazier (Ed.): *The Central Nervous System and Behavior.* New York: The Macy Foundation, 1960, pp. 33-126.

255. Mandelbaum, D. G.: *Selected Writings of Edward Sapir in Language, Culture, and Personality.* Berkeley: University of California Press, 1949.

256. Marcie, P., Hécaen, H., Dubois, J., and Angelergues, R.: Les troubles de la réalisation de la parole au cours des lésions de l'hémisphère droit. *Neuropsychologia* 3:217-247, 1965.

257. Marie, P.: *Travaux et Mémoires,* Vol. I. Paris: Masson et Cie, 1926.

258. ——, and Foix, C.: Les aphasies de guerre. *Rev. Neurol.* 24:53-87, 1917.

259. Marler, P.: Developments in the study of animal communication, Chap. 4. In P. R. Bell (Ed.): *Darwin's Biological Work.* Cambridge, England: Cambridge University Press, 1959.

260. ——: The logical analysis of animal communication. *J. Theoret. Biol.* 1:295-317, 1961.

261. Maspes, P.: Le syndrome expérimental chez l'homme de la section du splénium du corps calleux; alexie visuelle pure hémianopsique. *Rev. Neurol.* 80:100-113, 1948.

262. Matsubara, T.: An observation on cerebral phlebograms with special reference to the changes in the superficial veins. *Nagoya J. Med. Sci.* 23:86-94, 1960.

263. McCarthy, D.: Language development in children, Chapt. 9. In L. Carmichael (Ed.): *Manual of Child Psychology,* 2nd ed., New York: John Wiley and Sons, 1954.

264. McCarthy, J. J., and Kirk, S. A.: *Illinois Test of Psycholinguistic Abilities: Examiner's Manual.* Urbana: University of Illinois Institute for Research on Exceptional Children, 1961.

265. McCleary, R. A.: Type of response as a factor in interocular transfer in the fish. *J. Comp. Physiol. Psychol.* 53:311-321, 1960.

266. McDonald, E. T., and Aungst, L. F.: Studies in oral sensory-motor function. In J. F. Bosma (Ed.): *Symposium on Oral Sensation and Perception.* Springfield, Ill.: Charles C Thomas, in press.

267. McFie, J., and Zangwill, O. L.: Visual constructive disabilities associated with lesions of the left cerebral hemisphere. *Brain* 83:243-260, 1960.

268. McGaugh, J. L.: Effects of drugs on learning and memory. *Int. Rev. Neurobiol.* 8:139-196, 1965.

269. MacKay, D.: Discussion in J. C. Eccles (Ed.): *Brain and Conscious Experience.* New York: Springer-Verlag, 1966.

270. McNeill, D.: The capacity for language acquisition. Presented to the National Research Conference on Behavioral Aspects of Deafness, New Orleans, Louisiana, 3-5 May, 1965. To be published by Vocational Rehabilitation Administration, Washington, D.C.

271. McQuown, N. A. (Ed.), Bateson, G., Birdwhistell, R. L., Brosin, H. W., and Hockett, C.: *The Natural History of an Interview.* To be published.

272. Meier, M. J., and French, L. A.: Lateralized deficits in complex visual discrimination and bilateral transfer of reminiscence following unilateral temporal lobectomy. *Neuropsychologia* 3:261-272, 1965.

272a. Meyer, V.: Cognitive changes following temporal lobectomy for relief of temporal lobe epilepsy. *Arch. Neur. Psychiat.* 81:299-309, 1959.

273. ——, and Yates, A. J.: Intellectual changes following temporal lobectomy for psychomotor epilepsy. *J. Neurol. Neurosurg. Psychiat.* 18:44-52, 1955.

274. Miller, G. A.: Communication and the structure of behavior. In D. McK. Rioch and E. A. Weinstein (Eds.): *Disorders of Communication*. Baltimore: Williams and Wilkins, 1964.

275. ——: *Language and Communication*. New York: McGraw-Hill, 1951.

276. ——, and Nicely, P. A.: Analysis of perceptual confusion among some English consonants. *J. Acoust. Soc. Amer.* 27:338, 1955.

277. Milner, B.: Intellectual functions of the temporal lobe. *Psychol. Bull.* 51:42-62, 1954.

278. ——: Laterality effects in audition. In V. B. Mountcastle (Ed.): *Interhemispheric Relations and Cerebral Dominance*. Baltimore: Johns Hopkins Press, 1962, pp. 177-195.

279. ——: Psychological defects produced by temporal-lobe excision. *Res. Publ. Ass. Nerv. Men. Dis.* 36: 244-257, 1958.

280. ——: Some effects of frontal lobectomy in man. In J. M. Warren and K. Akert (Eds.): *The Frontal Granular Cortex and Behavior*. New York: McGraw-Hill, 1964, pp. 313-334.

281. ——: The memory defect in bilateral hippocampal lesions. *Psychiat. Res. Rep.* 11:43-58, 1959.

282. ——: Visually-guided maze learning in man: Effects of bilateral hippocampal, bilateral frontal, and unilateral cerebral lesions. *Neuropsychologia* 3:317-338, 1965.

283. ——, Branch, C., and Rasmussen, T.: Evidence for bilateral speech representation in some non-right-handers. *Tr. Amer. Neurol. Ass.* 91:in press, 1966.

284. ——, ——, and ——: Observations on cerebral dominance. In A. V. S. de Rueck and Maeve O'Connor (Eds.): *Disorders of Language*. Boston: Little, Brown and Co., 1964, pp. 200-214.

285. ——, and Kimura, D.: Dissociable visual learnind defects after unilateral temporal lobectomy in man. Paper read at 35th Annual Meeting, Eastern Psychological Association, Philadelphia, April, 1964.

286. Mishkin, M.: A possible link between interhemispheric integration in monkeys and cerebral dominance in man. In V. B. Mountcastle (Ed.): *Interhemispheric Relations and Cerebral Dominance*. Baltimore: Johns Hopkins Press, 1962, pp. 101-107.

287. ——, and Pribram, K. H.: Visual discrimination performance following partial ablations of the temporal lobe: I. Ventral vs. lateral. *J. Comp. Physiol. Psychol.* 47:14-20, 1954.

288. Morrell, F.: Electrophysiological contributions to the neural basis of learning. *Physiol. Rev.* 41:443-494, 1961.

289. Morris, C. W.: *Signs, Language and Behaviour*. New York: Prentice-Hall, 1946.

290. Moruzzi, G., and Magoun, H. W.: Brain stem reticular formation and activation of the EEG. *Electroenceph. Clin. Neurophysiol.* 1:455-473, 1949.

291. Mountcastle, V. B. (Ed.): *Interhemispheric Relations and Cerebral Dominance*. Baltimore: Johns Hopkins Press, 1962.

292. Myers, R. E.: Commissural connections between occipital lobes of the monkey. *J. Comp. Neur.* 118:1-16, 1962.

293. ——: Organization of visual pathways. In G. Ettlinger (Ed.): *Functions of the Corpus Callosum*. London: Churchill, 1965, pp. 133-138.

294. ——: Phylogenetic studies of commissural connections. In G. Ettlinger (Ed.): *Functions of the Corpus Callosum*. London: Churchill, 1965, pp. 138-143.

295. ——, Sperry, R. W., and McCurdy, N. M.: Neural mechanisms in visual guidance of limb movement. *Arch. Neurol.* 7:195-202, 1962.

296. Neff, W. D.: Neural mechanisms in auditory discrimination. In W. A. Rosenblith (Ed.): *Sensory Communication*. New York: John Wiley and Sons, 1961, pp. 259-278.

297. ——: Temporal pattern discrimination in lower animals and its relation to language perception in man. In A. V. S. de Rueck and Maeve O'Connor (Eds.): *Disorders of Language*. Boston: Little, Brown and Co., 1964, pp. 183-192.

298. Nielsen, J. M.: Agnosias, apraxias, speech and aphasia, Vol. 1. In A. B. Baker (Ed.): *Clinical Neurology*. New York: Hoeber, 1962, pp. 433-459.

299. Obrador, S., Carrascosa, R., and Corbonell, J.: Study of some motor syndromes (rigidity, tremor, spasticity and hemidecortication) by the carotid amytal test. *J. Neurosurg.* 18:507-511, 1961.

300. Ogden, C. K., and Richards, I. A.: *The Meaning of Meaning*. London: Kegan Paul, 1932.

301. Olds, J., and Milner, P.: Positive reinforcement produced by electrical stimulation of septal area and other regions of rat brain. *J. Comp. Physiol. Psychol.* 47:419-427, 1954.

302. Orton, S. T.: Specific reading disability, strephosymbolia. *J. Amer. Med. Soc.* 90:

1095-1099, 1928. Reprinted in *Bull. Orton Soc.* 1963.

303. Paterson, A., and Zangwill, O. L.: A case of topographical disorientation associated with a unilateral cerebral lesion. *Brain* 68: 188-212, 1945.

304. ——, and ——: Disorders of visual space perception associated with lesions of the right cerebral hemisphere. *Brain* 67:331-358, 1944.

305. Pavlov, I. P.: *Conditioned Reflexes. An Investigation of the Physiological Activity of the Cerebral Cortex.* New York: Dover Publications, 1960.

306. Penfield, W.: Functional localization in temporal and deep sylvian areas. In *The Brain and Human Behavior.* Baltimore: Williams and Wilkins Co., 1958, pp. 210-226.

307. ——: *The Excitable Cortex in Conscious Man.* Liverpool: The Liverpool University Press, 1958.

308. ——, and Jasper, H.: *Epilepsy and the Functional Anatomy of the Human Brain.* Boston: Little, Brown and Co., 1954.

309. ——, and Roberts, L.: *Speech and Brains Mechanisms.* Princeton: Princeton University Press, 1959.

310. Perez-Borja, C., and Rivers, M. H.: Some scalp and depth electrographic observations on the action of intracarotid sodium amytal injection on epileptic discharges in man. *Electroenceph. Clin. Neurophysiol.* 15:588-598, 1963.

311. Perria, L., Rosadini, G., and Rossi, G. F.: Determination of side of cerebral dominance with amobarbital. *Arch. Neurol.* 4: 173-181, 1961.

312. Pertuiset, B., and Arfel, G.: Evaluation par l'injection intracarotidienne d'amytal sodique de la valeur fonctionelle d'un hémisphère (conscience, motilité, langage, EEG).*Rev. Neurol.* 106:14-24, 1962.

313. Petit-Dutaillis, D., Guiot, G., Messimy, R., and Bourdillon, C.: À propos d'une aphémie par atteinte de la zone motrice supplémentaire de Penfield. *Rev. Neurol.* 90:95-106, 1954.

314. Pfeifer, R. S.: Pathologie der Hörstrahlung und der corticalen Hörsphäre, Vol. 6. In O. Bunke and O. Foerster (Eds.): *Handbuch der Neurologie.* Berlin: Springer, 1936, pp. 533-626.

315. Pichot, P.: Language disturbances in cerebral disease. *Arch. Neurol. Psychiat.* 74:92-96, 1955.

316. Pick, A. D.: Improvement of visual and tactual form discrimination. *J. Exper. Psychol.* 69:331-339, 1965.

317. Pierce, J. R., and David, E. E.: *Man's World of Sound.* Garden City, N. Y.: Doubleday and Co., 1958.

318. Piercy, M. F., Hécaen, H., and de Ajuriaguerra, J.: Constructional apraxia associated with unilateral cerebral lesions. *Brain* 83:225-242, 1960.

319. ——, and Smyth, V. O. G.: Right hemisphere dominance for certain non-verbal intellectual skills. *Brain* 85:775-790, 1962.

320. Porch, B. E.: Multidimensional quantification of gestural, verbal, and graphic responses of patients with cerebral pathology. Unpublished Ph. D. dissertation, Stanford University, 1966.

321. Purpura, D. P.: Further analysis of evoked "secondary discharge": A study in reticulo-cortical relations. *J. Neurophysiol.* 18: 246-260, 1954.

322. ——, and Cohen, B.: Intracellular recording from thalamic neurons during recruiting responses. *J. Neurophysiol.* 25:621-635, 1962.

323. ——, ——, and Marini, G.: Generalized neocortical responses and corticospinal neuron activity. *Science* 134:729-730, 1961.

324. ——, McMurtry, J. G., and Maekawa, K.: Synaptic events in ventrolateral thalamic neurons during suppression of recruiting responses by brain stem reticular stimulation. *Brain Res.* 1:63-76, 1966.

325. ——, and Shofer, R. J.: Intracellular recording from thalamic neurons during reticulocortical activation. *J. Neurophysiol.* 26: 494-505, 1963.

326. ——, ——, and Musgrave, F. S.: Cortical intracellular potentials during augmenting and recruiting responses: II. Patterns of synaptic activities in pyramidal and nonpyramidal tract neurons. *J. Neurophysiol.* 27:133-151, 1964.

327. ——, ——, and Scarff, T.: Properties of synaptic activities and spike potentials of neurons in immature neocortex. *J. Neurophysiol.* 28:925-942, 1965.

328. ——, and Yahr, M. D. (Eds.): *The Thalamus.* New York: Columbia University Press, 1966.

329. Riesen, A. H.: Plasticity of behavior. In H. F. Harlow and C. N. Woolsey (Eds.): *Biological and Biochemical Bases of Behavior.* Madison: University of Wisconsin Press, 1958, pp. 425-450.

330. Roberts, L.: Activation and interference of cortical functions. In D. E. Sheer (Ed.): *Electrical Stimulation of the Brain.* Austin: University of Texas Press, 1961, pp. 533-553.

331. Rootes, T. P., and MacNeilage, P. F.: *Coordinated Studies of a Syndrome of Impairment in Somesthetic Perception and Motor Function.* (Status Report on Speech Research [SR-1]). New York: Haskins Laboratories, 1965.

332. Rosadini, G., and Rossi, G. F.: Richerche sugli effetti elettroencefalografici, neurologici e psichici della somministrazione intracarotidea di amytal sodico nell'uomo. *Acta Neurochir.* 9:234-250, 1961.

333. Rosen, J.: *Phoneme Identification in Sensorineural Deafness.* Stanford, Calif. Stanford University Press, 1962.

334. Rossi, G. F.: A hypothesis on the neural basis of consciousness. *Acta Neurochir.* 12:186-197, 1964.

335. ——: Some aspects of the functional organization of the brain stem: Neurophysiological and neurosurgical observations. *Excerpta Med. Int. Congress Ser.* No. 93:117-122, 1965.

336. Rovit, R. L., Gloor, P., and Rasmussen, T.: Intracarotid amobarbital in epileptic patients. *Arch. Neur.* 5:606-626, 1961.

337. ——, Hardy, J., and Gloor, P.: Electroencephalographic effects of intracarotid amobarbital on epileptic activity. *Arch. Neurol.* 3:642-655, 1960.

338. Rudel, R. G., and Teuber, H.-L.: Crossmodal transfer of shape discrimination by children. *Neuropsychologia* 2:1-8, 1964.

339. ——, and ——: Decrement of visual and hepatic Muller-Lyer illusion on repeated trials: A study of crossmodal transfer. *Quart. J. Exper. Psychol.* 15:125-131, 1963.

340. Russell, R., and Espir, M. L. E.: *Traumatic Aphasia.* Oxford, England: Oxford University Press, 1961.

341. Saetveit, J. G., Lewis, D., and Seashore C. G.: *Revision of the Seashore Measures of Musical Talents.* Series on Aims and Progress of Research, Number 65. Iowa City: University of Iowa, 1940.

342. St. Augustine, *Confessions.* Cited in L. S. Hearnshaw, Temporal Integration and Behaviour, Chapter 20. In J. Cohen (Ed.): *Readings in Psychology.* London: George Allen and Unwin, 1964.

343. Schefleln, A. E.: The significance of posture in communication systems. *Psychiatry* 27: 316-331, 1964.

344. Schiller, F.: Aphasia studied in patients with missile wounds. *J. Neurol. Neurosurg. Psychiat.* 10: 183-197, 1947.

345. Schuell, H.: *Differential Diagnosis of Aphasia with the Minnesota Test.* Minneapolis: University of Minnesota Press, 1965.

346. Schultz, M. C.: Suggested improvements in speech discrimination testing. *J. Audit. Res.* 4:1-14, 1964.

347. Schwab, O.: Über vorübergehende aphasische Störungen nach Rindenexzision aus dem linken Stirnhirn bei Epileptikern. *Deutsch. Z. Nervenheilk.* 94:177-184, 1926.

348. Scoville, W. B., and Milner, B.: Loss of recent memory after bilateral hippocampal lesions. *J. Neurol. Neurosurg, Psychiat.* 20:-11-21, 1957.

349. Semmes, J.: Hemispheric dominance: A possible clue to mechanism. Paper presented at symposium on Man's Minor Hemisphere, meeting of the American Psychological Association, New York City, September, 1966.

350. ——, Weinstein, S., Ghent, L., and Teuber, H.-L.: Performance on complex tactual tasks after brain injury in man: Analyses by locus of lesion. *Amer. J. Psychol.* 67:220-240, 1954.

351. ——, ——, ——, and ——: *Somatosensory Changes after Penetrating Brain Wounds in Man.* Cambridge, Mass.: Harvard University Press, 1960.

352. ——, ——, ——, and ——: Spatial orientation in man after cerebral injury. *J. Psychol.* 34:227-244, 1955.

353. Serafetinides, E. A., Driver, M. V., and Hoare, R. D.: EEG patterns induced by intracarotid injection of sodium amytal. *Electreoenceph. Clin. Neurophysiol.* 18:170-175, 1965.

354. ——, and Falconer, M. A.: Speech disturbances in temporal lobe seizures: A study in 100 epileptic patients submitted to anterior temporal lobectomy. *Brain* 86:333-346, 1963.

355. ——, Hoare, R. D., and Driver, M. V.: A modification of intracarotid amylobarbitone test: Findings about speech and consciousness. *Lancet* 1:249-250, 1964.

356. ——, ——, and ——: Intracarotid sodium amylobarbitone and cerebral dominance for speech and consciousness. *Brain* 88:-107-130, 1965.

357. Shankweiler, D.: Defects in recognition and reproduction of familiar tunes after unilateral temporal lobectomy. Paper read at 37th Annual Meeting, Eastern Psychological Association, New York City, April, 1966.

358. Sharpless, S., and Jasper, H.: Habituation of the arousal reaction. *Brain* 79: 655-680, 1956.

359. Shelton, R. L., Jr.: Testing oral stereognosis.

In J. F. Bosma (Ed.): *Symposium on Oral Sensation and Perception*. Springfield, Ill.: Charles C Thomas, in press.

360. Sherrington, C. S.: Cutaneous sensations. In E. A. Schafer (Ed.): *Textbook of Physiology*, Vol. 2. New York: The Macmillan Co., 1898, pp. 920-1001.

361. ———: On nerve-tracts degenerating secondarily to lesions of the cortex cerebri. *J. Physiol.* 10:429-432, 1889.

362. Smith, K. U., and Akelaitis, A. J.: Studies on the corpus callosum: I. Lateral dominance in behavior and bilateral motor coordination in man before and after partial and complete section of the corpus callosum. *Arch. Neurol. Psychiat.* 47:519-543, 1942.

363. W. K.: The frontal eye fields. In P. C. Bucy (Ed.): *The Precentral Motor Cortex*, 2nd ed. Urbana: University of Illinois Press, 1949, pp. 307-342.

364. Sokolov, E. N.: Higher nervous functions: The orienting reflex. *Ann. Rev. Physiol.* 25:-545-580, 1963.

365. ———: Neuronal models and the orienting reflex. In M. A. B. Brazier (Ed.): *Central Nervous System and Behavior*. New York: Macy Foundation, 1960, pp. 187-239.

366. Sperry, R. W.: Cerebral organization and behavior. *Science* 133:1749-1757, 1961.

367. ———: Hemispheric interaction and the mind-brain problem. In J. C. Eccles (Ed.): *Brain and Conscious Experience*. Heidelberg: Springer-Verlag, in press.

368. ———: Neural basis of the spontaneous optokinetic response produced by visual inversion. *J. Comp. Physiol. Psychol.* 93:482-489, 1950.

369. ———: *Problems Outstanding in the Evolution of Brain Function*. (James Arthur Lecture.) New York: American Museum of Natural History, 1964.

370. Spitz, R.: *Hospitalism. The Psychoanalytic Study of the Child*. New York: International University Press, 1945.

371. Stengel, E.: Loss of spatial orientation, constructional apraxia and Gerstmann's syndrome. *J. Ment. Sci.* 90:753-760, 1944.

372. Stepien, L. S., and Cordeau, J. P.: Memory in monkeys for compound stimuli. *Amer. J. Psychol.* 73:388-395, 1960.

373. Sutherland, N. S.: Unpublished talks in the Neural Sciences Research Program and at the MIT Psychology Department, Fall, 1965.

374. Symonds, C. P.: Aphasia. *J. Neurol. Neurosurg. Psychiat.* 16:1-6, 1953.

375. Takahashi, K.: Slow and fast groups of pyramidal tract cells and their respective membrane properties. *J. Neurophysiol.* 28:908-924, 1965.

376. Tengsdahl, M.: Experiences with intracarotid injections of sodium amytal: A preliminary report. *Acta Neurol. Scand.* 39:329-343, 1963.

377. Terman, F. E.: *Electronic and Radio Engineering*. New York: McGraw-Hill, 1965.

378. Terzian, H.: Behavioral and EEG effects of intracarotid sodium amytal injection. *Acta Neurochir.* 12:230-239, 1964.

379. ———, and Cecotto, G.: Su un nuovo metodo per la determinazione e lo studio della dominanza emisferica. *G. Psichiat. Neuropat.* 87:889-923, 1959.

380. Teuber, H.-L.: Alterations in perception after brain injury. In J. D. Eccles (Ed.): *The Brain and Conscious Experience*. New York: Springer, 1966, pp. 182-216.

381. ———: Disorders of higher tactile and visual functions. *Neuropsychologia* 3:287-294, 1965.

382. ———: Effects of brain wounds implicating right or left hemisphere in man: Hemisphere differences and hemisphere interaction in vision, audition, and somesthesis. In V. B. Mountcastle (Ed.): *Interhemispheric Relations and Cerebral Dominance*. Baltimore: Johns Hopkins Press, 1962, pp. 131-157.

383. ———: Perception, Chapt. LXV, Vol. III. In J. Field, H. W. Magoun, and V. E. Hall (Eds.): *Handbook of Physiology*. Washington: American Physiological Society, 1960.

384. ———: Sensory deprivation, sensory suppression and agnosia. Notes for a neurologic theory. *J. Nerv. Ment. Dis.* 132:32-40, 1961.

385. Thorndike. E. L., and Lorge, I.: *The Teacher's Word Book of 30,000 Words*. New York: Teacher's College, Columbia University, 1944.

386. Thorpe, W. H.: *Bird Song: The Biology of Vocal Communication and Expression in Birds*. Cambridge, England: Cambridge University Press, 1961.

387. ———: The ontogeny of behavior, Chapt. 17. In J. A. Moore (Ed.): *Ideas in Modern Biology*. Proceedings of the 16th International Congress of Zoology, New York, 1965.

388. ———, and North, M. E. W.: Origin and significance of the power of vocal imitation: with special reference to the antiphonal singing of birds. *Nature* 208:219-222, 1965.

389. ———, and ———: Vocal imitation in the tropical bou-bou shrike (Laniarius aethiopicus) as

a means of establishing and maintaining social bonds. *Ibis* 108:432-435, 1966.

390. Tower, S. S.: Extrapyramidal action from the cat's cerebral cortex: Motor and inhibitory. *Brain* 59:408-444, 1936.

391. Trescher, J. H.: and Ford, F. R.: Colloid cyst of the third ventricle. *Arch. Neurol. Psychiat.* 37:959-973, 1937.

392. von Holst, E., and Mittelstaedt, H.: Das Reafferenzprinzip (Wechselwirkungen zwischen Zentralnervensystem und Peripherie). *Naturwiss* 37:464-476, 1950.

393. von Senden, M.: *Raum- und Gestaltauffassung bei operierten Blindgeborenen vor und nach der Operation.* Leipzig: J. A. Barth, 1932. English translation under the title *Space and Sight.* Glencoe, Ill.: Free Press, 1960.

394. Wada, J.: A new method for the determination of the side of cerebral speech dominance: A preliminary report on the intracarotid injection of sodium amytal in man. *Med. Biol.* (Tokyo) 14:221-222, 1949.

395. ——, and Rasmussen, T.: Intracarotid injection of sodium amytal for the lateralization of cerebral speech dominance: Experimental and clinical observations. *J. Neurosurg.* 17:266-282, 1960.

396. Waite, E. R.: Sympathetic song in birds. *Nature* 68:322, 1903.

397. Wall, P. D., Remond, A. G., Dobson, R. L.: Studies on the mechanism of the action of visual afferents on motor cortex excitability. *Electroenceph. Clin. Neurophysiol.* 5:385-393, 1953.

398. Walshe, F. M. R.: On the mode of representation of movements in the motor cortex with special reference to "Convulsions Beginning Unilaterally" (Jackson). *Brain* 66:104-139, 1943.

399. Wegener, J. G.: Cross-modal transfer in monkeys. *J. Comp. Physiol. Psychol.* 59:450-452, 1965.

400. Weinstein, E. A., Cole, M., Mitchell, M. S., and Lyerly, O. G.: Anosognosia and aphasia. *Arch. Neurol.* 10:376-386, 1964.

401. Weinstein, S.: Differences in effects of brain wounds implicating right or left hemispheres: Differential effects on certain intellectual and complex perceptual functions. In V. B. Mountcastle (Ed.): *Interhemispheric Relations and Cerebral Dominance.* Baltimore: Johns Hopkins Press, 1962, pp. 159-176.

402. Welch, K., and Stuteville, P.: Experimental production of unilateral neglect in monkeys. *Brain* 81:341-347, 1958.

403. Wenner, A.: Sound communication in honeybees. *Sci. Amer.* 210:116-124, 1964.

404. Wepman, J. M., Jones, L. V., Bock, R. D., and Van Pelt, D.: Studies in Aphasia: Background and theoretical formulations. *J. Speech Hear. Dis.* 25:323-332, 1960.

405. ——, and Van Pelt, D.: A theory of cerebral language disorders based on therapy. *Folia Phoniat.* 7:223-235, 1955.

406. Wermann, R., Anderson, P. J. and Christoff, N.: Electroencephalographic changes with intracarotid megimide and amytal in man. *Electroenceph. Clin. Neurophysiol.* 11:267-274, 1959.

407. ——, Christoff, N., and Anderson, P. J.: Neurological changes with intracarotid amytal and megimide in man. *J. Neurol. Neurosurg. Psychiat.* 22:333-337, 1959.

408. Wernicke, K.: *Der aphasische Symptomencomplex: Eine psychologische Studie auf anatomischer Basis.* Breslau: Cohn und Weigert, 1874.

409. Wever, E. G.: *Theory of Hearing.* New York: John Wiley and Sons, 1949.

410. Wilson, M.: Further analysis of intersensory facilitation of learning sets in monkeys. *Percept. Motor Skills* 18:917-920, 1964.

411. ——: Tactual discrimination learning in monkeys. *Neuropsychologia* 3:353-361, 1965.

412. ——, and Wilson, W. A.: Intersensory facilitation of learning sets in normal and brain-operated monkeys. *J. Comp. Physiol. Psychol.* 55:931-934, 1962.

413. Wilson, W. A.: Intersensory transfer in normal and brain-operated monkeys. *Neuropsychologia* 3:363-370, 1965.

414. ——, and Shaffer, O. C.: Intermodality transfer of specific discriminations in the monkey. *Nature* 197:107, 1963.

415. Winitz, H.: Language skills of male and female kindergarten children. *J. Speech Hear. Res.* 2:377-386, 1959.

416. Wolff, H. G.: Discussion. In V. B. Mountcastle (Ed.): *Interhemispheric Relations and Cerebral Dominance.* Baltimore: Johns Hopkins Press, 1962, pp. 199-203.

417. Yates, A. J.: Delayed auditory feedback. *Psychol. Bull.* 60:213-232, 1963.

418. Yoshii, N., Pruvot, P., and Gastaut, H.: Electroencephalographic activity of the mesencephalic reticular formation during conditioning in the cat. *Electroenceph. Clin. Neurophysiol.* 9:595-608, 1957.

419. Zangwill, O. L.: *Cerebral Dominance and Its Relations to Psychological Function.* Edinburgh: Oliver and Boyd, 1960.

420. ——: Discussion on parietal lobe syndromes. *Proc. Roy. Soc. Med.* 44:343-346, 1951.

Index of Speakers

A number in boldface type indicates a contribution in the form of a paper. Numbers in plain type refer to contributions to the discussions.

Index of Topics